Foundations of Health Care Management

Foundations of Health Care Management

Principles and Methods

BERNARD J. HEALEY

MARC C. MARCHESE

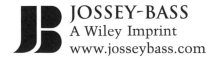
JOSSEY-BASS
A Wiley Imprint
www.josseybass.com

Published by Jossey-Bass

A Wiley Imprint

One Montgomery Street, Suite 1200, San Francisco, CA 94104-4594—www.josseybass.com

Jossey-Bass books and products are available through most bookstores. To contact Jossey-Bass directly call our Customer Care Department within the U.S. at 800-956-7739, outside the U.S. at 317-572-3986, or fax 317-572-4002.

Wiley publishes in a variety of print and electronic formats and by print-on-demand. Some material included with standard print versions of this book may not be included in e-books or in print-on-demand. If this book refers to media such as a CD or DVD that is not included in the version you purchased, you may download this material at http://booksupport.wiley.com. For more information about Wiley products, visit www.wiley.com.

Library of Congress Cataloging-in-Publication Data

Healey, Bernard J., 1947-
    Foundations of health care management : principles and methods / Bernard J. Healey,
Marc C. Marchese.
        p. cm.
    Includes bibliographical references and index.
    ISBN 978-0-470-93212-4 (pbk.); ISBN 978-1-118-22137-2 (ebk.); ISBN 978-1-118-23519-5 (ebk.); ISBN 978-1-118-25983-2 (ebk.)
    1. Health services administration—United States.   2. Health facilities—Administration.
3. Hospitals—Administration.   I. Marchese, Marc C.   II. Title.
    RA971.H3833 2012
    362.1—dc23
                                                                              2012020451

Printed in the United States of America

FIRST EDITION

PB Printing   10 9 8 7 6 5 4 3 2 1

CONTENTS

PART TWO

Managing the External Environment

PART THREE

Managing Human Performance in Organizations

TABLES AND FIGURES

Tables

Figures

THOSE IN CHARGE of the delivery of health services, and their managers, are facing massive changes in regard to how they deliver health care and the ways in which the outcomes of these services are evaluated. These changes are occurring as a result of health care reform, which has resulted from pressures exerted by health insurers, employers, government entities, health care professionals, and, most important, those who consume health services. The demand for change is not going away; it is in fact increasing as the amount spent on health care continues to rise every year. It is truly a time of crisis and tremendous opportunities for the U.S. health care system.

Since 1900 the length of life for most Americans has expanded, and the majority of individuals can expect to live into their eighties. Unfortunately, because of the epidemic of chronic diseases and their long-term complications, a very large percentage of these individuals will experience a decrease in their quality of life as they age. These diseases and their complications currently consume 80 percent of our scarce health care resources. Our inability to deal with this epidemic has resulted in the highest per capita expenditures compared with other industrialized nations for health care, even though the United States is doing very poorly in regard to health outcomes when compared with these other countries. These outcomes must change. We must make health care better and less expensive. The remedy will require improved management of every part of our health care system. It will also include a need for the organizations that deliver health services to learn how to empower those who actually deliver these services to their customers. For most of these organizations, this entails a movement from a bureaucratic management structure to a more decentralized organizational structure.

The current and future challenges health care facilities face in the changing world of health care today require better managers of scarce health care resources. These managers will need to rely less on the power granted to them by their position and more on their expertise and interpersonal skills to improve the quality of health services. The old bureaucratic system must be replaced by a more organic form of control that allows creativity and innovation to come forth to meet the demands of all stakeholders in the U.S. health care system. That is why a large portion of this text is devoted to the subject of creativity and innovation in the delivery of health services.

Our health care system needs to be organized better if we are to increase productivity, which will eventually result in reduced costs for improved care for large numbers of health care consumers. As many health care organizations improve their performance, others will follow their lead to remain competitive. To survive in and even exploit the changing health care environment, then, health care managers must have the requisite skills to motivate their employees to deliver extraordinary services on a daily basis. This health care management text will take current and future health care managers to new levels of knowledge, suggesting approaches that have been used in some of the most successful service delivery organizations in the world.

This book was written to address the need for new skill development for current and future managers of health care facilities. Health care managers should be trained in leadership skills, and should develop their ability to empower all employees to improve the quality of care and as well as outcomes for the population. Health care managers also require an understanding of change management and conflict management techniques, culture building abilities, quality improvement skills, communication skills, and an appreciation for team building and collaboration in the improvement of population health.

This book is separated into five parts, each of which addresses topics in health care management that seasoned managers and those preparing for a career in health care management must consider. Part One, Introduction to Health Care Management, offers the reader a chance to explore the critical issues that will affect the uncertain future of health care delivery in our country. The topics to be considered in this section of the book include the changing environment, new processes of health delivery, the current reform legislation, and the improvement of productivity in the delivery of health services.

Part Two, Managing in the External Environment, moves to the subject of the management of the external environment facing the vast majority of health care facilities in the United States over both the short and the long term. Specific discussion areas include the development of a health care organization's vision, mission, and business objectives, as well as the governance and management of the health care facility.

Part Three, Managing Human Performance in Organizations, spends a great deal of time discussing the various skills that health care managers need to develop as they attempt to improve their practice in regard to managing human performance. There is a great deal of attention paid to leadership development, as well as the process of change, the importance of motivating health care employees, the need for innovation in the delivery of services, and the development of culture in health care facilities. The need for managers to improve their communication skills is expressed as well. Finally, there is a special chapter devoted to the management of physicians, which is another component that requires attention when attempting to improve the efficiency and quality of health services.

Part Four of this book, Creating a High-Performance Workplace, considers several important issues in human resources management, such as recruiting and selecting new employees and improving the performance of existing employees. Among the other topics in this section are critical employee attitudes toward work, unions in health care, and performance appraisal.

Part Five, Special Areas of Health Care Management, covers the topics of marketing, finance, and ethical decision making as these pertain to health care managers. The chapters addressing these important components of health care management are followed by a final chapter that evaluates several of the important areas of change facing health care managers.

ACKNOWLEDGMENTS

We would like to begin by acknowledging the dedicated people who work in health care facilities across our country, and who despite limited resources have accomplished so much in making the United States a better place to lead a healthy life. This is really a book about how to better manage scarce health care resources in the face of the many challenges arising from health care reform.

During the process of writing this book we worked with many dedicated people who exhibited professionalism in everything they tried to accomplish. A number of the chapters were written by individuals with advanced education and experience in areas with which every manager of health care delivery should be familiar. These individuals include contributors Mark H. DeStefano, Tina Marie Evans, Dan F. Kopen, Kermit W. Kuehn, and Amy L. Parsons, We also thank Elizabeth "Lisa" Johnson, vice president of public relations and marketing at Blue Mountain Health System, for providing us with a health care advertisement for use in our chapter on health care marketing.

We wish to thank Fred Downs, Jim Goes, Michael Lin, Patricia Robbins, Victor Sower, and Susan L. Wilson, who gave us valuable feedback in the early stages of the manuscript's conception. Michael Lin, Patricia Robbins, and Victor Sower also offered thoughtful and constructive comments on the draft manuscript.

During the entire research and writing process for this book we were surrounded by intelligent, caring individuals who only sought to make our ideas better. We are very fortunate to have been given the opportunity to write a book for a national publisher, but we are equally privileged to have been able to work with such talent.

BERNARD J. HEALEY is a professor of health care administration at King's College in Wilkes-Barre, Pennsylvania. He began his career in 1971 as an epidemiologist for the Pennsylvania Department of Health, retiring from that position in 1995. During his government tenure he completed advanced degrees in business administration and public administration. In 1990 he finished his doctoral work at the University of Pennsylvania. Dr. Healey has been teaching undergraduate and graduate courses in business, public health, and health care administration at several colleges for over thirty years. He is currently the director of the graduate program in health care administration at King's College.

Healey has published more than one hundred articles concerning public health, health policy, leadership, marketing, and health care partnerships. He has also written and published two books about leadership in health care and children's high-risk health behaviors.

Healey is a member of the American Association of Public Health and the Association of University Programs in Health Care Administration. He is a part-time consultant in epidemiology for the Wilkes-Barre City Health

Department and a consultant for numerous public health projects in Pennsylvania.

MARC C. MARCHESE received his PhD in industrial and organizational psychology from Iowa State University in 1992. For the past seventeen years he has been a faculty member at King's College. He is currently a professor of human resources management and health care administration.

As a teacher, during his time at King's College he has taught a wide variety of human resources and health care courses, covering such topics as human resources management, quantitative business methods for health care, employee training and development, employment and labor law, employee staffing, and industrial psychology.

As a scholar, he has published numerous articles in academic journals. Some recent examples include "Tobacco: The Trigger to Other High Risk Health Behaviors" in the *Academy of Health Care Management Journal*; "Mentor and Protégé Predictors and Outcomes in a Formal Mentoring Program" in the *Journal of Vocational Behavior*; and "The Use of Marketing Tools to Increase Participation in Worksite Wellness Programs" in the *Academy of Health Care Management Journal*. He has also made numerous presentations at various national and international conferences. A few recent examples include "Three High Risk Health Characteristics and Their Consequences on Employees" at the 30th Annual Northeastern Association of Business, Economics and Technology Conference; "Is There an Ethical Way to Prevent Tobacco Use?" at the 134th Annual Meeting and Exposition of the American Public Health Association; and "The Use of Marketing Tools to Increase Participation in Worksite Wellness Programs" at the 2005 Allied Academies International Conference.

As a consultant, he has performed various functions for organizations. He has conducted training sessions on numerous topics (such as team building, the legal implications of employee training, and computer software skills) for local organizations. He has served as an expert witness in an arbitration hearing. He has been a statistical analyst for several projects (covering such topics as anger management, leadership effectiveness, and therapy alternatives, among others). He has designed and analyzed employee opinion surveys for a number of companies.

MARK H. DESTEFANO, a native of Southern New Jersey, earned a BS-BA with a concentration in accounting from Georgetown University in Washington, DC. Later, while working in the health care sector, he earned an MSHA from King's College in Wilkes-Barre, Pennsylvania. He is a certified public accountant in the State of Pennsylvania.

After graduating from Georgetown University's McDonough School of Business in 1989, he relocated to Northeastern Pennsylvania to work in the accounting and finance department of a third-generation, privately-held business, Pagnotti Enterprises, in which his family had an interest. At the time, Pagnotti Enterprises and its subsidiaries and affiliated entities had diverse interests in anthracite coal mining, banking, heavy and highway construction, worker's compensation, and cable television and broadband operations. He assumed various roles within the company and ultimately served as vice president and COO of the cable television operations, Verto Communications, until a sale of the business segment to Adelphia Cable Communications. He managed Adelphia's cable television and broadband properties in Northeastern Pennsylvania until 2006.

In 2007 he was hired by AllOne Health Group, a subsidiary of Blue Cross of Northeastern Pennsylvania, which had operations in the personal health and wellness, occupational health, and employee assistance programs, and in the small group health insurance space. He served as vice president of finance for AllOne Health Group until 2010.

He currently resides in Scranton, Pennsylvania; he has a controlling ownership in various entrepreneurial ventures in the retail and real estate brokerage sectors; and he serves on a number of corporate and community boards in Northeastern Pennsylvania.

TINA MARIE EVANS is associate professor and department head of the Applied Health Studies Department at Penn College. Dr. Evans is a 1998 summa cum laude graduate of Marywood University, Pennsylvania, with a bachelor's degree in sports medicine. Following her graduation from Marywood University, she completed her master's degree in health care administration at King's College in 1999. Evans taught at King's College in the Department of Sports Medicine for five years, and served as the interim director of sports medicine there before she accepted a teaching position at Marywood University for two years while completing her doctoral work. Evans was awarded the doctoral degree in December 2004 at Marywood University, specializing in health promotion.

She accepted a full-time faculty position at Penn College in fall 2005. She continues to be very active in grant writing; publishing scholarly manuscripts; and presenting on various allied health topics on the local, regional, national, and international levels. She is active in volunteer activities in her church and community. Outside of work, Evans enjoys the outdoors, swimming, golf, ballroom dancing, and spending time with her family.

ELIZABETH "LISA" JOHNSON is the vice president of public relations and marketing for Blue Mountain Health System in Lehighton, Pennsylvania. Ms. Johnson has more than twenty years of health care public relations and communication experience in small, community hospitals as well as large, tertiary hospital systems. She has received awards from the Hospital and Health System Association of Pennsylvania as well as awards for public relations, advertising, and marketing campaigns. She is serving her second term as an executive board member of the Public Relations Society of America's Health Academy and was appointed as co-chair for the Health Academy Conference in 2012.

DAN F. KOPEN is a practicing breast cancer surgeon with an office in Forty Fort, Pennsylvania. Dr. Kopen holds a BS in chemistry from Wilkes University and an MD from Penn State Milton S. Hershey Medical Center, and he did his surgical residency and fellowship at Barnes Hospital of Washington University in St. Louis. He has subsequently earned an MS in health care administration from King's College; a JD from Concord University in California, with an emphasis in the field of health care law; a master's certificate in Six Sigma health care from Villanova University; and a Six Sigma Black Belt certificate from Villanova University. He is a senior member of the American Society for Quality and a member of the Hastings Center, a nonpartisan bioethics research institute.

Kopen's interests include health maintenance and illness prevention; the provision of a healthful learning environment for our nation's children; and mitigating the deleterious effects on the quality of care that emerge at the interface of medical, business, and legal ethics. He provides lectures to the public and students ranging from grade school to college, graduate, and professional levels on topics including the importance of education and health maintenance, breast cancer screening and treatments, health care reform, and medical and legal ethics. He holds a board certification in surgery; is a fellow of the American College of Surgeons; and is a member of the American Society of Breast Surgeons, for which he serves as a national examiner for stereotactic breast biopsy certification and as chairperson of the Legislative Committee. He has published books for children in addition to the books *Understanding Health Care* (2002), for which he served as a coeditor and contributing author, and *Common Sense Health Care Reform* (2009, 2011), which he authored.

KERMIT W. KUEHN is a professor of management and entrepreneurship and the founding director of the Center for Business Research and Economic

Development at the University of Arkansas–Fort Smith. He has published research in general management, strategy, entrepreneurship, and health care.

A native of Nebraska, Dr. Kuehn earned his doctorate in 1993 in the area of management from the University of Nebraska. He also holds a master's degree in international management from the Thunderbird School of Global Management in Glendale, Arizona.

AMY L. PARSONS is a professor of marketing at King's College in Wilkes-Barre, Pennsylvania. She received the PhD in marketing from the University of Massachusetts, Amherst; an MBA from Syracuse University; and earned her BA at the University of California, Berkeley.

Her research has included buyer-supplier relationships, print advertising, internal marketing, health care marketing, and teaching issues. Her work has been published in the *Journal of Advertising*, *Journal of Advertising Research*, *Journal of Consumer Affairs*, *Journal of Supply Chain Management*, *Academy of Strategic Management Journal*, *Journal of the Academy of Business Education*, *Academy of Marketing Studies Journal*, *Journal of Marketing Education*, and *Journal of Internet Commerce*, as well as in *Health Marketing Quarterly*. She has also written book reviews in the *Journal of Consumer Marketing*, *Journal of Product and Brand Management*, and *Journal of Marketing Research*. She has presented her research at many international and national conferences, including the World Marketing Congress, the Academy of Marketing Science Conference, the Business & Economics Society International Conference, the Allied Academies International Conference, the International Academy of Business & Economics Annual Conference, the Teaching and Learning Conference, the International Applied Business Research Conference, and the Academy of Business Disciplines Conference. Her teaching interests focus primarily on the promotional aspects of marketing (advertising and selling) and consumer behavior.

PART 1

Introduction to Health Care Management

This book begins with an introduction to management principles, followed by an explanation of the various problems managers in the health care industry encounter. The two chapters in Part One address issues that are pivotal in determining the future of health care in the United States as well as the fundamentals of health care management. The intent of this first section is to give the reader an overview of the many issues facing those who work and supervise individuals in the delivery of health services. A secondary purpose of this Part One is to share the history, principles, and forces that affect the management of the largest sector of the U.S. economy.

Chapter One covers many of the critical issues confronted by both managers and nonmanagers who work in health care delivery. This chapter begins with a complete explanation of how the health care system will change as the effects of health care reform become evident. The delivery of effective and efficient health services is discussed at length, as is the role of the health care manager in making the necessary changes to the U.S. health care system a reality. Chapter One places a great deal of emphasis on the building of new processes in health care delivery that are capable of reducing costs while improving the quality of those services.

Chapter One also offers a comprehensive review of the changes made to the delivery of health services, many of which will affect the way health services are produced, delivered, and paid for. Managers will be given greater responsibility for making certain that the health care organization adheres to legal requirements and operates efficiently and effectively. Several of the current errors found in health care delivery are also discussed, along with recommendations for how better management can rectify them.

Chapter Two covers the fundamentals of health care management. This chapter starts with an overview of management theory that includes the history of management, along with a discussion of human relations theory and reengineering theory in particular. A great deal of the research found in the development of management theory is discussed in depth, all of which is then applied to the individuals who become managers in health care organizations.

The discussion then moves into management innovation as well as managerial skills and the functions of a manager. Chapter Two also discusses at great length, among other topics, system coordination and management of health care delivery. The management of technology, including electronic medical records and telemedicine, is also covered.

The goal of Part One is, in other words, to provide the reader with a sound understanding of the principles—and an introduction to the methods—of health care management.

1

Critical Issues for the Future of Health Care in the United States

Bernard J. Healey

LEARNING OBJECTIVES

- Understand the major problems found in the U.S. health care system
- Recognize the need for efficiency in the delivery of health services
- Understand the value of better management in the health care industry
- Become aware of the need to reform the present health care system
- Be able to explain how the problems of cost, access, and health levels in our health care system are interrelated

This is a book about the skills necessary to become a successful health care manager. It is a very special time in the history of health care—one in which we are faced with enormous change in the way health services are delivered to over three hundred million Americans. To deal with this never-ending environmental change, it is time for everyone responsible for those who deliver these very special services to better understand what these individuals need to consistently deliver quality health care to their patients. A health care manager must be able to improve the system of health care delivery while simultaneously helping his or her staff achieve personal growth in their chosen field of employment.

There are many problems found in our current health care system. Spending on health care has become one of the greatest predicaments to ever face our nation, and there is no definitive solution to this growing problem. This one category of spending has grown from an insignificant amount fifty years ago to almost 18 percent of GDP on an annual basis. In 1960 this spending represented a total cost of $26.9 billion, representing a per capita cost of $141. Today this cost has risen to $2.7 trillion, with $8,160 per capita expenditures. The Kaiser Family Foundation (Kaiser Family Foundation & Health Research & Educational Trust, 2010) reports that spending in health care will reach $4.3 trillion in 2018. In that year this expense will represent 20.3 percent of GDP, or $13,100 for each resident. This type of cost escalation for one category of spending is clearly not sustainable. There are many reasons for the cost escalation, but I believe that most Americans are far more interested in solving the problem for the future rather than blaming poor decisions that were made in the past. This book is about one very important potential solution to the problem: better management of scarce health care resources. We must consider the best way to improve the skills of the individuals chosen to manage these human and material resources.

Reform and improvement of the current health care system will require a greater emphasis on cost control. Costs continue to rise much more quickly than inflation, indicating that something is very wrong with productivity in the health care sector of our economy. These rates of increase cannot continue over the long term without doing very serious damage to our overall economic growth. Many years ago Victor Fuchs (1998) of Stanford University pointed out these major problems in our health care system: cost, access, and health levels. The rising cost of health care delivery—and the related problems of access for millions of Americans—are now leading factors in the recently passed **health care reform** legislation. As we analyzed the health care sector and compared it to other countries, it became very evident that our entire health care system was not performing very well: not only do we spend more on health care than any other country but also we are not very healthy as a nation. According to Fuchs (2009), coordinated care is necessary to get health care costs under control. Such coordination will require the three "I's": information, infrastructure, and incentives. To improve these components in health care delivery there is a need for better management of the entire health care system.

There is overwhelming evidence that improved information technology can enhance efficiency in businesses. The investment in information technology in the private sector is intended to improve bottom-line performance by reducing costs and increasing profits. However, the vast majority of health care facilities in our country have generally resisted making such an investment. There are many reasons for this resistance by special interest groups in health care, but this is no longer an acceptable strategy for health care organizations to follow as we implement health care reform efforts. In fact, a sizeable chunk of the new federal and state dollars going to health care is dedicated to the development of information technology to reduce costs, eliminate medical errors, and improve outcomes.

The infrastructure designed to deliver health services to consumers is in need of modernization. The world of work—including in the realm of health care delivery—is changing at a faster pace than anyone ever imagined. These changes are affecting workers and managers as they try to come together to deliver quality outcomes at a reasonable price. The majority of health care facilities are trying to deal with the rapid change in health care through better control by managers. They are also realizing that health care managers supervise the activities of employees, who serve guests of the health care facility. This puts the onus on managers to foster greater **empowerment** of the health care worker.

The rapidly changing health care system has made change very difficult, but I would argue that the changing health care industry is quite capable of exploiting this upheaval in ways that lead to a healthier population at a lower cost. This should allow wasted health care resources to be better used in satisfying unmet needs in other areas, such as education or environmental initiatives.

We need incentives to push managers to become catalysts in the process of bringing together new forms of technology used in the production of health services, resulting in lower-priced, better-quality health services being delivered to the buyer or consumer. According to Drucker (2010), management is the least understood of our basic tools required to improve outcomes. It is ironic that many large organizations are unaware of what management does or even what it is supposed to be doing. Of all the resources used in production, the only resource that is capable of growing on its own is human resources. Each human being determines what he or she will contribute to the production process.

New managers in health care are being recruited from pools of already-practicing health care professionals or new college graduates who have majored in health care administration or business administration. There are advantages and disadvantages to being from either of these two groups. Lombardi (2001) argues that a health care professional moves through numerous transition factors to become a health care manager. These factors, found in Figure 1.1, are very useful to show the new manager the transitions that need to take place as he or she moves into a managerial position in health care.

There are four basic transition factors: selfless service; circumstantial control; qualitative outcomes; and overall, comprehensive goals (Lombardi, 2011). These transitions involve moving from responsibility for only your own performance to responsibility for others, as circumstances rather than your own work flow determine your routine. Your output is now very difficult to measure, and your goals are now comprehensive rather than definite outcomes associated with your individual input.

Figure 1.1　Transition Factors
Source: Lombardi, 2001, p. 11. Reprinted with permission of John Wiley & Sons, Inc.

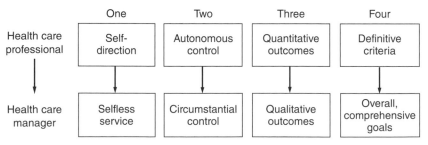

Although the future of cost-effective health care delivery is uncertain, there are tremendous opportunities presented daily for reducing costs and improving the quality of the health care experience. These opportunities are being found in both the private and public sectors as everyone is finally realizing that health care delivery has become the greatest problem facing all Americans. According to Oberlander and White (2009), the Obama administration continues to push for the cost savings from prevention, comparative effectiveness research, disease management, and improved information technology. These are all potential reforms that should reduce health care costs over the long term because they are investments in better health for the population. What is needed in the short term is better management of scarce resources. This book is designed to help both new and experienced managers in their crucial task of improving efficiency and quality in health care delivery, which will go a long way toward improving the health of all Americans.

As I have already stated, there is no question that the health care industry is in trouble. According to Shi and Singh (2010), the United States spends more than any other country on health care delivery, and costs continue to rise at an alarming rate. They note that despite our spending well over $2 trillion on health services, the outcomes resulting from this enormous expense do not do very well when subjected to cost-benefit analysis, and our outcomes have been worse than those found in every other industrialized nation. Serious infrastructure problems in health care delivery have increased costs while allowing the quality of health care to diminish. Buchbinder and Shanks (2007) argue that leaders as well as managers must reform this system: the leaders will provide the vision for a new health care system, and the managers will improve efficiency and patient satisfaction by making the best use of health care resources. Although numerous books published in recent years have addressed the importance of leadership in health care, there is still an overriding need for better management techniques. It is truly an exciting time as we explore new ways to improve the management of the largest sector of the U.S. economy.

Health care costs are going to continue to rise, despite our best attempts to control them. Managed care programs have sought to reduce costs in past years, and they were actually successful in decreasing the rate of cost escalation in health care delivery—for a short period of time. Most health economists are not very optimistic about controlling these escalating costs in the future. Their pessimism stems from two major triggers of cost increases: rising labor costs and new technology development. Callahan (2009) argues that 50 percent of the increase in health care costs each year can be attributed to the development and use of advanced technology. The cost of technology is projected to increase at least 6 percent per year into the distant future, leaving us with a perpetual cycle of cost escalation. Better health care management is our only hope of success in the battle to reduce the cost of health care delivery over the long term.

Management has been discussed, practiced, and written about since the beginning of time. Health care management as a separate discipline is of more recent origin. Management has become a popular topic in the delivery of health care because health care organizations are under tremendous pressure to produce better results. The entire health care system is being reformed, and the overriding concern is maximizing output while minimizing the use of limited resources. There is also a desire to improve the quality of health services. Improving the **efficiency** and **effectiveness** of health care delivery will require well-developed skills among managers—particularly those of unique importance to health services, such as communication and conflict management skills.

The changing health care system requires better management of people and things to accomplish assigned goals. This statement is true whether you are working in a hospital, providing health insurance, or managing an ambulatory care center. In fact, better management will be required everywhere in health care. According to Berry and Seltman (2008), health care is very different from other sectors of our economy. Health services are usually delivered to individuals who are not well, and therefore they become a need rather than a want.

Health care management involves certain functions and activities that must be performed to achieve the goals of a health care organization effectively and efficiently. These goals include effectiveness (or the ability to achieve goals) and efficiency (doing so with the minimum use of scarce resources). Griffith and White (2007) point out that the major demands of the health care market are better quality and reasonable costs, both of which fall under the heading of management and follower responsibilities. This is why better management of limited health care resources is so critical to the reform of health care delivery in this country.

Poor communication to staff and patients has become a very noticeable problem in the delivery of health services. In general, health care practitioners are held to a very low standard when it comes to communicating adequately with the consumer of health services—the patient (Halvorson, 2007). The health care system is a dysfunctional, disconnected network that does not provide linkage among caregivers. This system also provides very little feedback on the performance of service providers. It becomes the work of health care managers to improve the communication flow among managers, workers, and patients.

Gittell (2009) argues that despite having the best clinicians in the world, the United States is unable to provide cost-effective, high-quality health care. The U.S. health care system has consistently failed to improve the health of many Americans, having become consumed with a desire to cure rather than prevent illness. Unfortunately, the major causes of morbidity and mortality found in our country are a direct result of chronic diseases, which cannot be cured. These diseases can only be prevented, and a system that focuses on curing them is therefore doomed to fail. The failure to deal with the chronic disease epidemic has caused many people to question whether or not there is an appropriate system of delivering health care to Americans.

According to Black and Miller (2008), patients are demanding quality improvement. These researchers point out that there are three major reasons to improve health care delivery: patients deserve better, employees in health care deserve better, and our country deserves better. This improvement can only occur with better managers who appreciate their workers, treat them with respect, and empower them to make the system work. Such improvement is dependent on employees' delivering the care, which in turn is a reflection of those who manage these workers.

Hwang and Christensen (2008) argue that the major question posed in the health care cost escalation debate is, How can we make health care more affordable in this country? They point out that other industries have used cost-saving technology with innovative business models to offer more affordable products and services to consumers. Successful organizations throughout the world are very good at using the energy, creativity, and talent of their people to solve complex problems involving the cost and quality of their products and services. By unleashing their people, these companies have been consistently successful at reaching their predetermined goals at a reasonable cost. They are both effective and efficient because of the collaboration among managers and followers. Efficiency in the health care system entails the ability to produce what people want and need at the lowest cost possible. If a for-profit organization cannot give consumers the products and services they desire at a reasonable price, it is forced out of business, but this has not happened in the health care sector of our economy. The health care system is too important to go out of business, but it must be reformed—and that starts with better health care managers.

Berry and Seltman (2008) argue that bureaucratic, labor-intensive organizations—like those in the health care system—become less effective at goal achievement over time. These organizations begin using rules rather than common sense in dealing with the most important part of delivering health services: their employees. This usually results in a significant loss of commitment on the part of employees, causing the quality of care to diminish for patients. According to Collins (2009), many great enterprises follow a path of decline that usually involves distinct stages. It is interesting to note that the first stage of decline for these organizations involves arrogance and an entitlement mentality among leaders that are the result of previous success. This first stage of decline looks very much like where the health care industry is today. Collins points out that the solution to this decline can be found in **disruptive innovation,** a method by which companies learn ways to convert expensive, complicated products and services into simpler, less-expensive substitute products and services.

Managers of health care organizations, despite the unique services they produce, can learn to improve by looking at management from the for-profit business world (Langabeer, 2008). Health care organizations are very different from other business organizations, but there are also many similarities found among health care and the other business segments. For example, the management functions in all industries include planning, organizing, leading, and controlling. Any organization that is attempting to improve effectiveness and efficiency in delivering products or services must practice these functions.

HEALTH CARE REFORM LEGISLATION

The Accountable Care Act was signed into law by President Obama on March 30, 2010. This legislation is going to cause massive changes in the U.S. health care system. To respond to this new legislation, health care organizations need to change the way they do business.

This new law will force the secretary of health and human services to develop standards and rules designed to improve the efficiency of health plans, along with increasing the efficiency of the multitude of providers of health care. The law will call for improvement in the management of resources. A new Center for Medicare and Medicaid Innovation will be created to encourage new payment methods designed to support innovations in the organization of health care delivery.

A very promising part of the new law is the funding for **comparative effectiveness research (CER).** Nussbaum, Tirrell, Wechsler, and Randall (2010) point out that the new health care reform legislation includes an appropriation of an additional $500 million per year for the evaluation of medical procedures as part of CER. This should reduce the costs associated with wasteful medical tests and procedures, producing $700 billion in annual savings. This process represents an attempt to get runaway health care costs under control without reducing the quality of health care.

CER represents an intense evaluation of the varying treatment options for a given medical condition (Jacobson, 2007). The vast majority of countries that have reformed their health care system have included some form of CER in their final product (Mushlin & Ghomrawi, 2010). This was done in an effort to protect patients from harm while simultaneously improving quality and taming health care costs. This new legislation, and the resulting focus on CER, will produce an even greater demand for a new type of health care management.

ERRORS IN HEALTH CARE

We have to prioritize the elimination of errors in the health care system. Health care facilities must become obsessed with preventing these errors, or at the very least rapidly correcting them so that they never happen again. In the past a health care facility could mistreat a customer and not lose his or her business. Mistakes or medical errors could be made, and the facility would still be reimbursed for the defective service. In fact, the health care facility had a very good chance of being reimbursed twice for the same service. It could be reimbursed for the error, and then reimbursed again to correct the error.

An error is usually defined as an event that does not achieve its intended purpose. Every organization experiences occasional errors in what it is trying to accomplish. If the errors continue to occur, the consumer will usually respond by taking his or her business to the competition. In health care delivery there are two major types of errors: clinical errors and service errors. Clinical or medical errors have become epidemic in the American health care industry. Service errors will also need to be dealt with as the competition for patients' business becomes more intense in the future.

Excellent organizations are capable of both solving and preventing clinical and service errors (Fottler, Ford, & Heaton, 2010). These organizations understand that errors are the result of either human or system error. They are well prepared to diagnose the many possible causes of an error and, more important, to develop strategies to remedy the error or prevent it from occurring in the first place. Errors have become the norm in many institutions that deliver health care, but this is about to change because of health care reform and the resultant demand for efficiency and effectiveness in health care delivery.

The manager is responsible not only for counting things and improving efficiency but also for developing his or her staff. Because the management of health care requires the production of services, the development of the employees who deliver these services seems to be of the utmost importance. Too often the health care manager gets too involved in managing *things* and forgets about the importance of developing direct reports who deal with the customer on a daily basis.

Although in the past the health care facility had to pay attention to the demands of physicians and insurance companies, customers are now starting to fill the role of the demander of health services—and many health care organizations have not prepared their staff to respond appropriately. This can be a serious mistake because many of these new consumers will simply change health care providers if they feel that they are being ignored. Health care managers must be prepared to provide excellent services to every consumer, without fail.

CHANGING THE HEALTH CARE SYSTEM

The way business is done in health care facilities is in the process of change, which has been brought on by external forces. It seems that no one, except the providers of care, is happy with the current health care system. Even physicians are dissatisfied with what has happened to health care in America. What is more disturbing is the tremendous disagreement among most of the players in the health care system as to how the system should be changed to respond to its problems. Among the few areas of agreement are the need for improved efficiency, the need to reduce medical errors, and the need to control costs.

The U.S. health care system is simply not working very well. In fact, many health researchers and health policy experts are questioning if there is even a "system" present in the delivery of many health services. According to Swayne, Duncan, and Ginter (2008), a system is a set of elements that are related in some way to achieve the desired output. A simplistic way to look at a given system of delivering care within the broader U.S. health care system is found in Figure 1.2.

In this system, people and sophisticated technology become the input for the process of delivering health services. The throughput becomes the management of the process, which is designed to achieve the ultimate output

Figure 1.2   Simple System in Health Care

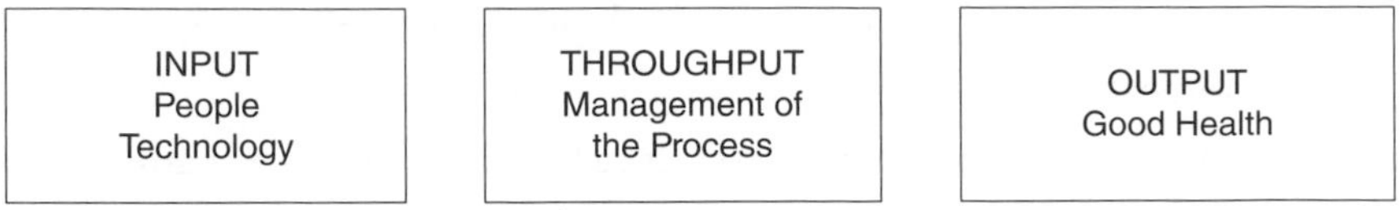

INPUT People Technology	THROUGHPUT Management of the Process	OUTPUT Good Health

or goal of the system—good health. Because our current health care system as a whole focuses on curing rather than preventing disease, its health outcomes are not good. The epidemic of chronic diseases suggests the U.S. health care system's failure to produce good health.

The simple model in Figure 1.2 works quite well when we are dealing with one provider, one disease, and one health care facility. The treatment of a communicable disease serves as an excellent example of how a given system of delivering care would function. In this case, the patient enters a health care facility or physician office with one disease, which is communicable and has an acute onset of symptoms. A method of treatment is prescribed, and after a few days the patient is usually cured, with no long-term complications. Here the system has worked well, and the patient, provider, and insurance company are all satisfied with the outcome. This is not the case with chronic diseases, because once acquired they have no cure—and they produce long-term complications that necessitate expensive treatment by many physician specialists. Although the diseases affecting Americans have changed, however, our system of health care delivery remains the same. The old health care system cannot deal with the epidemic of chronic diseases affecting most Americans as they grow older.

Because of multiple failures in the current health care system, the government and the various insurance companies paying for health services are demanding health care reform, which may result from the new legislation already discussed (Orszag & Emanuel, 2010). As part of this reform, enhanced horizontal coordination among providers, with a focus on much better monitoring of the patient, will lead to a change in infrastructure. Such new concepts as medical homes and greater accountability for resource use are definitely going to require drastic changes in our health care system's infrastructure. These changes will require further shifts in how health care managers and their staff deliver these services. They will also demand creativity and innovation from everyone responsible for health care delivery.

Health care institutions were originally designed as bureaucratic organizations because of the nature of the services delivered. The physician was in charge of the medical care for his or her patient and relied on medical expertise to control the system of health care delivery. Unfortunately for the physician, bureaucratic organizations do not fare well in times of constant change. A bureaucracy that is built on rigid rules and power is not capable of responding to change in a timely fashion. The health care environment is changing daily because of new technology, better-educated consumers, and shifting reimbursement patterns—in turn requiring a change in bureaucratic management. The physician no longer controls the delivery of health care and has been replaced by individuals possessing advanced managerial and leadership skills.

The new form of health care management requires a different set of managerial skills—skills that have worked well in many fast-paced organizations found in other economic sectors. Spear (2009) argues that high-velocity organizations use functional integration on a daily basis. These organizations are managed in such a way that all members of teams that are assigned work responsibilities collaborate to achieve proactive change in health care, and then attempt to turn that change into opportunities for company success and consumer satisfaction in terms of what services are delivered and how they are delivered.

Health care organizations must change radically in response to the various challenges the health care system faces. The mission statement of every health care organization in this country should address these challenges, which revolve around the quality of care and the improvement of health outcomes. The new mission statement of successful health care organizations will emphasize quality health services at a reasonable price. According to Griffith and White (2007), managers have the responsibility of properly implementing the mission, as developed by the board of directors and the leader of the health care organization. Therefore, meeting the challenges of providing quality services and achieving desired outcomes rests on the shoulders of health care managers, whereas the development of an appropriate mission statement to deal with those challenges is the responsibility of the CEO and the board of directors. The mission becomes the driving force of everything that the health care organization does and does not do.

There are many drivers of quality in regard to the health services an organization provides. Drivers of quality in health care delivery are both external and internal. Figure 1.3 offers a good overview of the various drivers, but the changing health care environment is continuously producing more of them. The manager must be aware of all of the drivers and be empowered to plan for them; he or she must also be proactive in responding to the demands they place on the organization. These drivers are so powerful that there is no going back to a bureaucratic management style, which would render rapid decision making impossible. The proactive and well-positioned health care facility can turn quality initiatives, spurred on by the drivers of quality, into opportunities through the use of better management techniques.

It has been almost impossible to convince health care organizations that they need to respond to consumer demands by developing different ways of delivering care. Moon (2010) argues that many organizations become so

---

Figure 1.3 Drivers of Quality
Source: Dlugacz, 2010, p. 4. Reprinted with permission of John Wiley & Sons, Inc.

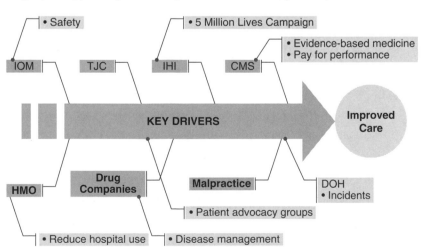

pleased with how they deliver services that they tend to forget what the consumer actually wants, instead delivering what they *think* the consumer desires. Physicians and health care facilities often have made the decisions about how and where care will be delivered, failing to realize that the consumer is the one who ultimately determines what will be produced, and where.

Senge (2006) points out that many of the problems we face today are a result of yesterday's solutions, a phenomenon that is a result of entrenched mental models concerning the best way to do business—deeply held images of how things work—that have formed over time. Many managers are afraid to change the business practices that worked well in the past, even when they realize change is necessary, and they fail to take new ideas into account because they are in conflict with the normal way business is done. This condemns the manager to failure in an environment of constant change: the old way of delivering health care simply will not work with the new diseases we face, and quite often the health care manager is the only one who does not understand this reality.

However, Senge (2006) also discusses the concept of personal mastery, which offers a potential solution to the restraints of a mental model developed in the past. This concept involves a learning process that brings employees together to form a different mental model that is better suited to the current situation. The new mental model requires the manager to work with people who are organized into effective teams devoted to improving the quality of care and obtaining better outcomes in health care delivery. Many health care organizations have as many as a hundred teams with a clinical and support focus in health care delivery designed to improve outcomes (Griffith & White, 2007). In numerous cases these teams have not worked well at the task of improving outcomes, and a given health care organization often does not do enough work to inspire winning teams. To be successful, all team members must openly question and evaluate their underlying assumptions about how health services should be delivered. The team needs to prioritize delivering what the patient wants and needs. The next step would involve consistency in the delivery of quality health services.

Collaboration among team members can go a long way toward improving both the quality and effectiveness of health care delivery (Buchbinder & Shanks, 2007). Better coordination of care should afford greater satisfaction for the team members while also improving patient outcomes and patient satisfaction. This team approach can work very well when treating chronic diseases, a process that involves multiple providers and therapies. The source of the cost and quality problems in our health care system is embedded deep within the work process of delivering health services (Gittell, 2009). It is management's responsibility to facilitate the development and progress of the team approach to delivering health care.

Love and Cugnon (2009) argue that all successful businesses have the unique ability to ignite the purpose and passion of their employees, especially when they work in teams. Such drive and enthusiasm are evident in successful and long-lasting health care organizations like Mayo Clinic. The management style of Mayo Clinic, which uses an empowered team approach to delivering health services, needs to be duplicated in other health care organizations to improve patient outcomes—particularly when dealing with chronic diseases.

Rae-Dupree (2009) argues that our country needs to use innovation to develop a very different business model that reduces costs while improving quality. This disruptive innovation includes a new method of management for an entirely different way of delivering health care. This new health care system will need to provide an incentive for prevention rather than obsessing over curing disease. A very good example of this concept is found in the medical home. Medical homes are facilities in which primary care physicians use evidence-based management practices that focus on the care of a patient over the long term (Shortell, 2010). This new concept incorporates both disruptive innovation and the development of a new mental model to give consumers of health services what they want.

Health care organizations needed to invest more in performance measurement, and they should place greater emphasis on evidence-based management. This entails prioritizing what is important in health care delivery. The first question to be answered is, Who determines what is important in health care delivery? Is it the patient, the provider, the government, the U.S.

health care system, or all of the above? The next question is, What will truly add value to the patient's health care experience? Once this question is answered, managers can prioritize what is to be accomplished, and then go about managing the organization to success.

EMPHASIS ON EFFICIENCY IN HEALTH CARE DELIVERY

Efficiency has become a critical concern of those who manage health services in this country. Managers are now being called on to improve services and reduce the costs associated with health care delivery, and they are going to require new skills and tools to accomplish this enormous task. The old rules of bureaucratic health care management need to be replaced with a management style that builds a thick culture, allows for effective communication between managers and employees, and nurtures employee personal growth. The health care manager must begin to realize how important his or her staff members are to improving the efficiency of the delivery of health services. Once this fact becomes part of the manager's style, it then moves into the culture of the organization.

According to Griffith and White (2007), leading health care organizations are spending an enormous amount of time building excellent services into their culture. In fact, fostering a thick culture among the various work teams in health care facilities has become the top priority of health care managers. The payoff will be increased efficiency, the elimination of waste, and the satisfaction of the patient as he or she consumes excellent health services. Shortell (2010) argues that the payment for health services will be moving away from a fee-for-service system to a system of payment that rewards cost-effective health care delivery. This change in payment will lead to the implementation of electronic medical records, the provision of better information for patients concerning treatment alternatives, and coordinated care by teams of primary care clinicians. This paradigm shift will require managers and employees to do things differently.

Such changes will foster the development of a learning health care organization in which employees are continually challenged to become masters of their profession. Senge (2006) offers the concept of personal mastery, mentioned earlier, as a major goal of the learning organization. This concept is based on the premise that organizations learn and grow through their employees' learning, growing, and being creative in their approach to how they do business. Exploring personal mastery goes way beyond competence and instead revolves around approaching life as a creative experience. This is exactly how we need to approach our problems in health care delivery. Health care organizations are not going to solve these problems; rather it is the health care workers actually delivering the health services who become problem solvers through their own personal mastery. It becomes the work of health care managers to create this environment for learning and growth.

The health care system has not been successful in keeping us healthy at a cost we can afford. Medical errors in delivery have become one of the leading causes of death, and costly technology is being used all too often with limited benefits. Most health care experts agree that this is clearly a systems problem that involves the use of wasteful and dangerous medical procedures. Senge (2006) argues that many organizations attempt to shift the burden when they encounter difficulty in achieving their goals, an effort that usually produces two stabilizing processes: symptomatic intervention and the development of a fundamental solution. The symptomatic response is a quick fix that usually offers a short-term solution, whereas the fundamental solution may take longer but results in a permanent solution. It is important for the health care organization and its managers to realize that goal achievement is totally dependent on the development and motivation of all employees in the organization. Solving problems requires a team effort to improve health care delivery for every patient, every day.

There are three indicators that the poorly defined problem of care under discussion is facing a shifting burden structure: the problem continues to worsen, the health of the system decreases, and a growing feeling of helplessness develops within the system (Senge, 2006). These indicators are evident in our current health care system. We have consistently attempted to solve the cost and quality problems in health care using systematic solutions (involving a change in inputs) or short-term solutions, which have not worked and have actually made the problems much worse. These solutions have almost always involved changing the way we pay for health services, but the problems we face go way beyond finances. The reduction in the quality of our health services is totally dependent on the individuals who deliver these services. The health care manager will therefore play a critical role in developing these employees and turning them loose to release their creativity and innovation in the interest of improving health care quality.

Hsieh (2010) may have given us a way to make a positive change in how an organization does business. In his new book *Delivering Happiness: A Path to Profits, Passion, and Purpose,* he talks about the qualities of excellent managers. These are individuals who believe that the best ideas and decisions are made from the bottom up, allowing them to devote time to removing obstacles that had heretofore prevented employees on the front line from delivering high-quality services. This very simple concept worked at Zappos, a company that has been achieving excellence in the delivery of services for years, and there is no reason to think that it will fail in the improvement of health care delivery. It requires a change in how health services are financed, managed, and consumed. The key to success begins with the manager and ends with the employees.

BUILDING A NEW PROCESS FOR HEALTH CARE DELIVERY

The per capita cost for health care is over $8,000 each year, and most other countries fare better than we do in both quality of care and life expectancy. The infant mortality rate in the United States is higher than that in most other industrialized countries in the world. We are wasting the scarce resources allocated to the delivery of health services and receiving very little if anything in return for the enormous cost (Shi & Singh, 2010).

This waste can only be eliminated through better management of the entire process of health care delivery. Black and Miller (2008) argue that waste is found in every organization, and that careful observation can provide a very real opportunity to improve organizational efficiency. The areas of waste and inefficiency will be found at the lowest level of the health care organization by empowered staff members who work together as a team.

These workers know where the waste and inefficiency can be found and, more important, what to do about it. The secret to success in managing health care facilities involves listening to your people and requesting their help in improving the organization's use of scarce resources. This requires the health care manager to spend a great deal of time communicating with staff and listening to what solutions to problems they have to offer.

The quality of service in the delivery of health care is primarily determined by the people working in teams toward positive patient outcomes. Achievement of these outcomes depends heavily on the successful management of the entire process. Figure 1.4 shows how information travels across facilities and cycles in a typical patient hospitalization. In this figure, the risk points at which mistakes in communication can be made include the admission cycle, the treatment cycle, and the discharge cycle. Communication errors occurring at any of these cycles can result in medical errors or a diminished patient quality experience, representing failure to that individual.

Figure 1.4   Risk Points in Communication
Source: Dlugacz, 2010, p. 45. Reprinted with permission of John Wiley & Sons, Inc.

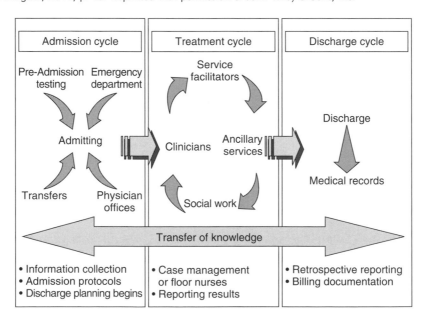

The manager must be aware of these risk points and be committed to reducing communication errors. He or she can accomplish this by better training all employees in protocols for transferring information concerning every patient. The payoff for implementing this training and securing employees' commitment to patient quality is an enormous competitive advantage for the health care organization.

According to Maxwell (2004), the change process takes time for acceptance by those who are experiencing it. In health care, the change process must be sustained over time to improve efficiency. The first step entails embracing information technology and the development and implementation of appropriate financial incentives for improved health outcomes and efficiency in their delivery. For these two things to occur, the payment system for health care delivery must change, shifting toward a focus on outcomes rather than activities. Halvorson (2009) points out that there are currently no billing codes for better outcomes or for care linkages. This seems to indicate that these goals are not that important—but they should be treated as paramount.

We need to develop an integrated health care system that produces coordinated care over time. This is very important for those individuals who develop one or more chronic diseases and want to avoid the complications that quite often result from them. The prevention of such long-term complications is a major challenge facing our health care system. These complications usually result in diminished quality of life for individuals as they age and enormous cost escalation that could have been prevented.

Chronic diseases are responsible for 80 percent of the $2.7 trillion currently spent on health care delivery (Remington, Brownson, & Wegner, 2010). These costs are only going to rise as the number of elderly individuals continues to grow and the expensive complications from these diseases continue to escalate. This alone would suggest the necessity of shifting resources from efforts to cure diseases to attempts to prevent chronic diseases and their complications.

Shortell (2010) wrote about restructuring health care organizations to encourage the integration and coordination of care, with a goal of cost reduction and improved quality. He believes that this goal can best be accomplished through the development and expansion of high-performing, patient-centered teams. These teams will need to be empowered to use information technology when seeking to gain an overall understanding of a patient's health condition.

Connectors that allow patients to move from one specialist to another are the key to real success in dealing with patients with multiple health conditions, better known as comorbidities (Halvorson, 2009). Comorbidities require the use of information technology to connect the multiple physicians caring for the patient experiencing them. The use of electronic medical records for a patient with comorbidities allows the many doctors to effectively practice as a team to improve the patient's health outcomes. The goal is the development of evidence-based medicine.

According to Chassin, Loeb, Schmaltz, and Wachter (2010), quality measures for use in improving the delivery of health services involve four criteria:

1. Research demonstrating that the measure, or process, does in fact lead to improved clinical outcomes.

2. There is proof that the evidence-based care has actually been given.

3. The process under observation leads to the desired outcome with few if any intervening processes.

4. The process has very few adverse consequences for the patient.

Following these criteria should improve health outcomes. This suggests that we need to carefully evaluate those who are advocating best practices in health care delivery when the proposed practices have not been completely evaluated. We have to look at what other successful organizations have done and try to follow their lead in giving patients what they desire. It becomes a very simple process to ask the patients what they want, and then consistently meet their demands. For this to happen, however, the health care manager and his or her team of professionals need to understand how valuable it is to have two-way conversations with patients about what they want from the health care encounter.

Goldsmith (2010) argues that the real key to quality improvement in health care delivery resides in better communication among health care professionals, a point discussed earlier in this chapter. He believes that information sharing will improve health outcomes while also increasing productivity for the clinical or administrative workforce by between 60 and 200 percent. This communication must become a dialogue between manager and staff and between staff and patient. At the risk of oversimplifying health care management, it quite often becomes a basic matter of spending time listening to direct reports and the consumers they represent. Satisfied customers lead to a wide variety of very positive results (Fottler, Ford, & Heaton, 2010). Satisfied customers are those who received exactly what they thought they were purchasing, combined with excellent services from the organization.

There is no question that a radical change in how we finance and deliver health services in this country has become mandatory if we are to save our health care organizations. On a macro level there are special interest groups that profit from the current poor management found in many health care organizations, and they will do everything in their power to block the required change. On a micro level, the individual health care organization needs to begin the change process by developing better managers, who will need training in new management techniques, including conflict management.

Health care managers using the old, bureaucratic management style would prevent conflict by establishing and enforcing targeted rules and regulations. Bureaucracies do not like conflict because it produces unrest and arguments that slow production. Today many organizations realize that conflict can be the result of creativity by workers, innovation, and rapid change in the process of producing goods and services. These organizations recognize that creativity, innovation, and change are desirable even if they produce conflict. This is especially true as our health care system responds to the demand for reform. Health care organizations need to train their managers to accept and manage the conflict that is inevitable in times of change.

However, health care managers will only be able to better manage the conflict produced by change if all employees are involved in the change process. Far too many health care facilities are looking for new leadership before they have restructured their management and prepared their employees for the radical change the future certainly holds. Strong leadership is always desirable, but better management is an absolute necessity for every organization as it responds to the changing environment.

Hammer (2007) points out that to redesign business processes and jobs, those in redesigned positions need additional training, and decentralized decision making at the lowest level of the organization should be encouraged. Redesigned organizations must also reward the process by providing incentives for excellence as well as its outcomes.

The **process audit** Hammer (2007) proposes is started by managers and supported by leaders. Implementing this audit will not be easy because health care organizations for the most part are bureaucratic, littered with rules and regulations that block change and resist innovation. It is going to require an evaluation of the process of delivering health care from the time the patient enters the facility until he or she leaves. It will require a team approach that fosters immediate communication among all team members, with the ultimate goal of successful patient outcomes and a satisfied health care customer. Health care organizations produce services, not products, and these are delivered by a team. The problems in health care delivery related to poor quality, accidents, and low customer satisfaction are all related to poor team performance. Health care managers need to spend a great deal of their time on developing a team approach to the delivery of health services.

It is important for health care managers to determine what consumers of health services want from a health care organization. They certainly do not want to be in a hospital, they do not want to be injured by the health care system, and they do not want to waste money on useless tests that produce very little if any value. They want the providers of these services to treat them with respect and help them with their health-related problems. They want high-quality services delivered by a dedicated team—services that they as consumers can evaluate.

This level of quality is not found in our current health care system. Caregivers in health care organizations do not link well to deliver care to the majority of patients (Halvorson, 2009), and this results in far too many patients experiencing poor outcomes. The health care manager is therefore faced with the daunting task of developing a team approach.

There are very few tasks that can be completed by one person in today's organizations (Zenger, Folkman, and Edinger, 2009). This is especially true in health care organizations, which require the expertise of numerous providers working together to produce successful outcomes for the patient. The more complex the health care procedure, the more critical the linkages among team members.

Health services are not prepared ahead of demand, so they must be evaluated as they are produced. If mistakes are made in the delivery of these services, therefore, it is too late to correct the faulty delivery, making it very important that systems be designed to prevent such errors before services are delivered. It is a fact in management that systems usually get precisely the outcomes they are designed to deliver, which is why our health care system must be designed to produce zero defects.

As already discussed, miscommunication among health care professionals is a major cause of medical errors, and addressing this is one of the greatest challenges health care managers face. How can the manager connect all of the individuals providing health services for the patient to achieve the best outcomes for each individual patient? Fostering team communication is the ultimate managerial responsibility in the delivery of cost-effective, efficient, quality care.

Solving this problem will require the development of a culture of safety in health care delivery. There is currently no real incentive to improve safety and thus the quality of care. Halvorson (2009) argues that the "non-system" of care in American medicine does a terrible job of connecting the required forms of care for patients with multiple diseases. These individuals make up a very large number of patients, and their comorbidities are responsible for 75 percent of the cost of health care. The issue of connectors of medical care for patients with multiple chronic illnesses has become a management nightmare for health care organizations in the United States. To see any improvement, according to Halvorson, the American health care system needs to develop a culture of continuous learning for all providers of health services.

PRODUCTIVITY AND PRIORITIZATION IN HEALTH CARE

The vast majority of the output of the health care industry consists of services delivered to consumers by health care providers. These services are produced when needed, so it is impossible to have an inventory of health services available for future consumption by patients. This creates problems for providers, who are faced with low demand for services at some points and very high demand at others. This also makes adequate staffing a major problem for health care managers. Fortunately, there are several other industries that deal with just-in-time production and have been able to produce excellent results. Health care managers need to look at how these industries deal with this type of unpredictable demand and attempt to duplicate their successful organizational design.

Shenkar (2010) argues that imitation needs to be viewed as a driver of innovation, not as a force that impedes it. He believes that productivity gains in business are not realized by innovation itself but by the improvements that result from it in the future. This is because the imitators do not have the enormous costs associated with an innovation, allowing them to view the innovation using multiple models. Imitators are less likely to become complacent because they realize how easy it is to duplicate the innovation, and they are therefore constantly trying to improve on it. Shenkar goes on to talk about the fusion of imitation and innovation to create a competitive advantage for a business. He calls this fusion "imovation," which may, if used properly, very well be required to solve many of our health care problems.

One of the possible side effects of just-in-time production in health care is medical errors. Champy and Greenspun (2010) argue that there are way too many steps in health care procedures that add little if any value to the patient's medical experience. Such procedures are not arranged in the best sequence, and they need to be redesigned to improve quality, safety, and cost. Let us look at a company—Alcoa—that should suffer from safety issues because of the nature of the products it produces. This producer of aluminum products has become the safest large manufacturing company in the United States.

The approach followed by Alcoa in reducing workplace injuries could be applied to address the epidemic of medical errors in the delivery of health services (Spear, 2009). Alcoa had problems with occupational safety until a new CEO prioritized safety as the company's most important goal. In 1987 Paul O'Neill, CEO of Alcoa, announced that his first goal for the company would be zero injuries in the workplace. O'Neill made safety problems reportable directly to him within twenty-four hours of their occurrence. He then designed a system with the ability to detect problems when and where they occur. These safety problems are then swarmed, which requires all involved to confront the safety issue using their specific skills at the time and place of occurrence. This makes it possible to gather information that would otherwise probably be lost over time. After a solution to the problem is discovered, the new knowledge is then shared with everyone who needs to know. This approach, used by high-velocity organizations, usually involves capturing existing knowledge and building in tests to reveal problems, swarming and solving problems to accrue new knowledge, and sharing the new knowledge gained throughout the organization.

In management circles it is well known that certain types of practices in the workplace result in higher levels of performance in an organization. There are many things that managers of scarce resources can do with their limited time on a daily basis. The health care manager needs to learn how to prioritize those activities that will produce the highest returns for the organization. According to Maxwell (2004), to become more effective a manager must prioritize his or her life and work and continue to manage priorities on a daily basis.

One of the most important skills required of the new health care manager is learning what to prioritize. It seems like a simple task, but when you are responsible for managing the delivery of health services daily prioritization can become complicated and demanding. It has been my experience that health care managers spend far too much time going to meetings and too little time being with the patients. Managers also spend too little time with the staff helping them understand what is and what is not important. Managers need to make communicating with patients and employees a high priority. Dye (2010) offers two excellent suggestions concerning the management of health care organizations. The first involves minimizing meetings, which are often unnecessary and keep the manager from doing more important work for the organization. The second relates to prioritization. The manager needs to write two separate lists on a daily basis: one list for personal affairs and one for work. The manager then should label the day's items as "urgent," "important," or "can wait." In health care, in the manager's work list, the patient needs to be labeled as "urgent."

Consumers demand excellent medical care and excellent customer service every time they visit a medical facility (Fottler et al., 2010). Meeting these demands is difficult, however, because every consumer of health services is different and therefore asks for varying degrees of clinical and customer service. It is very clear that consumers of health care do not want to be hospitalized, they do not want to be injured in the process of receiving health care, and they want to remain well as long as possible. Health care organizations and their managers need to learn how to respond to these consumer demands.

SUMMARY

The health care sector of our economy is undergoing tremendous change due to health care reform efforts introduced through government legislation. Health care facilities are not producing good outcomes for patients, even though the cost of these health services continues to increase every year. These problems require a drastic change in how health services are delivered and how they are reimbursed. There needs to be a tremendous reengineering effort, which in turn requires better managers and empowered followers to improve health outcomes while controlling costs.

The vast majority of health care facilities are still using bureaucratic management techniques that do not work very well in the face of enormous change. These organizations are still relying on rules and regulations that virtually eliminate any real attempts at creativity and innovation, which are so necessary in today's turbulent health care delivery environment. Organizations in the new health care system are in need of skilled health care managers who foster growth and development among their employees. A team of empowered employees should be delivering these vital services to consumers; and there needs to be a greater focus on the quality of health services, which requires a thick culture of excellence fostered by constant communication to all employees. This can only be accomplished through the development of health care managers who are capable of building new processes in health care delivery.

This health care reform effort is also creating opportunities for the health care system. The key to success is better management of scarce resources, which requires current health care managers to develop a multitude of necessary skills, including leadership and communication skills as well as the ability to empower lower-level employees to offer quality services to the consumer of health services. This book has been written for those who want the skills needed to be a successful manager of a health care organization during a time of great change.

KEY TERMS

comparative effectiveness research (CER)

disruptive innovation

effectiveness

efficiency

empowerment

health care management

health care reform

process audit

REVIEW QUESTIONS

1. Please name and explain the major problems in the health care industry, as outlined by Fuchs (1998). Do they represent isolated issues, or are they symptoms of much larger problems? Explain.

2. How might system redesign help address the efficiency issues found in the U.S. health care system?

3. Explain the reasons why the bureaucratic management structure will no longer work in the delivery of health services.

4. How will the new health care reform legislation affect the management of the health care industry in the United States?

2

Health Care Management

Bernard J. Healey

LEARNING OBJECTIVES

- Understand the major problems pertaining to the management of scarce health care resources
- Become aware of the functions of management
- Understand the value of better management of health services
- Be able to explain how management theory developed
- Understand the new theories of management as they relate to health care delivery

The health care industry has become the largest employer in the United States and is expected to continue to grow into the foreseeable future. This growth in health care employment will be the result of an increasing demand for health services caused by an expanding population, the aging of Americans, and a growing epidemic of very expensive chronic diseases (Shi & Singh, 2010). This growth in employment in the health care sector will require more managers of scarce health care resources, especially human capital. These managers will need better preparation that includes advanced training in interpersonal skills to be successful. Health care managers are responsible for people who deliver services to other people.

Kovner, Fine, and D'Aqila (2009) argue that for health care to be safe, efficient, and effective, managers and employees have to do many things right every day. To improve health care delivery, health care managers will require different skill sets along with continuing education for dealing with a constantly changing health care environment. They must be prepared to handle change on a daily basis as they attempt to deliver quality health services to demanding patients. It is important to note that they will be shouldering this new responsibility with very limited resources. The managers and the followers in health care organizations must be empowered by the administration to do what needs to be done to efficiently deliver health services while also avoiding errors in their delivery.

Management has usually been defined as getting things done through people. The process of management involves planning, organizing, and controlling people and things to deliver a product or service to consumers. Part of this process of management is leading and inspiring others to achieve the predetermined goals of the organization.

The study of management is so very important because change has become the norm, making it mandatory for managers to learn how to adapt to change as their organization evolves (Dyck & Neubert, 2009). Nowhere is this more evident than in health care organizations, which regularly confront monumental change. Health care managers face survival issues that include difficulty obtaining reimbursement, staffing shortages, rising costs, regulatory pressures, and increasing consumer demand for quality (Johnson, 2005). These challenges will only get worse as health care reform is fully implemented. The change that is all around us as the health care system reforms requires leaders with vision—but it will also require better management of scarce resources, especially human resources.

Health care is most certainly the ultimate service industry, requiring very special people with special skills to deliver services. Blanchard (2010) argues that empowered employees are even more important than customers because the employees are the ones providing the superior services that keep customers loyal. This is especially true with patients in health care. The management of health services requires special training, including instilling the realization that the vast majority of managerial decisions have effects on employees and patients rather than on machines and products. Halvorson (2009) points out that to achieve the majority of health care goals we will need to use the right tools. This book was written to supply health care managers with the right tools, including new theories of management, to improve our current health care system.

MANAGEMENT THEORY

For better managers to be prepared for the difficult challenges ahead, they need to understand past and current theories of management. **Management theory** is a collection of observations about how the process of managing people and things occurs in our world. Management theory has been around since the very beginning of time, and it has evolved over the centuries. Throughout the years specific schools of management thought developed, and various theories of management were practiced with great success in the workplace. As the environment changed, old theories did not work as well and new theories emerged and were reluctantly embraced. Recycling old management theories and changing them to deal with the current environment became the normal way to address management concerns. In fact, Johnson (2005) has identified four theories of management that have been under continuous discussion in recent years: scientific management, bureaucratic management, human relations theory, and reengineering theory.

Even though management thought has been around for hundreds of years, it is only within the last hundred or so years that the study of management has developed a well-researched theoretical base. A very large number of management theories are now available in introductory management texts. This chapter will cover some of the older management theories and then move into some of the newer ones, leading into a discussion of management functions and skills, team-based management, and the role of innovation in regard to the newer thoughts about the management process. One must keep in mind that, as already mentioned, new theories of management are developed in response to the old theories' failure. Only recently have health care facilities started to realize that bureaucratic management no longer works in health care, primarily because consumers play a role in obtaining their own health care. It is interesting to note that the majority of health care facilities still cling to bureaucratic management techniques because they are still operating using legitimate power bases. Those in charge of managing health care facilities are frightened of losing power and are fearful of changing the management structure.

Figure 2.1 shows the major branches represented in the classical approach to management, which has offered great insight into production and administration. These branches are well represented by scientific management, administrative principles, and the bureaucratic organization. The theories that resulted from the classical approach have been used by many of the most successful organizations in America since the beginning of time. They were developed by Frederick Taylor (scientific management), Henri Fayol (administrative principles), and Max Weber (the bureaucratic organization), with all of these scholars placing efficiency as the ultimate goal of any organization. How could anyone argue with that underlying goal?

According to Goldsmith (2011), management is concerned with productivity and efficiency, but it is also concerned with the motivation and leadership of people. The question posed by this definition of management revolves around the importance of each component: productivity and profits versus the personal growth of the employee at work and at home. One of

Figure 2.1 Major Branches in the Classical Approach to Management
Source: Schermerhorn, 2010, p. 28. Reprinted with permission of John Wiley & Sons, Inc.

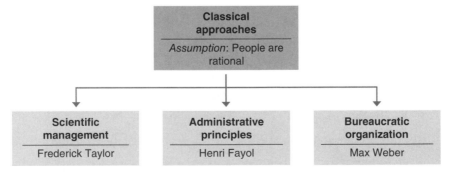

the first schools of management thought is usually referred to as the classical approach, which was an outgrowth of the Industrial Revolution and an attempt to discover the best way to perform and manage work activities. Dating back to the early 1800s, the classical approach was primarily concerned with efficiency and effectiveness, and was not as oriented toward the individual employee. In fact, by being efficient and making profits, people had work that supplied them with purchasing power and allowed them to grow through their efforts. There was no time for human concerns in the workplace, only greater emphasis on production. The fact that profits increased and organizations grew seemed to validate the classical approach to management.

The theory of scientific management was developed by Frederick Taylor. In 1911 Taylor published "The Principles of Scientific Management," which focused on increasing worker productivity (Taylor, n.d.). This theory focuses on the study of the process of work in an attempt to improve output from that work—to find the best way to perform a given job. The major focus of this management theory is on the improvement of operational efficiency through a comprehensive examination of work rules and standards. In other words, we scientifically study the process of work to determine the optimal way to complete each part of that process. For scientific management to work today, a complete mental revolution would be necessary on the part of workers and managers, who would have to unite to better perform the tasks at hand.

Taylor's theory also required scientific selection of workers for the job, managers' cooperation with the workers, and the division of the work equally among workers and managers. Work would be divided according to the level of skill possessed by each worker, enabling specialization of work that would ultimately increase productivity. This would allow each worker to produce more, lower production costs, and ultimately increase profits. Even though everyone did not agree with scientific management techniques, the theory seemed to work very well at increasing productivity and profits for employers.

The theory of administrative principles was another addition to the classical approach. This theory, which involves principles of managerial duties and methods of managing developed by Henri Fayol, revolves around the belief that management as a discipline can be applied to all organizations. The administrative principles Fayol developed resulted from his actual experiences as a manager working in the mining industry in the early 1900s. According to Schermerhorn (2010), Fayol proposed five rules or duties of the manager:

- Foresight
- Organization
- Command
- Coordination
- Control

Fayol has been given the title of the father of modern organizational theory because the duties he outlined resemble the functions of management that are taught in most management courses even today. He believed that a generalized theory of management could be taught to others, but that the major emphasis needed to be that at any point any employee may take on duties that require managerial decisions. Although he stressed authority and the control of employees, he did communicate ideas that showed flexibility and adaptation. His greatest contribution to management theory involved his principles of effective management.

The theory of bureaucratic management, which was also an outgrowth of the classical approach, focuses on the development of rules as the basis for efficiency. According to Borgatti (1996), the architect of this theory of management was Max Weber, a German philosopher who believed that bureaucracy was an appropriate framework for attaining the greatest degree of efficiency in any organization. The bureaucratic organization, which has become the dominant model for organizations throughout the world, is structured around logic, order, and legitimate authority. Schermerhorn (2010) points out that the characteristics of a bureaucracy include a clear division of labor and hierarchy of authority, formal rules and procedures, an impersonal relationship among managers and employees, and careers based on merit. These characteristics have combined to become the normal organizational form for the large majority of businesses over thousands of years of evolution. These bureaucratic organizations increased their efficiency and made profits, which defined success for organizations.

Weber, in his study of organizations, found that bureaucracy and rationality were identical when it comes to running a business enterprise. According to Weber, rules and regulations, along with a very clear hierarchy of authority, need to be present in a business to defeat the competition. Management is necessary to make businesses efficient, and a bureaucratic structure enables managers to accomplish the efficient delivery of goods and services to consumers. Establishing a bureaucracy seemed to Weber a logical way for a business to increase its efficiency and, therefore, deliver profits to the owners and payments to workers.

Weber believed that forming a bureaucracy required the development of highly trained managers. These managers needed to be selected and trained for their specific duties, and they also had to make decisions according to the rules and regulations promulgated by the organization. In addition to the need for clear lines of authority within the organization's power hierarchy, there had to be a respected, logical chain of command for making decisions. Management, according to Weber, was to be very impersonal and should focus on the goal of efficiency in the production process.

Lombardi and Schermerhorn (2007) argue that many times an organization with a bureaucratic structure will be successful in specific arenas. Unfortunately, this mechanistic form of organization does not do very well when the environment is unstable and rapid change has become a constant force that managers must confront. In the twenty-first century change and conflict have become a way of life for almost every business worldwide, requiring a movement from a mechanistic design to a more organic structure that can be proactive rather than reactive to new threats and opportunities.

Figure 2.2 shows the shift from rigid, mechanistic, bureaucratic organizations to adaptive organizations characterized by an organic design. Organizations need to become more agile and more capable of rapidly responding to change and actually turning it into a business opportunity. The adaptive organization shown on the right side of Figure 2.2 is decentralized; there are fewer rules, and there are wider spans of control and a more personal way

Figure 2.2   Continuum of Organizational Alternatives, from Bureaucratic to Adaptive Organizations
Source: Lombardi & Schermerhorn, 2007, p. 70. Reprinted with permission of John Wiley & Sons, Inc.

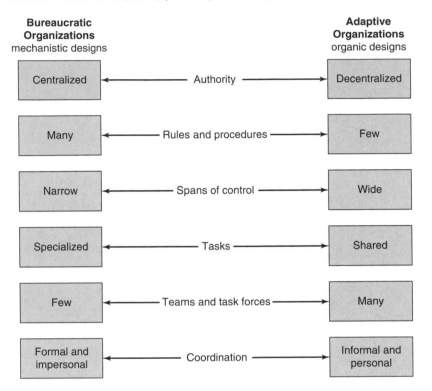

of coordinating the work process. Adaptive organizations thrive on teamwork and employee **empowerment** to accomplish their goals and objectives. An adaptive structure requires the empowerment of all employees, which entails a great deal of trust and a loss of control on the part of managers.

Figure 2.2 shows the most important components of the adaptive organization, which has the type of organizational structure that is capable of dealing with the most important problems faced by the health care sector of our economy. As depicted in the figure, the adaptive organization has an organic design that is decentralized; there are few rules; and shared tasks, team problem solving, and informal and personal coordination are the norm. These are the exact characteristics needed in health care organizations.

Empowered health care employees must handle the changes in health care today by working in teams to respond to consumer demands.

The classical approach, especially the building of bureaucratic organizations, worked fine until it didn't work anymore. The business environment had changed, but management principles remained the same. Bureaucratic organizations were comfortable for numerous managers, but many businesses started to realize that bureaucracies did not function very well in a changing world. Beginning to question the underlying assumptions of the classical approach, they started to actively explore other management theories that might allow them to respond more rapidly to shifting consumer demands for quality products and services. There were so many management theories developing that it became very confusing as to what theory the top businesses were actually using.

It suddenly became very important to focus on the people that make the product or deliver the service. Managers want to have enthusiastic, motivated, and productive workers, but they are usually confused about how to acquire and keep workers who possess these qualities. It became evident to management researchers that a bureaucratic organization was not where these workers would want to spend their career. The new world of work was in dire need of engaged workers and inspirational managers.

Branham and Hirschfeld (2010) define employee engagement as an increased emotional and intellectual connection between an employee and his or her work or place of employment. Engaged employees have totally dedicated themselves to what they do at work, making them extremely productive. This is exactly the type of employee that we have to find to improve our health care system.

The cost escalation and quality issues in health care are found deep in the work process of delivering health services (Gittell, 2009). The majority of health care facilities in our country are bureaucratic, and many of these have disengaged a large number of employees, producing lower productivity, medical errors, and poor quality in the delivery of services. Survey after survey of health care employees finds low morale, insufficient motivation, and job dissatisfaction.

Muzio (2010) points out that as management theory continued to evolve through the 1950s there was a much greater interest in people rather than just efficiency and increased productivity. This emphasis on the human side of management ushered in human relations theory. One of the first individuals to advocate paying attention to the people part of production was Robert Owen, a textile mill manager in Scotland who was more concerned with the treatment of individuals than with the machinery used in the production process.

The catalyst leading to the creation of the human relations approach to management was the famous Hawthorne studies, which were completed at a Western Electric Company plant in Illinois in 1924. These studies involved experimentation with several factors, such as workplace illumination and wage incentives, to motivate employees toward increased productivity. The conclusion from these experiments was that there were social aspects of managing workers as well as economic factors. This research concluded that human behavior, workers' attitudes concerning work, and the informal work group are all important contributors to worker motivation.

This work also brought about the theory developed by Abraham Maslow involving a hierarchy of human needs, which was published in 1943 (Maslow, 1998). The motivators of employees begin with lower-level needs, called basic and security needs, and then can progress to higher-level needs, such as social, self-esteem, and self-actualization needs. According to this theory, to continue to motivate individuals the manager has to consider more than money as a primary motivator.

Maslow's work was followed by the work of Douglas McGregor, a researcher from MIT, whose theories were labeled Theory X and Theory Y. McGregor's research consisted of a set of assumptions that managers hold concerning their employees. Theory X involved mostly negative assumptions about employees, including the fact that they were usually lazy and needed to be watched while at work. Theory Y involved positive assumptions about employees, including the fact that most employees are interested in more responsibility, are naturally creative, and enjoy work (McGregor, 1957).

The workplace needed managers who could empower their workforce as well as workers who wanted to be empowered. Hammer (2007) introduced the concept of the process audit in 1990, focusing on helping companies plan and execute process-based transformations. This new management focus concentrated on the redesign of the entire work process of a given business. It required the total redesign of jobs such that decision making could move down to lower-level employees, who would be rewarded for the work process and work outcome. Although the new form of management was very difficult to implement, it led to tremendous improvements in speed, quality, and profitability for organizations that used the process audit to redesign their internal production process. The redesign effort had to be supported by increased training for all members of the organization.

Hammer and Champy (2003) point out that reengineering does away with the old assumptions of how business is done and moves to a radical redesign of business processes, concentrating on cost, quality, service, and speed in delivery. During this management process the business starts over in an attempt to rebuild itself to better serve the customer. Managers simplify existing business practices by starting with the desires of the customer and working backward. Lower-level employees, who are usually closer to the customer, especially when delivering a service, are empowered to act immediately. This new form of management essentially eliminates bureaucratic control, affording employees greater freedom to deliver quality to the consumer. The process also requires the development of a team approach that handles the entire process of work.

Champy and Greenspun (2010) argue that there are three major components of reengineering health care delivery in this country: technology, processes, and people.

- Technology is becoming the enabler of reducing costs and improving quality. It is a tool that must be used to gather necessary data about the various processes performed in the delivery of health services.

- Processes in health care have not responded to the changing environment facing the health care sector. The consumers of health care want to be healthy, not to be allowed to become ill—but health care organizations today focus on curing rather than preventing illness. Reimbursement focuses on activities, not on outcomes. This must change.

- People are the most important component in the delivery of high-quality health services at a cost we can all afford. The dedicated individuals who deliver health services are ready to become empowered so that they can help improve health care delivery.

Muzio (2010) points out that if leadership requires the ability to inspire others to facilitate change at all levels, then managers require leadership skills. In an environment of fast-paced change, managers must exhibit many of the same skills found among leaders of a business enterprise. This concept assumes that the organization has moved away from a bureaucratic organizational structure to a more organic form of management.

MANAGEMENT INNOVATION

In *The Future of Management,* Gary Hamel (2007) challenges traditional management theory. This book points out that new realities in the world of work require new organizational and managerial capabilities. Many of the underlying assumptions of the classical approach to management are no longer applicable to the changing work environment and the changing wants and demands of consumers. According to Hamel, the new problems managers face in the twenty-first century require new theories of management. The new theory developed in this book is called management innovation, which encourages managers to address challenges in a way that improves the total performance of their organization.

The foundation of any organization trying to compete in today's turbulent environment depends on the organization's mission, vision, and values. The problem is that the goals of the organization of today cannot be achieved using old bureaucratic theories of management. As already mentioned, the rigid rules and regulations of a bureaucratic organization stifle the innovation and creativity so necessary to beat the competition.

It is extremely difficult to change the bureaucratic structure of management because it has worked so well in the past. Another reason not to move away from the bureaucratic model is that when power is concentrated in the hands of a few, especially if they benefit from the current organizational structure, they are capable of obstructing change. The vision of the organization, along with the power to achieve that vision, must be shared. Such empowerment will not occur, however, when the manager is fearful of losing power and blocks the necessary change.

Muzio (2010) points out that a service delivery organization is nothing more than a group of people joined together with other resources to produce value for the consumer. This definition makes output or value the endpoint in the production process. How we get there is up to the manager and other members of the team. Muzio also cautions that how we get there must not come at a cost so high that it results in the loss of critical human capital.

There has been a great deal of discussion about the use of new management practices, going back as far as the famous Hawthorne studies in the 1920s. Unfortunately, this talk has led to very little real change in the practice of management. We all know that a bureaucratic organization is not a fun place to work, but this organizational structure does increase efficiency and improve the bottom line, and it is protected by those who profit from its existence.

The rigid rules and regulations of a bureaucratic organization do not allow the manager to be innovative. In fact, in this type of structure it is very doubtful whether management innovation is even possible. This is especially true in regard to the managerial thought process of health care delivery. Most health care managers see themselves as pragmatic doers, not as process innovators. Management innovation is not really expected in health care delivery. That is about to change.

Fottler, Ford, and Heaton (2010) argue that those who work in health care delivery want their job to offer fun, fairness, interesting work, and importance. Obviously they also need competitive compensation packages, but they want much more from the occupation to which they have chosen to devote all or a portion of their working years. Monetary rewards only motivate for a short period of time, but other nonmonetary aspects of work are capable of pushing individuals to constantly try to improve performance. The manager then needs to be the one who establishes a workplace that encourages fun, fairness, interesting work assignments, and a feeling by employees that they are an important part of the health care team—an atmosphere that is not present in a bureaucratic health care organization.

These same nonmonetary rewards of work are important in the encouragement of creativity and innovation in the workplace. To improve the delivery of health services, employees have to be encouraged to break the rules and regulations found in a bureaucracy and begin to add value to the customer's health care experience. For this to happen, the health care manager also has to break rules and start inspiring the most important component of excellent service in health care—health care employees. The new rules of health care delivery have to prioritize consistent, value-adding service.

MANAGERIAL SKILLS

Most managers, including those who manage health care facilities, usually have developed special skills that allowed them to be appointed to a managerial position. The skills most frequently associated with management include technical skills, human skills, and conceptual skills, which are usually associated with work expertise or good people skills.

Technical skills may be found in all managers but are most important for those occupying lower-level managerial positions, especially in health care facilities. Individuals usually develop these technical capabilities after a long time of perfecting their work skills before moving into a managerial position. They include expertise in a specific area of work, allowing the individual to be promoted to a managerial position supervising those with lesser skills in that particular area. Individuals with excellent technical skills are promoted into managerial positions to share these work skills with their direct reports.

Human skills allow one to appreciate the value of coworkers and work well with others. These skills are known as interpersonal, and they include the ability of the manager to communicate effectively with workers, both orally and in writing. Those exhibiting human skills can get along with people and are usually capable of motivating them to work harder. Drawing on this skill set can be very useful in deciding how to motivate lower-level employees to complete the task assigned. Human skills have become so important in modern management, even when compared to production and efficiency, that a new theory was introduced: human relations theory.

Conceptual skills come into play when a manager needs to be able to both understand complex tasks and reduce them to a level at which solutions can be applied. Johnson (2005) points out that conceptual skills allow the manager to better understand the complex interrelationships that exist in the workplace. These are higher-level skills that are usually found in higher-level managers. They involve the manager's ability to see the organization as a whole. Managers who possess conceptual skills are capable of looking way beyond the problems of today and focusing more on the opportunities of the future.

The emphasis in health care has always been on technical skills, and the managers of health care employees were usually developed and promoted into managerial positions because of their advanced technical skills. The patient was seen as a passive entity in health care delivery who was only concerned with technical superiority and motivated by basic needs. The managers of health care organizations today, however, need to develop technical, human, and conceptual skills in their pursuit of quality and productivity in the evolving health care system.

MANAGEMENT FUNCTIONS

Certain **management functions** are fundamental to any organization that is attempting to provide goods or services efficiently and effectively to its customers. Research has shown that most managers use the functions of planning, organizing, leading, and controlling. These same functions are required of health care managers as they endeavor to provide health services efficiently and effectively to a variety of customers. Figure 2.3 shows the various functions of a manager and their interrelationships. Different managers place different value on the importance of each specific function.

The **planning** function in health care delivery is concerned with the development of goals and objectives along with the strategies designed to achieve them. Barton (2010) argues that planning in health care can occur at an organizational level, at a project level, or at a program level. The problem with planning for reaching long-term goals at any level is the volatile environment the health care sector faces. Planning is susceptible to

Figure 2.3 Functions of Management
Source: Lombardi & Schermerhorn, 2007, p. 17. Reprinted with permission of John Wiley & Sons, Inc.

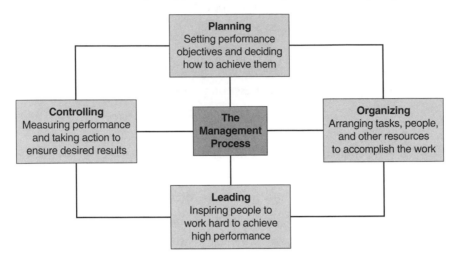

macro and micro environmental influences on a daily basis. Despite this confusing environment, however, managers must develop a plan of action for their health care facility. According to Swayne, Duncan, and Ginter (2008), the management of plans requires agreement on objectives, the evaluation of performance based on the attainment of those objectives, and the application of corrective action if objectives are not met. Because the only constant in health care delivery is constant change, planning is one of the most difficult functions for the health care manager (Fottler et al., 2010).

The **organizing** function entails designing positions and grouping them into departments that ultimately carry out the organization's plans. To achieve the goals set forth in the planning process, it is critical that positions within the organization be organized for maximum efficiency. Although we tend to dislike the bureaucratic organizational structure, most successful organizations began with a bureaucratic design, whereby the power flows downward from the top of the management hierarchy.

The organizing function in management involves the appointment of individuals to positions that are designed for one purpose: the accomplishment of goals in an efficient and effective manner. Components of the organizing function include communication, the achievement of synergy, avoiding the duplication of resources, and the establishment of lines of authority. This internal function requires that managers pay attention to the division of work, assigning employees to specific duties and departments and developing working relationships among employees. This function of management allows individuals to work together to achieve goals that they could not achieve individually. An organization usually retains its structure as long as it is successful in the achievement of the goals established in the work plan.

Leadership in an organization represents the power to inspire others to achieve and surpass the goals set forth in the mission statement. Although there is no universal definition of leadership, it is generally accepted that it involves the power to persuade others to follow. The success or failure of the organization is usually determined by the leadership found in the organization. It is a given that all leaders manage and all managers lead. Therefore, leadership has become a very important function in today's environment of constant change.

The leading function in health care delivery involves influencing others to achieve organizational goals. Everyone in a health care organization, especially managers, must be involved in leadership. The manager must lead employees to service excellence (Fottler et al., 2010). Lombardi and Schermerhorn (2007) point out that effective leadership in health care involves empowering lower-level employees so that they are more willing to make decisions to better serve their customers. This leading function is critical for the manager in the empowerment of employees to produce excellent services for their patients. This ability to make decisions without prior approval to better meet patient needs helps employees grow in their position, also offering them the motivation to continue to grow. Such an opportunity for personal growth is not usually present in a structured, bureaucratic organization, which is why the decentralization of decisions and actions is so very important in service delivery organizations.

The **controlling** function in health care delivery consists of various activities designed to ensure that employee actions lead to the achievement of organizational objectives. According to Lombardi and Schermerhorn

(2007), this function consists of evaluating the performance of work, comparing the actual output of employee performance with desired objectives, and then taking corrective action as necessary. The controlling function is meant to be a positive rather than a negative force. It is meant to improve the performance of employees, and must be critical but constructive in its intent. There is an old saying in management that workers respect what managers inspect. This is crucial in health care delivery, in which medical errors are capable of causing patient disability and even death.

SELF-MANAGED WORK TEAMS

Health care has traditionally been delivered in a bureaucratic format, with the physician in charge of almost every aspect of medicine. Physicians had a monopoly over a patient's demand for health services and never really looked at medicine as a team process. Thanks to the ongoing reform of health care delivery, however, the future of health services will include a team approach that involves many health care providers bringing a variety of health care skills. Members of a health care team might include, for example, case managers, nurses, physician assistants, medical practice managers, secretaries, pharmacists, telephone counselors, and external evaluators. This collection of providers needs to become a self-managed work team that is charged with delivering services efficiently and is measured by the health outcomes of its patients.

The management of human resources is a fundamental function of any organization, particularly in the management of health services, which are delivered by people to people. Health care managers are primarily responsible for the delivery of very important services that are difficult to measure in terms of their quality. Making matters even more challenging is the fact that almost all health services are delivered by more than one provider. It becomes almost impossible for anyone to manage a team other than the team itself. This is why self-managed work teams are so popular and in most cases so efficient in the delivery of services. The use of self-managed work teams to control the work process is actually a form of management innovation.

Hamel (2007) argues that management innovation fosters value-creating changes in the structure of the organization as well as in the role played by the managers. The goal of achieving a competitive advantage is met, according to Hamel, when one or more of the following three conditions occurs in the work process:

1. The new innovation in management challenges current beliefs.

2. The proposed innovation involves systemic change that includes process and method.

3. The innovation includes a continuous process of rapid invention that compounds over time.

An example of the successful use of management innovation using team-based management is found in W. L. Gore and Associates, a company built by Bill Gore in 1958. This extremely successful company generates $2.1 billion in annual sales and employs more than eight thousand workers worldwide. It produces thousands of innovative products, and avoids bureaucracy at any cost. Gore's management structure includes no supervisors, and workers are free to choose what they want to do at work. The operating unit of this business is the small, self-managed work team. Each work team hires, fires, rewards, and even chooses a team leader, all without the supervision of a manager. Employees in this company are responsible to their team leader.

This company's products are developed during a discretionary half day a week of free time called "dabble time," which allows employees to be innovative and create new products. W. L. Gore and Associates has found its way to success by purposely avoiding the trap of bureaucratic management, instead using team-based management that leads to the development of new products and increased profits every year.

This same concept was transplanted to the delivery of health services by Mayo Clinic in three metropolitan areas: Rochester, Minnesota; Scottsdale, Arizona; and Jacksonville, Florida. The clinic began as a single, small outpatient facility over 140 years ago, and later became the first integrated group practice in this country. Mayo Clinic now employs over seventeen thousand physicians and is well known for achieving high-quality care at a very low cost. Mayo Clinic has used meeting the needs of the patient as its primary approach, and has been named by *U.S. News & World Report* as among the "best hospitals" for twenty years. They did this by practicing team-based management of patient services. Mayo Clinic attracts employees who like to practice delivering medicine to patients as a team (Berry & Seltman, 2008). The clinic searches for team players, and then supports the team approach by using communication technology. Managers of health care organizations must also learn how to work with teams as they seek to improve the quality of care. Berry and Seltman point out that teamwork in health care delivery is no longer optional. Mayo Clinic has united all staff members to work together in a complex organization, with the aim of improving care for all patients. This is not by individual choice, but by organizational design.

Mayo Clinic uses an all-salary approach rather than a fee-for-service approach to compensating their physicians that encourages quality health care while discouraging wasteful and potentially dangerous testing. The staff are immersed in serving the patient and working together as a team. The clinic culture encourages respect among patients and providers. According to Berry and Seltman (2008), the two principal values of Mayo Clinic are as follows:

1. The needs of the patient are the primary concern of all employees of the clinic.

2. Medicine should be practiced as a cooperative science involving all members of the team.

These two principles are appropriate for adoption by all facilities delivering health services to their patients. The patient, as the real consumer of health services, needs to be respected and communicated to, just like any other consumer of services would be treated. All of the available research supports the assertion that if the patient is involved in his or her own health care delivery, clinical outcomes improve, costs are reduced, and the health care facility gains a competitive advantage.

The team of health care professionals must be working together with one overriding goal: obtaining the best health outcomes for individual patients. According to Dlugacz (2010), the use of patient-focused health care usually results in greater efficiency and effectiveness in the delivery of health services. This occurs because the environment is right for two-way communication between patient and provider. Such communication can result in uncovering nonmedical issues that may have a tremendous impact on health outcomes.

Coordination among employees that results in shared goals and knowledge as well as mutual respect improves the chances for solving complex problems in the workplace (Gittell, 2009). This relational coordination is capable of reducing medical errors and improving the overall health care experience for patients. It can also result in bolstered employee commitment.

A large number of health care organizations have fostered work practices that encourage divisions among employees. This is the result of a bureaucratic structure that does very little to promote communication. Improving the quality of health services goes beyond commitment and skilled employees because health care providers have to coordinate their work with one another in the delivery of health care.

HEALTH SERVICES MANAGEMENT

The management of services is very different from the management of products delivered to customers. According to Thomas (2010), services are difficult to conceptualize because they are so personal and intangible. This description implies that services do not take a concrete form and are evaluated in various ways by different individuals.

A major challenge in managing health services is the difficulty the patient has in evaluating the quality of the services delivered. That is changing in a dramatic way. Lee and Mongan (2009) argue that patients actually hold the power necessary to shape the entire health care system in this country. These consumers of health care are becoming more demanding as they learn more about their health thanks to advancements in technology. The news media is also supplying a great deal of health-related information to consumers on a daily basis. In addition, the government is providing consumers with information, as evidenced by the Institute of Medicine's report (2001) on the epidemic of medical errors.

In addition to the problem of incorporating patients in the management of their own health care, the costs associated with health care delivery are increasing so rapidly that the entire health care system is in crisis, causing more and more individuals to become uninsured. Lee and Mongan (2009) argue that the reason behind cost increases is found in the progress being made in health care. Although progress is needed, the system that delivers the progress needs to be better organized, and to be forced to stop the waste of scarce health care resources—which will require better management of these resources. Finally, the current health care system is obsessed with curing rather than preventing illness. This has placed too much power in the hands of the physicians who do the curing and the insurance companies that decide whether or not to pay for the cure.

According to Fottler et al. (2010), health care managers have been more concerned with patients' clinical needs than with their wants and expectations, which has resulted in patient dissatisfaction. It is becoming increasingly clear that health care managers and workers need to pay much more attention to what patients want to keep them satisfied, or these patients will take their business to the competition.

The U.S. health care system is dysfunctional. The major problems found in health care delivery, including cost escalation, decreasing quality, and poor outcomes, are symptoms of a system that is not working very well. These problems are not unique to health care and have been solved in other industries through disruptive innovation that changes the process of delivering products or services to the customer.

One cause of the ever-growing problems in health care delivery is a lack of system coordination. It is not a new problem in health care, and it is not unique to the U.S. health care system. To improve this problem, managers of health care facilities need to spend more time and effort in the job design process. Those who work in health care delivery want empowerment to improve their patients' experience. Such employee empowerment is necessary to deal with the current epidemic of medical errors found in most health care facilities. The reduction in medical errors will not occur with the use of, or by using, bureaucratic rules and regulations. The right process will need to be developed and implemented by empowered employees who know how to reduce errors and are free to do so.

A focused job design process has the ability to improve coordination among providers while enhancing the quality and efficiency of patient care (Gittell, 2009). Shortell and Kaluzny (2006) argue that managers of health care organizations are responsible for defining strategic goals to ensure survival and growth.

Managers have a great deal of responsibility for building and sustaining a strong culture among their workforce. Companies that exhibit a strong, thick, and positive culture are usually very successful in coordinating the delivery of health services. Further, organizations that employ and promote individuals whose personal values are aligned with organizational values have increased productivity and reduced employee turnover (Atchison & Carlson, 2009). These organizations also foster increased employee satisfaction, which is associated with increased patient satisfaction.

Christensen, Grossman, and Hwang (2009) believe that the best integrator of a disruptive value network will be able to come up with a formula that makes money while keeping the population healthy. A disruptive value network would improve health care delivery in a way that is not expected—for example, with a focus on health outcomes rather than business activities. It will include an emphasis on long-term investment in wellness and quality improvement in health care, with an understanding that the payoff for this investment will not occur in the short term.

The special ingredient in the improvement of health care quality and cost reduction is primary care. The primary care component of our health care system has fallen on hard times. We need more doctors choosing primary care as their specialty, and we need to make better use of—and empower—such nonphysician primary care providers as nurses and physician assistants. The payoffs of this long-term investment are well worth the cost.

We also need to pay more attention to waste in the delivery of health services. Summer (2011) points out that lean thinking consists of an uninterrupted, value-adding process in the flow of work as the product or service is being produced. This process does not foster wasteful, non-value-adding elements like waiting time and hospital readmission. These are items that can be fixed in the short term. The extraordinary change resulting from the new health care reform legislation is producing opportunities to improve the quality and reduce the cost of the delivery of health services to more people.

According to Halvorson (2009), the perfect system of health care delivery would be capable of disseminating all of the necessary information about every patient all of the time. The availability of this medical information to each patient and physician can improve the quality of medical care, should lower the rate of medical errors, and will go a long way toward reducing wasteful duplication of tests and procedures.

Finally, MacGillis (2010) questions the increase in size of the majority of health care organizations in this country. He is interested in whether they produce better care for patients or whether they have just become monopolies. There is no question that health care organizations have grown in size, which should reduce their fixed costs and then lower prices for the health services delivered. However, despite the growth in size of health care facilities, the costs have continued to rise. Growing larger to increase the economies of scale and reduce cost escalation usually forces the development of a bureaucratic organizational structure. This in turn forces rules and regulations, destroying employee empowerment and thereby reducing innovation and creativity in the delivery of health services.

The management of scarce health care resources has developed over the years according to managerial theories from the private sector. A number of health care facilities cling to many of the outdated features of bureaucratic management. The ways in which health services have been delivered seemed to work well with a top-down management structure, but this was before chaos became the norm in most health care organizations in the United States. With the insurer demanding efficiency and lower prices and the consumer demanding quality, layers of management are unable to satisfy the wants and desires of those who pay for health services.

Lee and Mongan (2009) argue that a more efficient, reliable, and safe U.S. health care system is in the beginning stages of development. Even though this mammoth change will initially be chaotic, it will ultimately result in a better-organized system of health care delivery. Shifts in organization and management in various facilities across the United States will not be accomplished with bureaucratic management techniques. Decision making has to be fast, necessitating decentralization along with the development of self-managed work teams. A team approach will require a movement toward newer management techniques that foster worker empowerment, which will enable employees at the lowest levels of the organization to make decisions and respond directly to change. Management innovation must become the norm in these rigid health care facilities.

Beeret (2009) points out that the most important challenge faced by contemporary organizations is the ability to remain relevant and, therefore, continue to be supported by their top management. To remain relevant an organization requires management innovation capable of exploiting the changes being wrought by environmental chaos. This in turn requires managers to learn new ways to manage human resources because, as already stated, bureaucratic management techniques will no longer work.

This chaotic health care environment is producing competition that many health care organizations have never seen. To compete effectively in terms of quality and price, and as part of remaining relevant, health care organizations must develop a competitive advantage. Lepak and Gowan (2010) argue that in the past employees were not considered a competitive advantage, only an expense. This has changed in recent years, especially in service-producing organizations. In fact, in health care organizations the employees delivering the services may very well be the most important part of staying ahead of competitors.

Health care organizations must become aware of their new reality to remain creative, adaptive, and innovative in the delivery of health services (Beeret, 2009). Even though this is very difficult to do, it is mandatory if an organization is going to survive. Managers need their followers' help to understand the changing reality their organization faces and to develop ways to deal with it.

Health care managers must also learn how to motivate a vast array of individuals with varying degrees of educational attainment and experience. Many of these employees are better educated and have more experience than the manager. It is critical that the health care manager gain the respect of all of the team members he or she is supervising. According to Pyzdek and Keller (2010), a well-designed management system operated by motivated employees is capable of continually delivering superior products and services to customers. The superior services that result from happy employees become the organization's competitive advantage.

A very good example of management innovation in health care delivery is found in a new role for pharmacists in the United States. The pharmacist is the key player in the detection of overlapping prescriptions or dangerous drug interactions. Pharmacists also are a source for advice on the use of cheaper generic drugs. What is more, pharmacists are being enlisted by health insurers and large employers to help with a major problem that increases health care costs and produces bad health outcomes: half of U.S. patients do not take their medications as prescribed (Abelson & Singer, 2010). This represents an innovative use of pharmacists' skills and makes them a very important part of the health care team.

MANAGEMENT OF TECHNOLOGY

We need to have up-to-date information to improve the quality and reduce the cost of health services (Halvorson, 2009). The improvement of quality in any business has never been achieved without the availability of necessary data. In health care, bad data, especially in terms of financing decisions, have prevented such improvement. These bad data have led to a fee-for-service payment system, which has produced too many medical activities of limited or no value that have failed to add value to patients' health outcomes. Many of these reimbursement issues will be improved as new information technology is developed and used in third-party reimbursement for health services.

The rapid development of technology, particularly information technology, is providing many opportunities for health care managers to improve the efficiency and the quality of health care delivery. Health care managers need to welcome these opportunities, more of which are becoming available every day. The advancement of cutting-edge and very expensive technology is also a major cause of the chaos that is so very evident in health care today (Lee & Mongan, 2009). The available technology is capable of solving the vast majority of present and future problems in health care, but it requires better organization and management. This is a distinct function for the health care manager that requires a whole new set of managerial skills. It requires the manager to have an appreciation for the value of technology in health care delivery and a vision of how to use the technology to improve health outcomes. Over the last few years most policymakers in health care have realized that technology must become a major player in the changing health care industry.

Technology can be classified as medical equipment, pharmaceuticals, medical devices, medical processes and procedures, and a means of organizing health information (Williams & Torrens, 2008). Technology needs to be further developed and managed for efficiency and effectiveness, and it should be considered a major investment with little or no immediate return. If managed properly, such an investment can yield profits for the health care facility and reduce health care costs while improving the quality of health care for large segments of our population. Two of the most promising forms of information technology are electronic medical records and telemedicine.

Electronic Medical Records

Electronic medical records (EMRs) are not new, but in recent years they have been being pushed to wider adoption by several funding sources. These are computerized medical records used in a health care facility or a physician office. EMRs would eventually replace redundant, wasteful paper records, providing a more sophisticated virtual record of each patient's health history. In 2003 the president of the United States started a national push for all Americans to have EMRs (Williams & Torrens, 2008). The American Recovery and Reinvestment Act of 2009 may accelerate the pace of EMR adoption by health care providers because it includes funding to promote the use EMR systems. Halvorson (2009) argues that EMRs are among the most important tools, and can make health care a great deal better for a large number of patients. Physicians who order tests using an EMR should be able to arrive at a safer and higher-quality health outcome (Lee & Mongan, 2009).

Although EMRs are capable of supplying real-time medical information for health care providers, they are only one tool or connector necessary for the improvement of patient care. They will improve the system of health care delivery only if they are connected to additional computer tools capable of elevating the general standard of health care.

According to the Institute of Medicine (2003), EMRs are designed to enable health care professionals to

- Collect and store health information on individual patients over time

- Allow immediate electronic access to authorized users

- Provide decision-making support to help manage the safety, quality, and efficiency of health care delivery

- Support efficient processes within health care organizations

If EMRs succeed in executing these functions, and if patient confidentiality is guaranteed, a number of the barriers to exemplary patient health care will be eliminated, allowing for improved quality at a reduced cost. To meet the true potential offered by EMRs, health care managers need to be trained in their use and potential abuse. Halvorson (2009) points out that data become the key ingredient when the goal of the health care facility becomes actual health care improvement. It is the management of data that makes the whole improvement process work for the patient.

EMRs should improve efficiency and the quality of medical services for most patients, and should do very well in a cost-benefit analysis. By managing health information appropriately, the health care facility can virtually guarantee that patients' needs are met or exceeded (Fottler et al., 2010). The needs of the providers of health services are also met through the use of EMRs. It seems that technology, along with better management of this technology, is a win-win situation for patients and providers.

Telemedicine

Telemedicine, also called distance medicine, employs the science of telecommunication for medical diagnosis when the patient and the provider are separated by distance. This computerized patient care has many uses, which include providing medical care for rural residents and bringing specialists' diagnoses to distant locations. Health care reform and technology are inter-acting in ways that are making the expansion of telemedicine a very real possibility.

There are many new uses of telemedicine, such as patient home monitor-ing, that may very well represent a new way to reduce costs and improve the quality of patient care (Shi & Singh, 2010). There is also a role for telemedicine in the provision of health education and health promotion activities designed to prevent disease from occurring in the first place. This type of innovation in health care delivery is especially appropriate for dealing with the epidemic of chronic diseases in the United States. The use of infor-mation technology to educate large segments of the population about chronic diseases, such as heart disease, lung cancer, and diabetes, can reduce the incidence of these expensive diseases and their complications. These educa-tion programs can be made available to schools, workplaces, and the general public at a very low cost, thereby serving large parts of the population.

SUMMARY

As the expanding health care industry, the largest employer in the United States, continues to increase the number of employees required to deliver health services, there is a greater need for health care managers with the requisite skills to deliver quality health services to demanding consumers. These managers will be faced with constant change as they deal with reform efforts in the health care sector.

There is a real need for health care managers to move away from old theories of management and begin to embrace new management theories that focus more on leadership, change management, conflict resolution, and building culture. The old theory of bureaucratic management has failed in health care because this sector is dealing with enormous change and can no longer function as a bureaucracy. The new world of health care delivery requires managers who are well versed in the attributes of a more organic means of managing employees.

An adaptive organization with an organic design focuses more on the people delivering the services than on rules and regulations. Managers now need greater interpersonal skills to acquire, develop, and retain the type of health care employee necessary to deliver quality services while reducing the costs associated with health care delivery. There is now a much greater demand for the health care manager to become proficient in human relations theory and ultimately reengineering theory, which involves supervising empowered employees.

The new health care manager has to develop and work with self-managed work teams in the delivery of health services. This manager will also have to encourage creativity and innovation among all members of the health care team. Success in managing teams requires the health care manager to develop a whole host of new managerial skills, the most important of which is the ability to gain the trust and cooperation of the employees who actually deliver these vital services.

Many health care facilities in the United States are in desperate need of disruptive innovation to remain relevant. The competitive health care environment is producing rapid change that can only be handled by managers who have learned how to respond to change through their empowered employees. These managers must realize that their employees are their most important source of competitive advantage. A change in the management of health care employees will enable health care organizations to exploit all of the opportunities that have become available in the new world of health care delivery.

KEY TERMS

controlling

empowerment

leading

management functions

management theory

organizing

planning

REVIEW QUESTIONS

1. Please name and explain the major functions of a health care manager.

2. Please describe the different types of managerial skills, and explain how they can be useful to health care administrators.

3. Discuss the value of teamwork in the delivery of health services.

4. What role does the management of technology play in improving the quality of health services and in reducing the cost of delivering these services?

PART 2

Managing the External Environment

Part Two of this health care management text consists of just one chapter, Chapter Three, which deals with strategy and structure on the path to achieving success. The turbulent external environment of the health care system in general or of individual health care facilities is a critical component in the success of any health care organization today. The health care manager must pay particular attention to strategy development and the structure and design chosen to achieve that strategy.

This chapter pays a great deal of attention to the governance and management of the entire health care organization. Such an organization views the external environment as a source of consumers, suppliers, and, of course, employees. There are numerous strategies that can be considered once the mission, values, and overall objectives of the health care organization have been put forth. Therefore, the board of directors and CEO along with managers, employees, and consumers need to be involved in developing the mission statement the organization will follow.

This chapter also looks at the operating environment within a health care organization, with the aim of helping future health care managers understand the value of the organizational vision, mission, goals, and objectives and how they all work together to define success for any organization. A discussion concerning strategy development and organizational design is a very important part of this chapter.

Every health care facility has specific strategic choices and subsequent processes that are designed to achieve success for the facility itself and perhaps for the U.S. health care system as a whole. Chapter Three pays significant attention to organizational structure in relation to organizational design.

3

Strategy and Structure
Choosing the Path to Success

Kermit W. Kuehn

LEARNING OBJECTIVES

- Understand what strategy and structure are and the relationship between them
- Describe the strategic management process
- Discuss various aspects of environmental scanning in the strategic management process
- Understand the importance of the Five Forces Model in analyzing an industry
- List and describe the main issues of organizational design and the general options available to the manager

The health care industry is perhaps one of the most dynamic sectors of our economy, and one of the most influential in terms of its portion of gross domestic product. Factors from every direction drive the changes we currently see and certainly will experience in the future. Whether we look at the economic factors, or a host of other forces, such as technology, societal expectations, and changes in public policy, their combined effect makes for immense strategic challenges for managers in the health care sector.

There are few organizational leaders today who would not be able to at least speak of their organization, customers, and markets in strategic terms. Being able to understand strategic concepts and speak in the language of strategy has become more and more important to leaders, whether the organization is public or private, for-profit or nonprofit. Developing and managing effective strategy is an essential ingredient in successful health care organizations.

In many ways health care organizations were late to the game when it came to thinking in strategic terms. Such business concepts as markets, target groups, efficiency, and competition are relatively new to the health care industry's vocabulary. I recall in the mid-1990s being invited by a regional VA hospital to introduce its senior administrators to strategic concepts and to facilitate discussions on formulating a strategic plan by which the institution would be judged. Prior to that, no one had thought of their work in such terms. Today, however, developing and managing strategy is one of the most important roles of a health care organization manager.

STRATEGIC MANAGEMENT AND STRUCTURE

Strategic management involves several activities that rest on an appropriate infrastructure to support the chosen strategy. Issues related to organizational design and the development of goals, policies, and procedures; job design and incentives; and supporting organizational values and culture are important parts of this infrastructure. A discussion of organizational design and structure will follow an overview of the processes and tools used in strategic management.

Strategic management encompasses managerial decisions and actions that determine the long-term performance of the organization. It is an ongoing process whose focus is on formulating, implementing, and controlling broad plans for the organization.

Managing Strategy

As individuals, to succeed at anything we need to think about our end goal—call this our objective. We can then consider how we are going to achieve our objective, determining what strategies we are going to use. In sum, objectives and goals are about what we intend to achieve, whereas strategies and tactics are about how we're going to achieve them. Even after we have established these goals and strategies, certain things are necessary for us to achieve the result.

Consider a guy who wants to lose ten pounds within two weeks. He sets the objective, to lose ten pounds in two weeks. He then determines a strategy to make this happen, deciding to exercise regularly. So we have the "what" and the "how." But there is much more that is needed to be successful. There is a better chance of success if he puts certain things in place to support his weight loss program. Call this his infrastructure, or simply his support structure. Its purpose is to make possible the accomplishment of the objective. He decides to sign up for a gym membership and even requests the help of an on-site trainer to help him with his routine. He sets up a schedule to meet with this person three times a week, and even asks his friend to hold him accountable to this commitment.

What is important to note in this example is not only the importance of setting objectives and strategies and putting together a support structure but also that an essential part of success rests in pulling these elements together to yield a cohesive and integrative process to deliver the desired objective. These are the essential ingredients of any good plan, whether for an individual or for an organization. This is the essence of successful strategic management. Although the management process may be much more complex for organizations than it is for an individual, the process is similar in many ways.

Strategic management, then, is about those decisions and activities that will position an organization to confront the future. Strategies reflect the decisions management makes to bring the organization into that future reality, ideally accompanied by great success. Strategy involves a way of thinking—call it "big picture" and future oriented. Such terms as *strategic vision* and *strategic thinking* are used to emphasize this particular mind-set.

Strategic thinking involves a set of skills that allows the decision maker to grasp the organization and its context as an integrated whole, generally referred to as systems thinking, and to comprehend the shape of the future that is unfolding. The result is an articulated future for the organization, called a strategic vision. The strategic vision, then, reflects top management's aspirations for the company as to future direction, a rationale for the chosen direction, and the identity for the organization that is to result (Thompson, Gamble, & Strickland, 2008).

Strategic management, to be effective, requires an organization's management to have a clear understanding of what the organization is about. Strategic management entails a clearly defined sense of purpose, which is captured in a mission statement and reflected in the goals and strategies set by the organization. It is the distinctive mix of these ingredients that has the potential not only to make an organization unique in the industry but also to be a source of competitive advantage in the immediate market context.

Who Is Responsible for Organizational Strategy?

Strategic management is a primary responsibility of the governing board and senior administrators of the health care organization. It is the responsibility of all who work for the organization to understand their respective parts in fulfilling the strategic direction set by leadership and to support them through their daily activities. That is easier said than done.

Organizations are complex systems with a lot of moving parts, both human and nonhuman. This is the context of strategic management and the exciting challenge that greets managers each day as they walk in the door. Strategic questions are never fully and finally answered, they're just continually asked: What are we doing? How are we doing it? Why are we doing it? How can we do it better?

Before looking more closely at this critical process that will determine organizational survival and success, let's consider the decision makers involved. Organizations in the end are more than mission and vision statements, strategies, and structures with people employed in them. They are really stewards of aspirations and resources that are expected to deliver a desirable end result. This is certainly the case in the health care field, in which the loftiest aims are pursued: the health and well-being of a community or specific constituency within a community.

Who is tasked with ensuring that this stewardship is maintained in a manner that aligns with the aspirations of the many stakeholders connected to the organization? In most health care organizations, governance is viewed as the responsibility of two distinct groups—governing boards and senior administrators. Their roles are distinct, yet they do overlap and should complement each other.

A governing board, variously labeled a board of trustees, a board of directors, or something similar, is the first entity established to determine the purpose, vision, and values of the health care organization. This board typically comprises key stakeholders of the proposed entity. In the case of a community hospital, for example, board members might include representatives from physician groups; members of a funding foundation, if there is one; employees; recognized leaders of the business community; as well as representatives of groups to be served by the hospital.

The governing board is also responsible for hiring and working with the senior administrator of the organization, typically the CEO or president. The board's role is one of oversight of the entity to ensure that the organization maintains the key purpose, vision, and values that are to guide it. Practically speaking, this means the board approves strategic choices proposed by senior administrators and the annual budget allocated to carry out the mission. The board also monitors results for compliance.

Administrators are the day-to-day managers of the health care organization who are authorized to make decisions consistent with the mission, vision, and values set by the governing board. The terms *managers* and *administrators* are used interchangeably throughout this chapter and typically refer to the senior leadership team of the organization. It is not uncommon for an administrator, particularly the CEO, to be a voting member or director on the governing board. It is also possible for the CEO to chair the board.

Previously I discussed leadership's role in the pursuit of strategy and the maintenance of organizational structure. Governance and management, involving the application of organizational policy, pertain very much to the roles of leaders and tend, even, to define those roles.

Strategic management focuses organizational efforts on finding ways to move a company forward and, in doing so, considering the impact of current decisions on the achievement of organizational goals (Drucker, 1974). Let's now look at how this process proceeds.

THE STRATEGIC MANAGEMENT PROCESS

As stated earlier, strategic management is a process whereby organizational leadership determines the "what" and the "how" of decisions that will guide all members toward a positive future. Figure 3.1 outlines the four components of this process. At the outset it should be noted that although the process is depicted as very orderly and sequential, it is actually quite different in practice. The presentation in the figure is helpful for the purpose of this discussion, but in practice the process is more likely to be in both directions and iterative, with findings in a subsequent component resulting in changes to an earlier component. The more dynamic the competitive context, the more likely it is that this will occur.

Strategic management begins with an assessment of the environment, followed by the formulation of a strategy with measurable objectives, the execution of the strategy, and the ongoing control and evaluation of the process.

Environmental Scanning

Environmental scanning, often referred to as situational analysis, is a systematic analysis of the current external reality facing the organization in its

---

Figure 3.1   Strategic Management Process

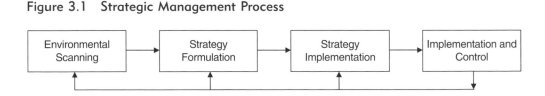

market, an internal assessment of the relative strengths and weaknesses of the organization in light of this reality, and an examination of potential opportunities and threats the organization will face going forward. To conduct such an analysis an organization selects the types and sources of information it will monitor to keep abreast of what is happening in its operating context.

This is a formidable task. There is an overwhelming amount of data that could be collected, but the relevant information to be drawn from these data is often ambiguous and difficult to extract. Then the challenge is to turn these data into meaningful information that can be acted on by organizational managers. Finally, there are numerous and diverse interests operating in the environment on the part of stakeholders, all of which need managerial attention as well.

Stakeholders are individuals and groups who care about what the organization is doing and how it is doing it. For a health care provider, stakeholders can range from patients and physicians to investors and insurers, and may include numerous special interest groups focused on very narrow issues, such as how the organization disposes of medical waste. The list of interested parties can be substantial, but not all are worthy of equal attention.

The environmental scanning process helps organizational managers sift through these data and the interests of the many stakeholders to arrive at actionable choices. A common approach to conducting an environmental scan is through what is referred to as a SWOT analysis, whereby the strengths, weaknesses, opportunities, and threats are systematically examined.

Once the environmental scan is complete, managers must be able to do the following:

1. Understand the reality in which the organization currently operates

2. Have a good sense of the reality it is likely to face in the future

3. Know well the organization's capabilities, good and bad

4. Be able to devise and execute a plan that will enable the organization to survive, and even prosper, in that future environment

A SWOT analysis is a tool to help deliver these outcomes.

The first thing to notice in this discussion is the assumption that the environment is not static or even stable. It assumes that dynamism is the normal state of things and that the forces operating in the environment are constantly changing. Few people in the health care field need to be convinced of this assumption.

As already noted, analyzing the current situation requires the organization to examine both its external and internal environments. Figure 3.2 illustrates the scope of this analysis. The external environment is viewed in two parts: a general, or macro environment and a more immediate, or task environment.

First we'll take a look at the general environment, which reflects the broad context under which all organizations operate in the industry. We'll follow this with a closer look at the immediate environment, which deals with the day-to-day operating context of the organization and its markets. We'll conclude our discussion of environmental scanning with a brief look at the internal environment, which addresses the culture and structure of the organization itself.

The **general environment** affects all organizations in the health care sector. Each organization typically has an indirect influence on what happens in this broader environment. This means that although the organization is affected by forces in the general environment, it has a limited ability to control or manipulate these forces. A hospital in Kentucky will have little influence over an economic recession, for example, but it will need to respond to it.

As can be seen in Figure 3.2, typically included in this type of analysis are economic, political-legal, sociocultural, and technological factors. Table 3.1 summarizes the types of issues within the four areas, each of which is examined as part of a SWOT analysis to determine the emerging issues, if any, and the potential for harm to the organization as well as for new opportunities. For example, the aging of the baby boomer population reflects a major societal shift, a trend that falls under the sociocultural heading. Another example is recent legislation to reform the U.S. health care system,

Figure 3.2   Environmental Factors

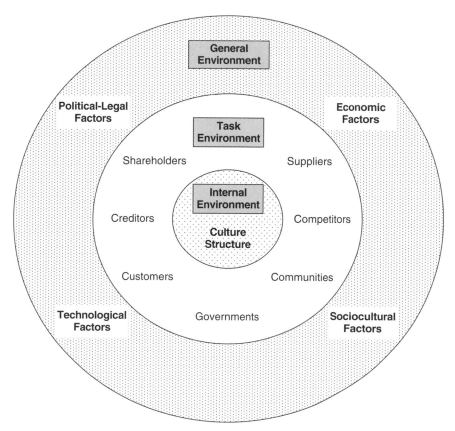

a driver under the political-legal heading. Reform efforts affect every person and every organization that operates in the United States.

What issues do these shifts or trends bring out? Are these opportunities or threats to the organization—or both?

The **immediate environment,** also called the task environment, refers to the industry within which the organization operates. It is called the immediate environment because it is the organization's day-to-day context. A health care organization, for example, spends every day of its existence in the health care industry, a loose collection of organizations that face a similar operating environment consisting of rules, practices, and constraints. This

Table 3.1   Typical Factors Analyzed in the General Environment

Economic	Political-Legal	Sociocultural	Technological
Inflation rates	Antitrust laws	Population size and makeup	Intellectual property protections
Interest rates	Taxation laws	Age structure of the population	Investments in research and development
Trade and budget deficits or surpluses	Regulatory environment	Geographic shifts in the population	Technology infrastructure
Currency exchange rates	Labor laws	Birthrates and life expectancy	Product adoption rates in society
Income distribution	Stability of government	Work attitudes and lifestyle trends	Technology transfer regulations
Employment levels	Social welfare policies		
Gross domestic product	Property rights		

includes the organization's specific operating context—the geographic locations and communities it serves. The immediate environment is a context in which the organization has considerable control over its destiny.

An industry is much like a sport. There are rules, players, referees, coaches, and teams. In any sport, some teams are better than others, as is the case with players and coaches. How do we determine who is relatively better at the game than others? Through some form of competitive assessment we determine rankings and, ultimately, champions.

A similar process takes place with organizations in any given industry operating in a market. Organizations compete for customers, for resources, and even for survival. Although many organizations in the health care sector are legally classified as nonprofit, the same basic rules apply. They must demonstrate a capacity to service a market with a limited amount of resources and be judged effective relative to certain standards of performance. In the health care field, these performance criteria might be based on customer satisfaction scores, regulatory standards, mortality rates, or quality metrics, to name a few.

One of the tools used to assess the competitive character of an industry is Porter's Five Forces Model (Porter, 1980). We will take a closer look at this tool following the discussion of environments.

Analysis of the **internal environment** involves a thorough examination by organizational members of their competencies and capabilities relative to the needs of the future and the competitors with whom the organization will eventually contend.

Competencies give an organization potential capabilities, which allow an organization to provide goods and services successfully in its market. Think of competencies as skills and abilities that permit the organization to deliver specific services or goods in a superior manner. Unique competencies combined in novel ways can endow an organization with competitive advantages that can be sustained over long periods of time.

Take an example of a hospital that has a well-regarded cancer treatment center and is the only treatment center of its kind in the region. This is a service capability that gives the organization potential competitive advantage relative to other hospitals in the region. Having such a capability could be listed as an organizational strength. Will this matter in the future? Or will current progress in treatments and cures render much of this capability irrelevant?

Organizational strengths are capabilities that are superior relative to those of immediate competitors and are valued in the market. Weaknesses would reflect relatively inferior capabilities in an area the market values.

Strengths can be derived from many areas. Having nationally recognized physicians in certain specialties within a clinical setting may be a strength, as might being able to recruit and retain quality nurses in key areas. Perhaps a capability is centered on an efficient operating structure that keeps costs low while delivering top-quality outcomes. Further, it could be unique partnerships that make the institution more capable.

Although strengths may be more appealing to talk about, an internal assessment must also look at what the organization doesn't do particularly well. The inability to recruit and retain physicians in key specialties is one example of a shortcoming. Or perhaps there are administrative weaknesses, such as inefficient process controls. Low morale among nursing staff is another internal factor.

In the end, it is about *relative* strengths and weaknesses, which means that a strength or weakness is thought of in terms of the capabilities or deficiencies of competitors. It is a comparative strength or a comparative weakness. Moreover, it is possible to have relevant competencies to deliver particular goods or services but to not be able to combine competencies in a manner that is economically viable.

Finally, strengths and weaknesses are examined in light of the opportunities and threats observed in the external environment. Organizations will seek to match strengths with opportunities to be exploited and attempt to address or offset threats. Particular weaknesses are targeted for solutions that upgrade capabilities or deflect the impact of a threat.

As discussed earlier, assessing the external and internal environments allows organizational decision makers to make informed choices as to the future direction of the organization. Important to this process is understanding the degree of competition in an industry. It has been demonstrated that high levels of rivalry among competitors in an industry reduce the average profitability of that industry, and thus the return on investment for the industry's firms (Porter, 2008).

Porter's Five Forces Model is a typical framework used to examine this more immediate context and includes the following dimensions, each discussed in turn: (1) the threat of new entrants, (2) the threat of substitutes, (3) the bargaining power of suppliers, (4) the bargaining power of buyers, and (5) competitive rivalry. Some analysts add a sixth force, the bargaining power of other stakeholders (interest groups, donors, community organizations, government entities, and so on), as a separate and increasingly important factor.

Each force helps shape the nature of an industry. The more forces affecting an industry and the degree to which each force does so will determine the level of rivalry among competitors. The six forces are discussed in turn in the following paragraphs.

The *threat of new entrants* to an industry increases the capacity of goods and services provided by the industry, and a new entrant will seek to gain market share to establish its presence. To do this, the new entity may use any combination of competitive pricing, cost advantages, and promotional activities to establish and extend the business.

The threat of new entrants depends on how high the barriers are to entry. Barriers may include the costs associated with establishing a presence, which can include the actual cost of physical assets; regulatory hurdles; and existing competitor responses. For example, if existing competitors can and are willing to make a new entrant pay dearly for entering, then it is less likely that there will be many new entrants.

Notice the number of new restaurants or retail stores in your community. The barriers are quite low to entry, and as a result many newcomers enter. Contrast this with the likelihood of a new regional hospital entering your neighborhood. Or consider even more challenging industries, such as commercial aircraft manufacturing or even automobile manufacturing, in which the costs of entry are prohibitive.

The *threat of substitutes* involves an indirect competitor that provides essentially the same function as the industry's product or service, but does so in a different manner. If switching costs are low and the threat of substitutes is high, the industry is limited in its options as far as pricing, and thus profitability.

Switching costs refer to the ease by which a customer can change to another supplier. If the restaurant doesn't offer tea, for example, I can readily switch to coffee at very little cost.

Downloading a digital copy of a DVD or a book substitutes for going to the video store or bookstore. Bicycles substitute for cars, as cars do for airplanes. Using WebMD or even YouTube might substitute for a doctor's appointment. Overseas experimental or alternative treatments or medications may substitute for traditional in-house and approved approaches.

The *bargaining power of suppliers* pertains to organizations that provide the labor, capital, goods, and services the industry requires. Suppliers, which have the ability to pass on higher prices, define the character or quality of a product or service, or force costs on the industry, possess significant power.

Industries that have a limited number of suppliers and limited substitutes, and that are dependent on the supplier firms for key inputs, are vulnerable to suppliers' flexing their muscles.

Unions that are able to pressure industries for more wage and benefit concessions, or oil producers that can pass higher costs on to auto service centers, are examples of suppliers exhibiting strong bargaining power. A health insurer passing premium increases on to employers or the insured is another. An airline attempting to raise airfares, only to have to reduce them again, is an example of a supplier with weaker bargaining power.

The *bargaining power of buyers* examines the ability of customers to force industry participants to reduce prices, offer better quality, or provide more services. Buyers are able to do this by playing one seller off of another, thus negotiating a better value for themselves. Buyers unable to negotiate better outcomes for themselves are considered weak.

Individual consumers and businesses may have bargaining power relative to industry producers. Cell phone companies face constant pressure to price better, offer more features, and develop new models. Within the health care industry, increasingly standardized services are beginning to be marketed with prices quoted. Laser surgery, treatment for cataracts, and many dental services are examples of procedures for which consumers shop for the best deals.

Competitive rivalry is evident in any number of ways in an industry, such as in price discounting, the proliferation of products and services being offered, and advertising. The power of the competitors in an industry as well as the degree of pressure they exert on other industry players affect the intensity of rivalry among competitors. Porter (2008) views rivalry in terms of both the intensity of the competition and the dimensions on which the competition is focused. The basis of competition, these dimensions, will significantly affect industry profitability. If price is the sole dimension on which all industry participants compete, then the rivalry will be economically quite damaging to overall industry profitability—an ugly scenario.

The *bargaining power of other stakeholders,* our sixth force, is determined by those interest groups, donors, community organizations, and government entities that may have strong influence over certain aspects of—and specific organizations within—an industry. They assert influence because they control access to resources, such as donor organizations; or a stakeholder may be a special interest group pressing for discontinuation of the use of incinerators for medical waste disposal. The list of stakeholders and their impacts can be quite lengthy, given the increasing variety of these groups and their growing effectiveness in pressing their respective agendas.

Strategy Formulation

After conducting the SWOT analysis, it is necessary for the organization to determine which actions it will take to capitalize on its strengths or competencies, or that allow it to focus on developing the capabilities it deems necessary for future success in its market. The organization then considers strategic options and makes decisions accordingly, all of which are reflected in the vision, mission, and strategic plan, to be implemented over a window of five to ten years.

Strategy formulation involves activities and decisions that result in a clear sense of organizational purpose. Through this process the organization must not only state in clear terms its purpose for existing but also specify the foundational principles and core values by which it will operate. This purpose and supporting operating philosophy are reflected in the vision and mission statements and flow into action through the objectives set and strategies developed to put them into effect.

Organizations will invariably make some statement as to their mission, which they may call a statement of purpose. For this discussion, we will view statements of purpose and mission statements as essentially the same thing.

A *mission* is "a broadly defined and enduring statement of purpose that distinguishes a health care organization from other organizations of the same type and identifies the scope of its operations in product, service, and market (competitive) terms" (Swayne, Duncan, & Ginter, 2008, p. 162). That is quite a mouthful, but the definition highlights some key aspects of a mission statement.

Although most organizations will make some statement as to why they exist, many will not explicitly create a *vision* statement. Often organizations attempt to create a mission statement that will carry the load of both a vision statement and a mission statement, confusing both concepts in the process. Let's look more closely at this distinction.

For example, Celgene is a multibillion-dollar global biopharmaceutical firm with distinct vision and mission statements:

> *Vision:* At Celgene, we seek to deliver truly innovative and life-changing drugs for our patients.

> *Mission:* Our mission as a company is to build a major global biopharmaceutical corporation while focusing on the discovery, the development, and the commercialization of products for the treatment of cancer and other severe, immune, inflammatory conditions.

An even simpler example and illustration of the difference between a mission statement and a vision statement comes from CVS Caremark, a Fortune 500 retail pharmacy and health clinic chain:

> *Vision:* We strive to improve the quality of human life.

> *Mission:* We provide expert care and innovative solutions in pharmacy and health care that are effective and easy for our customers.

It might help to think of vision and mission in this way. Vision tends to be more focused on the future and will reflect the aspirations of the institution in a way that inspires commitment. It is an ideal, and as such lifts the human spirit and stirs the imagination. It is short and clear, it strikes to the heart first and the mind second, and it tends to be less concrete. It is "heaven," not "earth." (Perhaps a vision reflects a desire to make a dream a reality.)

Mission statements are earth first, with heaven as a backdrop. A mission statement defines the organizational footprint in the marketplace today: what the organization is, what it does, and how it does it. It is also short, concrete, and practical.

If having a vision is to lift your eyes to the horizon, then having a mission is to direct your eyes to the ground directly in front of you. In summary, the organization will keep one eye on its dream to remain inspired and hopeful, the other on the road immediately in front of it to navigate its daily course.

From a managerial perspective, objectives are used to translate vision and purpose into specific performance targets—the outcomes and results the organization seeks to achieve. *Objectives* are goals, specified in concrete terms, that the organization wants to accomplish within a particular time frame. For our purposes here, objectives and goals are used interchangeably.

Objectives are what the organization will measure when evaluating its performance, and all decisions and activities will flow from these few selected outcomes and targets. Objectives should reflect a balance between purely financial targets and nonfinancial or strategic ones. Research has supported the argument that healthy organizations pursue a balanced approach (Crabtree & DeBusk, 2008).

One approach that has gained considerable acceptance in organizations that think strategically is called the balanced scorecard (Kaplan & Norton, 2000). The balanced scorecard methodology divides organizational objectives into two broad categories—financial and strategic. Financial objectives might include targets for after-tax profits, cash flows, the use of capital assets, or revenue increases. Strategic objectives would include targets for market share, competitive positioning, brand strength, or the quality of the products or services offered in relation to those of competitors. Although the balanced scorecard was originally developed for use by for-profit enterprises, government and nonprofit organizations have also found the tool helpful in defining strategic objectives (Niven, 2008).

To be effective, objectives need to possess certain characteristics that will permit the organization to assess how well it is doing in achieving them. They need to be quantifiable, or measurable, and they must specify a time frame in which they are to be accomplished. Good objectives push the organization to go beyond its current capabilities, forcing it to stretch to achieve them. And big, long-range objectives will have to be broken down into short-term goals, which must be set for all levels of the organization.

Whereas an organization's vision, mission, and objectives reveal why the organization exists and what it intends to do, strategy determines how the organization goes about achieving these things. In essence an organization's *strategy* is the basic way it seeks to position itself in the market to gain a sustainable competitive advantage.

Generally speaking, an organization has three basic options when it comes to its approach to its market. It can set out to (1) grow, (2) remain static, or (3) shrink the business. Whichever approach it selects, strategies are central to delivering the desired outcome.

Although there are a number of recognized perspectives as to how an organization might approach the formulation of its specific strategy (see Miles & Snow, 1978), only one will be discussed here. Porter (1980) argues that any organization operating in any given industry has a limited set of options from which to choose when it comes to positioning itself relative to competitors. He refers to these options as generic strategies. His framework includes three generic strategies: cost leadership, differentiation, and focus.

An organization implementing a *cost leadership* strategy seeks to ensure it is the low-cost provider in its industry. Walmart is an example of an organization that has successfully executed this strategy. Organizations that choose a *differentiation* strategy seek to be unique among competitors in their industry. For example, and in contrast to Walmart, Saks Fifth Avenue is a retailer offering a differentiated product. Although both Walmart and Saks Fifth Avenue are in the retail business, often selling items in similar product categories, such as clothing or women's accessories, they've positioned themselves in the market in very different ways. A differentiation strategy often allows an organization to charge more for its products or services, as these are unique or distinctive.

These generic strategies are also used in the health care industry. Pfizer pursues a differentiation strategy as a pharmaceutical manufacturer. Its highly successful cholesterol drug, Lipitor, is one of the many products with which it seeks to establish a unique position in the market. The medication has been under patent protection for a number of years, allowing Pfizer to enhance the brand and charge a premium for this product. That protection has come to an end, however. Contrast Pfizer with Watson Pharmaceuticals, a generic drug manufacturer negotiating for rights to produce a generic version of Lipitor. Watson uses a cost leadership strategy to produce low-cost pharmaceuticals.

An organization using a *focus* strategy is really pursuing a cost leadership or differentiation strategy within a more narrowly defined customer segment of a market. For example, some clinics pursuing a focus strategy concentrate only on low-cost delivery of cataract surgery, and some clinics may seek to differentiate their services by only offering "high-quality" Lasik refractive surgery. Organizations that use a focus strategy are not, as the name implies, trying to please everyone interested in a particular product or service, but rather those who seek specific experiences or benefits, such as low-cost offerings or quick turnaround.

Once an organization has established objectives and determined its basic strategy, it has largely completed the planning part of the strategic management process. The process then moves toward implementation of the strategic approach and the development of details that support the successful execution and evaluation of the strategic process.

Strategy Implementation

The process of strategy implementation requires an organization to establish objectives (preferably annual objectives) and devise policies. The strategic objectives must be followed up with policies that encompass a wide range of issues, from employee incentives to resource allocation priorities, to ensure that the objectives can be executed properly.

Organizations must develop initiatives that will be used to reach specified objectives and that are consistent with the strategic direction set for the organization and its subunits. These decisions typically permeate the structure and activities of the organization. Specific programs are developed, budgets are determined, processes and procedures are defined, and performance metrics are set.

Evaluation and Control

The evaluation and control aspects of the strategic management process involve the measurement and evaluation of not only individual program initiatives but also the organization's overall performance relative to its strategic objectives. It is the responsibility of senior management to ensure that systems are in place to measure and evaluate progress toward these objectives. As stated earlier, strategic management is an ongoing and iterative process, and the control function informs relevant decision makers as to their success in achieving objectives.

As we conclude our discussion of strategic management, it must be noted that there is little doubt of the pressure the health care industry faces from many sides. There have been numerous attempts at reform, and still the level of industry performance lags behind expectations in terms of innovation, lower costs, and better quality, all of which have typically been experienced in other industries. Costs continue to rise, and quality and access issues continue to frustrate legislators and the public at large (Porter & Teisberg, 2004).

The concepts discussed here provide managers of health care organizations with a useful framework by which to examine the industry and the forces at work therein. Now we turn our attention to the designing of organizations and the structures necessary to support organizational strategies.

ORGANIZATIONAL DESIGN AND STRUCTURE

Early on in the life of the organization, organizational decision makers made design choices that resulted in the organization's appearance today. If you've ever walked into a doctor's clinic or a hospital, you have been immediately affected by these choices. The people you encounter; the departments you see as you walk down the hallways; and the policies, rules, and procedures that must be followed, and even the layout of the physical space, are all a result of this design process. We take it for granted and as a given in any organization, but this structure is intentional.

Organizational structure dictates the manner in which an organization divides up the tasks to be done, assigns them to people, and then coordinates among them to accomplish objectives (Hodge, Anthony, & Gales, 2003). **Organizational design** is the process that results in this formal structure, but it is a concept that involves a host of other details that permit the organization to function as a cohesive unit. Design issues include the technology used, communication systems, unit size, control systems, policies and rules, and degrees of decision making authority within and across units and levels.

There are several design options that when integrated into a whole will result in an organizational structure that has certain capabilities as well as limitations. Think of design in terms of a person deciding what to wear for a given day. This person will select from different options of clothing and accessories that, when combined, ideally will result in an appropriate and effective combination that meets the requirements of the day. Working in the backyard requires a different combination of attire than would going to a symphony.

In the same way, health care organizations can be expected to have structures that are different from consumer retail organizations. Yet we can expect that they will have some commonalities as well. The discussion later in this chapter refers to design and structure interchangeably.

The resulting structure is formally depicted in an organizational chart, although many details of actual organizational functioning are not revealed in this rather simplistic graphic format (see Figure 3.3 for an organizational chart of a small hospital). We do glean much from the organizational chart. In most cases, we see immediately the relationship among people and departments in the organization. We see a hierarchy of authority, a depiction of who reports to whom. We see the position of the board of directors relative to the organization and its managers. This is important information, and it

Figure 3.3 Simplified Organizational Chart for a Small Hospital

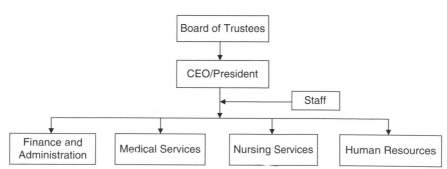

is management's formal statement in regard to organizational structure. It defines what the organization looks like.

Before we go into more detail as to the concepts and principles that guide organizational design, let's take another moment to understand the relationship between strategy and structure.

Strategy Versus Structure

Early on in the study of organizations, there was considerable debate as to which came first, structure or strategy. More specifically, which one had the greatest influence on organizational character and direction? The proponents of the primacy of structure argued that industries comprised organizations that had successfully developed structures with which to compete. These organizations looked essentially the same from a structural perspective. As a result, organizations could and should only develop strategies that were compatible with existing structural configurations.

The argument was that a structure exists in an industry because the requirements and priorities in the core technology or processes of that industry are the same for all industry participants. For example, if you are a petroleum refinery, the processes used to produce minimally acceptable outputs, such as unleaded fuel of a certain octane level that meets government standards, require high-cost and sophisticated technology and a highly skilled workforce. This reality limits, even determines, the strategic options of each and every organization involved in refining petroleum.

From this perspective, industry "rules" determine strategic options. That is, the external environment, not organizational decision makers, determines strategy. Strategic objectives that are inconsistent with these rules will fail.

Those who support the primacy of strategy over structure argue that no organization is determined by the external environment, at least not entirely. There is plenty of evidence of "rule breakers" who are redefining their industries. What has Amazon done to Barnes & Noble? Or Netflix to Blockbuster?

Leadership, by definition, is responsible for the effective management of the organization within its operating environment, and that includes the organization's intentions concerning the future. According to this view, organizations choose which products, customers, and lines of business they will target; which ones they will abandon; and which new ones to consider. The assumption, when considering strategy to be of primary importance, is that decision makers make choices that really make a difference in their environment, while not ignoring the constraints of that reality.

This means that although organizational design and structure are essential, and although there are always constraints on an organization's options, strategic choices have an immense potential to influence the organization, whether positively or negatively.

Broad Design Considerations

Earlier we discussed management's responsibility to specify the formal structure of the organization. I noted that this is depicted in the formal organizational chart. The reality of social systems, organizations being one class of human social system, is that people don't just operate within their formal roles or assignments. They naturally establish contacts and maintain relationships with individuals outside their designated team, department, or division.

These relationships are part of what is referred to as the informal structure. People move across boundaries to verify information or simply to get things done that are being frustrated by the formal structure. According to the simplest logic, why ask my boss to do something that he or she may not be all that interested in doing when I could call the person I know in the relevant department and just ask him or her directly? Or get a favor from that person? Or resolve a conflict through "back channels"? That is the practical and political value of the informal structure, and it has the potential to create headaches as well.

The reality is that the organization relies on the informal structure to get work done. Not all contingencies are answered by the formal system, and even if there is a mechanism for addressing a particular contingency, it isn't always efficient for getting things done. So the informal structure remains an important facet of the modern organization that management not only must be aware of but also must be able to manage to some degree. An organization's informal structure is primarily a communication system, often used to spread gossip and rumors but also to pass along managerial views and the reasoning behind what internal critics consider illogical or unfair.

It is not my intention here to deeply analyze this informal structure, but rather to use this discussion as a backdrop for looking at the formal design choices with which the organization must wrestle. Two concepts are central to the process of designing the basic structure from which the organization will operate: integration versus differentiation and decentralization versus centralization.

Integration Versus Differentiation

At the outset of this discussion about structure, one might ask why we would spend so much time and effort in delineating the relationships among the activities associated with health care and the innumerable details involved. The simple answer is that management is the discipline of planned action, and therefore managers seek to conduct their activities in the most efficient and effective manner. *Effective* means that we want to be doing the right things, and *efficient* means we want to be doing the right things right.

Hence it is not effective to be doing the wrong thing in a given circumstance, or to arrive at the wrong result. The wrong treatment or a wrong diagnosis is not effective health care. It is not efficient to have to do a thing twice that should have been done once, or to have two people doing that which one could do.

Effective and efficient management systems then seek to make sure that the right people are doing the right thing consistently in the right way. With that objective in mind, managers must wrestle with what is necessary in design terms to get this end result—effectiveness and efficiency. These two words are at the root of many of the challenges we face in modern health care.

We begin our discussion of design choices with the concepts of integration and differentiation, which reflect the tension inherent in managing modern social systems. Recall from our earlier discussion of organizational structure that the design process involves dividing up tasks and determining who will undertake them. This is formally called the division of labor.

Quite simply, we determine all the things we need to do to fulfill our mission, or purpose for existing; we divide them into logical packages called jobs; and we assign people to these jobs. Why must we do this? It is a reality of modern organizational life that one person cannot do all the tasks required in an effective and efficient manner.

This division of labor into manageable units is called differentiation. The result is that people are focused on a more narrow set of tasks for which they are responsible. They become specialists in their assigned area. The modern hospital has moved far along the road of specialization, a clear example of differentiation at work. Physicians specialize in rather narrow areas of expertise, such as oncology, pediatrics, and cardiology. And think of the specialties that exist for technicians and nurses.

The benefit of this differentiation is that you can have specialists across many important areas who have developed expertise and a language for conducting their work and describing their priorities in regard to what is done and how. The end result for the organization is that people are different from one another. This diversity is both good and bad, in this case.

On the one hand, the specialist is the best in his or her area of specialization; on the other hand, the specialist is not all that knowledgeable about the many other units operating in the organization. Further, he or she often has little reason to even care what is going on in other units. This is the challenge of the division of labor. You gain the advantages of specialization, but at a price for the whole organization.

Integration is the process by which an organization coordinates the differentiated units to produce a cohesive and desired result. The organization that split up work into narrowly defined tasks is the same one that is trying to tie these units back together in a way that will ensure healthy patients, or any number of desired outcomes.

This is the tension that exists between these two concepts, and management must work to strike the right balance between these two forces for the good of the organization and its customers.

Up to this point in our discussion of differentiation we have looked at the division of labor assuming that the workers were on the same occupational level. That is, with the example of physicians' being divided into specialties, we were assuming that all physician specialties were essentially on the same level of task demand, responsibility, complexity, and so on. In essence, these specialties were on the same horizontal plane or level. This form of differentiation is referred to as horizontal differentiation. There are others, however.

Vertical differentiation involves the hierarchical division of work, which is based on health care professionals' responsibility for and authority over the tasks being performed. We often refer to this as the chain of command. Here the emphasis is on the vertical levels involved in dividing up and overseeing the specializations created. The number of levels vertically is influenced by the degree of direct control managers feel is appropriate for the units created. Fewer levels of hierarchy reflect a flatter structure, whereas more levels will define a taller structure. There are strengths and weaknesses of each, but in today's fast-moving and dynamic environment flatter structures are the general trend.

Shorter or flatter structures tend to be able to adapt more quickly to a changing reality because they have fewer levels between the relevant decision makers and those actually in need of a response. As more and more industries become unstable, facing constantly changing market demands, there is pressure on organizations to adapt while maintaining high levels of performance. This is particularly true in the health care industry, in which the rules by which these organizations must operate—and the manner in which the health care organization is paid for its work—keep changing.

Decentralization Versus Centralization

Health care administrators must gauge organizational responsiveness to the constantly changing criteria that define success. The number and seriousness of the questions in regard to changes to health care regulation that need to be answered continues to grow as the complexity of the operating environment increases. In this context of uncertainty, who should be making the decisions is always under review. How can you ensure that your decision makers are asking the best questions—questions that will result in timely responses to the demands on the organization, whether these are from patients, employees, or vendors?

This is the essence of the debate surrounding centralization versus decentralization. How much decision making authority should be pushed down to lower levels of the vertical hierarchy? An organization cannot be described as centralized or decentralized when it comes to decision making authority. It is really more a question of degree. All organizations operate with some level of decentralization, so the question to be asked is more about how much decentralization is present in an organization relative to how much is needed to achieve the objectives being pursued.

Organic Versus Mechanistic Structures

As managers have wrestled with implications of the integration-differentiation and centralization-decentralization design options, the structures created result in organizations that are either more organic or more mechanistic. Organic organizations tend to have flatter structures, be more flexible and adaptive, and have more decentralized decision making. Mechanistic organizations tend to have taller structures, be more rigid and bureaucratic, and have more centralized decision making. These organizations have many levels in the decision-making hierarchy, with relatively more rules, procedures, and policies to govern decision making in every situation (high standardization); they are more attentive to maintaining the vertical relationships therein; and they are more methodical and slow-moving.

Flatter structures tend to be described as more organic in nature. These have fewer levels of decision-making hierarchy; they are more dependent on employees at lower levels of the hierarchy to make decisions (low standardization); they value the horizontal relationships that form to achieve tasks; and they tend to be more responsive and quick to adapt to changes in the environment.

Although organic structures in general seem most appropriate for the reality of the current health care environment, each type has its strengths and weaknesses. Organizations seek to use some elements from both types to achieve desired results.

The question of what is the appropriate level of differentiation or centralization is a complex one. What is important to grasp at this point is that managers have an array of decisions to make, only a few of which I have touched on so far, in the pursuit of a management system that can deliver the desired outcomes consistently over time.

Let's now take a brief look at some of the general structural types an organization might select in its attempt to design an effective performance system.

General Structural Types

If we were to examine the organizational charts of several organizations, we would find that they vary considerably—and we might conclude that all organizations are structured differently. Although this may at first seem to be the case, the reality is that there are relatively few structural types or templates. The following paragraphs detail three main hierarchical designs, and a fourth that is an emerging variation: functional, divisional, matrix, and hybrid.

Functional Structures

In a **functional structure**, tasks and people are grouped based on what they do (the functions they serve) for the organization. For example, people who work in human resources–related tasks are grouped together and labeled the Human Resources Department. The same could be done with accounting, legal, surgery, pediatrics, or any other department made up of individuals performing similar functions for the organization.

A key advantage of this type of structure is that it puts related tasks and the experts who do these tasks in the same department. The department thus becomes the center for this knowledge and expertise. This structural type also reduces the need to provide these functions in each department throughout the organization. For example, accounting tasks are an essential activity throughout a hospital. By directing these tasks to one central group there is greater efficiency in that the unit has at its disposal all the necessary skills needed to handle any accounting assignment.

This approach also allows for the recruitment and development of more people with ever-increasing expertise in the area. Having seasoned accountants and fresh graduates working together increases the overall capability of the organization in this skill area. This is true in other departments as well.

The downside of functional structures is that focusing on specialization fosters a narrow functional view of the organization. That is, accountants see the organization in terms of accounting values and priorities, and as a result may not understand or value other functional views or even the broader organizational perspective. Further, promotion is typically vertical and within the functional department, resulting in mid-level and senior functional heads with limited exposure to general administrative experience. This vertical emphasis creates functional silos that can weaken coordination and communication across functional groups.

Divisional Structures

A **divisional structure** groups people and their task assignments according to some common focus. This focus could be a particular product, customer, or geographic location. A large health care organization might have several products it offers, such as insurance, hospitals, and specialized clinics. Or it might align its people according to particular clients, such as children or those undergoing cancer treatment. Or it might choose to group people based on location, such as by western, central, and eastern regions of the U.S. market. In fact, it may choose to use all three divisional forms at the same time.

A divisional structure is often used by larger enterprises to segregate large sections of the company's business into groups that are semiautonomous; mostly self-managed; and, as already mentioned, focused on a narrow aspect of the company's products, clients, and markets. Each division has its own accounting, human resources, and marketing functions, along with any others necessary to perform its role. In essence, each division may largely be able to stand as an independent unit.

General Motors, with its Chevrolet and Cadillac divisions, is product focused. Bank of America uses a structure revolving around customers, with retail, commercial, investing, and asset management divisions. McKesson, a global provider of pharmaceuticals and health care technologies, is a U.S.-based company that focuses on both product and geographic location.

One of the drawbacks of a divisional structure is that it becomes more difficult to operate from a unified and consistent image in the marketplace due to the unique demands of each of the divisions and the relative autonomy each division has to operate its "businesses." In addition, unlike the functional design, the divisional design has considerable duplication of functions and services across units. Finally, the divisional design encourages increased competition among units for organizational resources.

Matrix Structures

A **matrix structure** combines a functional structure with a divisional structure as a way to address short-term projects or programs. Notice how in Figure 3.4 the top of the matrix reflects a typical functional design, with departments, such as marketing and finance and accounting, reflective of task groupings based on related activities. Along the left side of the matrix are the units or projects that require functional representation.

Figure 3.4 Matrix Structure

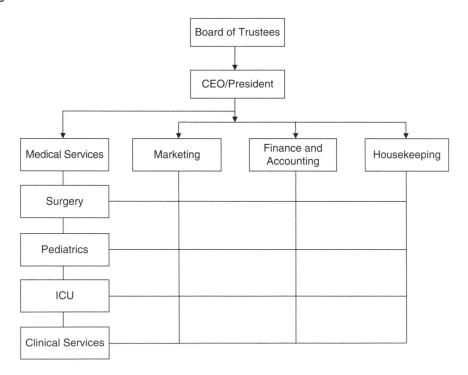

One of the advantages of the matrix design is that functional expertise can be assigned to a project or task to the degree that it is needed for the duration of the project. For example, a project labeled ICU Quality could reflect a desire to define, assess, and implement a quality initiative in the intensive care unit of a hospital with a matrix structure similar to that depicted in Figure 3.4. The structure might pull people from accounting, the administration, and medical services to carry out this project. Each of the participants would be temporarily assigned to the team, which is headed by a project or program manager.

Once the project is completed, participants return to their respective functional departments. In the meantime, however, they may be assigned only part-time to the matrix team, and in fact may be formally assigned to more than one matrix team at a time, depending on project requirements.

The key advantage of such a design is that it permits the organization to be more responsive to environmental pressures while using scarce resources more efficiently. It allows the organization to make sure it has the right people at the table for the issue at hand. Units to address special problems or issues that come up can be promptly organized and staffed to deliver a desired outcome. Specialists, rather than being confined to a department that may use them only from time to time, are assigned as necessary to units and then returned to their primary department when not needed.

The challenge with the matrix structure starts with the "two bosses" problem. A person assigned to a matrix team has both a functional boss and a project boss. This inherently violates a basic principle of management called the unity of command, whereby each person has only one boss. Conflict is more likely with this design. The skills to function within a matrix design are more diverse because the structure is more complex. Being able to handle the increased ambiguity of roles, and being able to negotiate for clarity and for necessary resources, are important skills for members of organizations using a matrix structure.

Hybrid Structures

As organizations grow and become more complex, a single basic design cannot meet the varied needs of the organization. Many health care organi-

Figure 3.5   Hybrid Structure

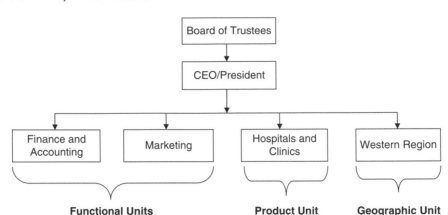

zations will use a combination of these general structural types to form a **hybrid structure** (see Figure 3.5).

Further, organizations often use more informal, or "soft" structures to achieve the necessary levels of cooperation and coordination among units to accomplish various tasks. These structures overlay the formal structure and focus on lateral relationships over vertical ones, taking the form of cross-functional teams, ad hoc committees, cross-departmental liaisons, information systems, and organizational culture to further integrate the differentiated organizational structure.

We can see that organizational design is an important management activity requiring managers to adopt appropriate structures to achieve organizational objectives. No single solution fits all the demands placed on a health care organization and its members.

PHYSICIAN ORGANIZATIONS: A CLOSER LOOK

Managers have a wide range of tools available to them as they seek to execute the mission and chosen strategies of their health care organization. A key relationship in the health care organization is between the organization and those who deliver patient care—the physicians.

To this point we've approached the management of the health care organization much like we would that of any other organization, which has allowed us to simplify the task of grasping the basic concepts that underpin any organization. However, this simplistic approach also ignores certain unique features that affect how the health care industry functions and the specific forces that have a bearing on how organizations operate therein.

One such unique feature is the development and evolution of independent physician groups, whether called physician networks or physician organizations. The power and influence of these groups have a considerable impact on the health care organization in general and administrative decisions in particular. Economic pressure has squeezed industry participants and moved them to create cooperative alliances that are intended to reduce costs and thereby maintain income for both hospitals and physicians. The emergence of managed care in the 1980s resulted in business models, such as HMOs and PPOs, that sought to contain costs in the delivery of health services. This was a critical evolution in the physician network model, as it increased the negotiating power of physicians relative to these managed care organizations.

Any alliance must provide the partners with something of value for their participation. Physicians and hospitals sought to create alliances to offset the power of the managed care organizations (Olden, Roggenkamp, & Luke, 2002). Physicians want access to first-rate facilities, high-quality nursing care, appropriate insurance, efficient administrative support, and assistance in such areas as marketing of services. Hospitals want to gain access to essential physician services, share the risks associated with such services, and reduce costs.

This negotiated relationship is evident in many hospital organizational charts in which physician groups not only are represented on the governing board but also may in some cases report directly to the board. In the end, physicians continue to act as independent contractors while forging essential partnerships with community health care organizations to maintain access to the many benefits they seek. And health care organizations invest considerable resources to recruit, retain, and educate physicians to maintain organizational capabilities.

TECHNOLOGY AND STRUCTURE

A discussion on structure and design would not be complete without mentioning the role that technology plays in how the health care organization looks and operates. Technology, broadly defined, is anything used to perform a task. This means that the processes and methods, tools, machines, information, skills, and materials used in doing its work make up an organization's technology.

Using this broad definition, think of the things made possible in modern medicine via innovations in technology, particularly as they affect the organizational design and work flow of the modern health care organization. Consider first the old technology, such as e-mail, and how it changed communication and the administrative structure of organizations. Reflect on the structural changes as more and more procedures are done on an outpatient basis, for example, the impact on the number of hospital beds required to serve a community and how these beds are used. Or consider the development in Internet-based technologies, such as telemedicine, that confer the ability to examine, diagnose, and prescribe treatment remotely.

Technology is a constant force for change in health care organizations, and it presents some of the greatest challenges to health care managers. Technology can be expected to bring even greater opportunities in the future.

SUMMARY

The health care sector is facing unbelievable strategic management challenges as the effects of health care reform work their way through health care delivery. Health care organizations have been very slow to respond to these strategic challenges because this sector was protected by passive consumers and third-party payers of health care bills. This has all changed because costs have continued to rise, consumers are now paying some or all of their health care bills, and health outcomes have not improved. We are now in real need of strategic management.

Success in the delivery of health services requires realistic goals, backed up with effective strategic management practices. Health care managers need to develop a clear vision of what their health care organization is all about. This business process usually starts with environmental scanning, moves to vision development, and then shifts to strategy formulation, followed by the execution and evaluation of the choices made during the process. Strategic management has become a necessity in ensuring the survival and growth of the many organizations that deliver health services in our country.

Health care organizations must also give a great deal of attention to organizational design and structure. The structure of a health care organization consists of the way it divides up the tasks that are to be completed in delivering superb services to customers. Organizational design, the process that leads to the development of the organizational structure, focuses on such aspects as communication, policies, and rules; control systems; and decision-making authority. To be successful in the future, health care organizations must delegate decision-making authority to lower-level employees, which will require a change in thought process among most health care managers.

Flatter organizational structures in health care delivery, as well as greater decentralization, enable health care organizations to respond better to the changing health care environment. The expanding use of technology in health care, especially in information services, has become a necessary adjunct to dealing with rapid change. The design of new and innovative structures that support a swift response to change and the exploitation of technology will ensure that health care facilities remain relevant in the emerging world of health care delivery.

KEY TERMS

divisional structure

environmental scanning

functional structure

general environment

hybrid structure

immediate environment

internal environment

matrix structure

organizational design

organizational structure

Porter's Five Forces Model

strategic management

REVIEW QUESTIONS

1. Define strategy and structure, as well as the relationship between them.

2. Describe the strategic management process and the components that make up that process.

3. Discuss the various aspects of environmental scanning in the strategic management process.

4. Describe Porter's Five Forces Model. How can it help managers assess the dynamics of an industry?

5. What is the difference between organizational design and organizational structure?

6. List and describe the main issues involved in designing an organization. What are the general design options available to the manager?

PART 3

Managing Human Performance in Organizations

The central theme running throughout this entire management text is that your most important resource in an organization is your people. This is especially true in health care management, because health services are delivered by people to people. This section of the textbook includes four chapters all focusing on human resources and their importance in the delivery of health services.

Topics covered in this section include leadership, change, motivation, innovation, communication, and physician management. The authors attempt to show the role managers play in relation to these very important people-related topics.

The first topic discussed in Part Three is leadership (Chapter Four). The discussion begins with the basics of leadership theory and moves into explanations of behavioral theory, situational leadership, and transformational leadership. The author then addresses some of the newer theories in leadership development, such as servant leadership and employee empowerment, among others. The discussion then moves to quality issues that include health outcomes and medical errors.

After a very thorough discussion of leadership, this book takes you through the change process in health care delivery (Chapter Five). This chapter covers the fundamentals of implementing change, and continues with a deep discussion concerning how to motivate employees to offer excellent services to every customer who comes to their health care organization. This is followed by an exploration of the process of innovation and how it should fit into the culture of excellence in health care delivery. The next chapter contains an in-depth discussion of the need for better communication among health care employees and their managers (Chapter Six). The communication process, along with the various communication skills that are required of every health care manager dealing with change and innovation in the workplace, are covered in detail.

The last topic discussed in Part Three is the management of physicians (Chapter Seven). This chapter describes the changing environment for physicians and addresses physician management, physician reimbursement, and patient care quality concerns. Among other topics, there is quite a bit of discussion concerning ethical concerns and management models that involve physicians.

4

Leadership as Plural

Bernard J. Healey

LEARNING OBJECTIVES

- Understand the use of leadership skills in the improvement of health care facilities

- Recognize the need for the empowerment of workers to deal with the major problems in our current health care system

- Understand the value of team development in the delivery of health services

- Be able to explain the need for leadership development programs for all health care professionals

Our health care system is in the process of unbelievable, breathtaking, and escalating reform. These reform efforts are challenging every health care organization to change the way it does business. A change of this magnitude will require leaders in health care with special skills, including abilities in regard to communication, conflict management, and building a culture of trust and a desire to help lower-level employees grow and develop. These leaders will have to recognize that the whole reform effort is meaningless if we do not understand the importance of followers, who are the ones actually delivering services to the patient or customer.

Leaders and leadership development are needed to improve the quality of health care delivery and to reduce the cost of these services. Buchbinder and Shanks (2007) argue that leaders differ from managers in that the leaders keep the organization on course with the **vision** and remove obstacles, whereas managers usually focus more on efficiency in day-to-day operations. Having followers is a necessary prerequisite for an effective leader. In fact, the ability to inspire followers is probably a good leader's most important characteristic. It seems that many of the qualities that are found in a good leader are also found in a good manager or a good follower. For health care facilities to survive and prosper in the reforming health care industry, leadership needs to emerge everywhere in every health care facility. This is going to require the collaboration and involvement of all health care employees.

The leader's central responsibility in any organization is to provide a vision of the future that supplies the organization with positive and **sustainable momentum** (Lombardi & Schermerhorn, 2007). Sustainable momentum is usually provided by the leader and the vision of the organization, allowing the organization and the employees to continue to grow. This function is much different from the management function. The leader must delegate the day-to-day activities of managing to his or her empowered managers. This affords the leader the valuable time necessary to prepare the organization for the changes brought about by the reform of the entire U.S. health care system. The leader needs to provide the health care facility with the vision necessary to improve efficiency and reduce costs. This complex task can only be completed through the use of a team approach that embraces and is prepared to exploit change for the opportunities it often brings. That is, anyone responsible for any part of the process of delivering health services requires leadership abilities.

Figure 4.1 demonstrates the leading function's relationship to all of the other management functions found in any organization at a given point in time. This diagram points out the importance of the leading function as the **inspiration** for the entire management component of the organization, which is very much the case in health care facilities. The health care leader

Figure 4.1   Leading Viewed in Relation to Other Management Functions
Source: Lombardi & Schermerhorn, 2007, p. 245. Reprinted with permission of John Wiley & Sons, Inc.

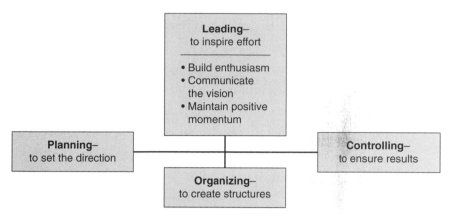

inspires others to do extraordinary things by helping the health care team perform. Zenger, Folkman, and Edinger (2009) believe that inspiration may be the most important leadership ingredient, and that it is necessary for any successful organization. Their research suggests that inspiring staff members can motivate them toward goal achievement and the accomplishment of the organizational mission in all types of occupations, including health care.

Who gets listened to in an organization has taken on great significance because of health care reform. According to Hamel (2007), the power in an organization is found among the top administrators, but unfortunately the wisdom, imagination, and creativity are more likely to be found among the lower-level employees. This holds true in health care organizations, in which health services are delivered by nonadministrators who have a much better grasp on the best ways to deliver these services. Listening to your followers in health care delivery has taken on tremendous importance because of the need to reduce medical errors, improve health outcomes, and at the same time lower the costs associated with the delivery of health services.

Hamel (2007) argues that organizations are not adaptable but individuals are—and that leaders have to concentrate their efforts on one follower at a time. He believes that most individuals are not resistant to change, but instead welcome change for the new experiences and challenges it brings. This is where leaders can excel in providing individuals with the chance to change, be challenged, and achieve personal growth. This change is the responsibility of leaders and empowered workers dedicated to service excellence.

A leader's effectiveness can be measured according to the extent to which the organization is successful in the achievement of its goals (Yukl, 1989). This definition is appropriate for the challenging world of health care. Blanchard (2009) argues that **high-performing organizations** concentrate their efforts on three very important areas of concern: being the provider of choice, the employer of choice, and the investment of choice. For a health care organization to achieve its many important goals, there is a great need to employ individuals who are capable of delivering quality health services. If the organization becomes the employer of choice for great employees, it will usually become the provider of choice because of the excellent services those employees deliver. At least for now, leaders of health care facilities need to spend all of their time on guiding their organization to become the employer of choice.

LEADERSHIP BASICS

Leadership is one of the most important functions of managers, but not all managers are capable of performing this function. There is no universally accepted definition of leadership, even though the concept has been discussed since the beginning of time. This is probably because there is ongoing research concerning the topic, with new results being published almost every day. The only agreement among the many researchers of leadership is that good leaders are capable of influencing large numbers of people through the use of some type of power. The various forms of power seem to allow individuals to assume the leadership role at different times, in different places, and in different situations. Power can originate from one's position in an organization or from one's personal power, as shown in Figure 4.2.

The various sources of power, as depicted in the figure, include the following:

Figure 4.2 Sources of Power
Source: Lombardi & Schermerhorn, 2007, p. 248. Reprinted with permission of John Wiley & Sons, Inc.

Power of the POSITION: based on things managers can offer to others.	Power of the PERSON: based on the ways managers are viewed by others.
Rewards: "If you do what I ask, I'll give you a reward."	**Expertise:** as a source of special knowledge and information.
Coercion: "If you *don't* do what I ask, I'll punish you."	**Reference:** as a person with whom others like to identify.
Legitimacy: "Because I am the boss, you *must* do as I ask."	

- *Legitimate power.* This type of power usually is granted by the organization, and can be taken away by the organization. It generally involves a title, high status, and supervisory authority over other individuals, and it comes with the ability to influence lower-level employees. A manager is given legitimate power by the organization and has the ability to exercise influence over his or her direct reports.

- *Reward power.* This type of power, which flows from the legitimate power granted to a manager by the organization, involves the ability to grant rewards to individuals for their work or support. A reward could be a pay increase or a promotion granted to an employee by a manager. Reward power usually has to do with the manager's position in an organization, and it can be taken away by the same organization.

- *Coercive power.* This type of power, which is part of the legitimate power granted to a manager by the organization, involves the ability of a manager to apply some type of discipline to a lower-level employee. It represents a negative form of influence and usually requires the use of fear.

- *Expert power.* This type of power involves the expertise or perceived competence of the individual holding a position of influence. A manager gains expert power through his or her superior knowledge, skills, or understanding of something the organization and its employees value. Expert power is quite often acquired by the individual through advanced education and training; it belongs to that individual, not the organization. Because this power comes forth from the individual, it cannot be taken away by the organization. If individuals with expert power leave the organization, they take this form of power with them.

- *Referent power.* This type of power, which is also called charisma, involves the communication skills or likeability of the person wielding influence. It is usually a result of the admiration for or interpersonal skills of the manager, which he or she has usually fostered over time. It offers a great source of influence by one person over others. This type of personal power can be developed and improved over time, and cannot be taken away by the organization.

It is interesting to note that although many people spend a great deal of time gaining the power of their position, they never really own this type of power. By contrast, however, personal power can be developed and expanded by the person, and he or she owns it forever. Personal power is quite often associated with excellent leaders, and it is crucial in empowering employees and developing them into the organization's future leaders. In times of great change in an organization's surrounding environment, personal power is usually the most important in leading followers. A leader, to empower his or her people, needs to share any of the five sources of power with them. A successful leader usually learns how to help develop personal power in his or her employees, and also shares with them the power granted by his or her position.

DuBrin (2007) believes that leadership involves the ability to acquire the respect and support that are necessary to accomplish organizational goals. The health care manager must work very hard to gain the respect of his or her followers. It becomes more important for this manager to listen to employees and help them to clear roadblocks to attaining their personal and organizational goals. Employees listen to what the manager says, but they also watch what he or she does.

Health care managers have the additional responsibility of not only discovering the company's culture but also working to foster a thick and positive culture—one in which all employees are moving in the right direction and that is devoted to improved health services. A bond must develop between managers and workers. Rice (2007) argues that leaders need to be able to go beyond competence, building the bonds with employees and customers that develop trust and thus make great things happen.

As already mentioned, leaders must share power with every worker in the company if the business is to accomplish its primary goals. This is a very difficult task for those who have spent their whole career trying to gain power. They usually do not trust their followers enough to in effect give away their precious power, even in the interest of goal accomplishment.

There is an overwhelming need for leadership development in health care organizations as they respond to the changes brought on by health care reform. Dye and Garman (2006) argue that on top of responding to reform efforts, leaders also have to deal with the problems associated with running a multifaceted organization. Health care facilities are complex entities that can completely exhaust both their employees and their managers. This is the major reason for the development of health care leaders, who will be tasked with creating the vision that replenishes the energy of those who provide health services and those who manage this most important service industry.

The components of excellence in the delivery of services include focusing on the needs and desires of the consumer, treating the consumer as a guest, and managing the total health care experience (Fottler, Ford, & Heaton, 2010). These components require the health care manager and his or her employees to understand what patients want and to make certain they receive what they desire from the health care facility. The concept of treating the patient as a guest is a research area on which many of the world's most successful companies are currently focusing. It seems like an excellent idea to incorporate this new leadership thought process in the delivery of health services. To treat patients as guests in health care, however, the entire health care system must be changed. The starting point for this major change is the complete empowerment of all employees, which would allow them to begin serving their guests.

LEADERSHIP THEORY

There is nothing new about the concept of leadership—it has been around since the beginning of time. If you look at the history of civilization, you will discover that in times of conflict there have always been individuals who rose to the challenge and were called leaders. These individuals were capable of influencing others to join their cause, and usually the conflict was resolved. The special characteristic that seemed to make these leaders successful was a charismatic way of gaining influence over others.

Leadership theory began to develop in the early 1900s as a study of the elite—individuals who, having been born to the right parents, had inherited genius or gifts that prepared them for a career in politics, finance, the military, and other areas of influence. These chosen individuals were capable of seizing power because of their status in life, earned through their birth into wealth and power.

One of the most influential books about management and leadership, *Functions of the Executive,* was written by Chester Barnard in 1938. Barnard offered his own insight as an executive on the various roles of a manager. He believed that leadership was one of the most important functions performed by a manager, and argued that leadership, to be effective, had to be perceived as legitimate by followers. Introducing a systems approach to the organization, Barnard brought the motivation of employees as well as collaboration among members of the organization to the forefront of managerial thinking.

There are many theories of leadership that can easily be applied to the health care industry. Leadership theory is nothing more than a collection of thoughts that may be able to help us better understand the practice of leading. There are probably thousands of books that provide great insight into what it requires and means to be a leader, many of which explore how best to lead a health care facility. I would like to briefly discuss the following theories as a potential basis for learning how to lead health care facilities: behavioral theory, situational leadership, transformational leadership, and servant leadership. I have chosen these theories because they involve followers in their explanations of leadership effectiveness, and because they are service oriented in their application.

Behavioral Theory

Behavioral theory started to develop in the 1950s as researchers began concentrating on what leaders do rather than on their common traits. This approach to leadership, which sparked interest in the various styles of leadership, focuses on the behaviors exhibited by the leader in the workplace. This research showed that one's chosen leadership strategies are strongly influenced by one's assumptions about human nature.

Behavioral theory supports the assertion that individuals can learn to be leaders through readings, education, and training programs. This research opened up a great deal of interest in leadership consulting for businesses trying to provide leadership development for their managers.

Northouse (2010) argues that a leader can exhibit two types of behaviors: behaviors that focus on tasks, and behaviors that focus on relationships with and among employees. Both areas are important for a leader to be effective in attaining organizational goals, but relationship-focused behaviors seem to promote employees' acceptance of the leader and their now common goals. Moreover, the leader recognizes that it is important for employees to be satisfied with his or her behavior.

A book written by Douglas McGregor in 1960, titled *The Human Side of Enterprise,* introduced us to Theory X and Theory Y managers. The Theory X manager, on the one hand, has several negative assumptions about employees, including that they dislike work, they need to be controlled at work, and they will avoid responsibility. The Theory Y manager, on the other hand, believes that employees like responsibility, they have self-control, and their potential is only partially used in the workplace. According to these assumptions, a Theory X manager would exhibit more bureaucratic behavior, and a Theory Y manager would have a more participative style.

Situational Leadership

The situational or contingency school of leadership has focused its research on how a leader functions in different situations. According to Pierce and Newstrom (2008), the theory of situational leadership, introduced by Fred E. Fiedler in 1967, posits that some situations are more favorable to leaders than others. This theory looks at the leader's orientation to others, the situations the leader faces, and how the leader reacts to these situations. It stands to reason that different situations will require different styles of behavior from the leader.

Fiedler (1967) argued that there are three specific situation variables capable of affecting the leader's success:

- *Leader-member relations.* This involves how well the leader gets along with his or her followers.
- *Task structure.* This involves the degree to which the leader's job is structured.
- *Position power.* This involves the amount of power available to the leader.

In addition to the situation, whether the leader is task oriented or relationship oriented comes into play. These variables offer a number of scenarios whereby a manager possessing certain traits or behaviors could be successful or could fail. The real value of this model is found in its analysis of how a leader may require a particular style to be successful in a given situation.

The theory of situational leadership offers very useful information for leaders involved in the delivery of health services. This is because there are so many different situations that can confront health care managers at different times and in different locations in a health care facility. For example, the situation in an emergency room is best managed by an individual with a task-oriented style of leadership. In other parts of a health care facility, such as medical records or discharge planning, a relationship-oriented style may be more successful. The situational variable in health care delivery is a critical concern for providing leadership in the changing health care environment.

Transformational Leadership

The work process in delivering health services to customers is undergoing dramatic change, which is being ushered in by customers, third-party payers, providers, and the U.S. government. Strong leadership and employee empowerment, as well as a commitment to excellence from all health care professionals, are needed to compete in these turbulent times. This is also going to require a specific type of leadership style—usually transformational, which helps employees with the process of change. **Transformational leadership** involves an exceptional form of influence that moves followers to accomplish more than what is usually expected (Malandro, 2009).

What the patient wants in health care delivery is essentially a process change that will require everyone on the health care team to work together. Leaders need to begin the process of changing the culture in the organization, rendering its members capable of undertaking new tasks and accepting change as an opportunity for growth. Followers need help in understanding the need for this change, and they require support to change the work process.

Northouse (2010) discusses two types of leadership: transactional and transformational. Transactional leadership, which is frequently used in organizations, revolves around exchanges that occur between the leader and the follower. An exchange can range from praise of the employee to an increase in pay in an attempt to motivate that individual to improve his or her performance. On the other side of the leadership continuum is transformational leadership, which places greater emphasis on the followers' being inspired by the leader's personal power to do more than what is expected of them at work. This approach by the leader, strongly supported by recent literature, pushes the follower to seek satisfaction of his or her higher-level needs (Trompenaars & Voerman, 2010). Transformational leaders express genuine understanding of and compassion for followers.

According to Lussier and Achua (2010), transformational leaders are capable of transforming the needs of followers from desires revolving around their own self-interest to wants that focus on collective organizational issues. To accomplish this goal there is a need for trust building, which will take a great deal of the leaders' time and energy but is well worth the effort. Lussier and Achua (2010) point out that the successful process of transformation requires the involvement of all of the company stakeholders, who must embrace and improve on the shared vision. The key concept that is brought forth by this leadership style is a shared vision along with shared values. These gifted leaders are aware of what holds personal meaning for them, and they practice this through what they do in their leadership role. Lussier and Achua define having a sense of personal meaning as knowing the degree to which one's work is worthy of one's energy and commitment. This is a gift that the leader can give to others in the organization.

Northouse (2010) argues that a transformational leadership style is one of the most important components of worker motivation, which is vital to the attainment of organizational goals. According to Lussier and Achua (2010), the transformational leader endeavors to make a convincing case for change in the process of work, and then provides effective leadership in the process of change. This is the approach that health care managers need to follow as they attempt to improve health outcomes for their patients. The transformational leader has a very clear vision of where the organization should be in future years. In health care, such a vision might require followers to focus entirely on what customers want from their health care experience. A transformational leadership style fosters a bond between leader and follower in the achievement of a common goal: patient satisfaction.

The transformational leader attempts to raise the process of work to a higher level by appealing to higher ideals and employees' moral values (Burns, 1978). Transformational leadership abilities may be found in employees at any level and any type of position. Followers are elevated to their better selves in their service to others. Lombardi and Schermerhorn (2007) point out that transformational leaders understand the value of enabling followers to gain power and thus allowing them to make decisions to serve the customer. What better time to use transformational leadership than when dealing with individuals who are in their most vulnerable state— when they are ill, maybe very ill.

Possessing emotional intelligence and interpersonal skills is essential for anyone attempting to be a transformational leader. Barrett (2011) defines emotional intelligence, or the emotional quotient, as the ability to identify and use emotions in ourselves and in those for whom we are responsible in our role as a leader. This emotional intelligence allows us to communicate effectively with our employees, which is particularly important with self-managed work teams delivering health services.

Hesselbein and Shrader (2008) point out that the most important component of leading others is aligning teammates around a shared vision and then empowering these followers to lead. Figure 4.3 offers a useful way to see how the transformation from "I" to "we" can become reality for a business. The transformational leadership style allows health care managers and employees to essentially become one as they approach the delivery of quality health services. Probably the most important characteristic of the health care manager as he or she attempts to improve services and get all employees tuned in to the same vision is the ability to communicate with all stakeholders the importance of positive change. There will be much more discussion about the importance of communication throughout the organization in Chapter Six.

Figure 4.3 Transformation from "I" to "We"
Source: Hesselbein & Shrader, 2008, p. 47. Reprinted with permission of John Wiley & Sons, Inc.

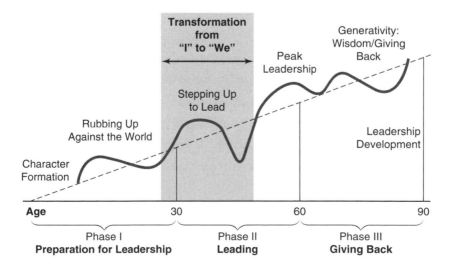

Servant Leadership

Trompenaars and Voerman (2010) point out that in 1970 Robert Greenleaf completed an essay titled "The Servant and Leader," which started a revolution in how we think about leadership (Greenleaf, 1996). His essay called for a change from organizational bureaucracy and hierarchy to an organization based on teams—on decentralized decision making with a new focus on the personal growth of employees. This type of leadership, which is actually an extension of many of the concepts found in the transformational style, is a refreshing change from models that rely heavily on power as the basis of leadership.

Servant leadership occurs when serving and leading are in harmony, and the two concepts merge in one or more people (Trompenaars & Voerman, 2010). It also represents an entirely new way of motivating individuals to grow and achieve greater self-actualization. The individual who is a servant leader has a greater desire to serve employees and customers than to lead. This inclination to serve has been associated with excellent leadership because followers want to be part of the goal achievement process. Because the servant leader places customers, employees, and the community above gaining more power, he or she is capable of obtaining the respect and trust of employees, allowing them to build the positive, thick culture that is so very necessary in delivering excellent services.

According to Greenleaf (1996), some of the more important characteristics found in the servant leader include abilities in regard to listening, empathy, healing, awareness, persuasion, conceptualization, foresight, and stewardship, as well as a commitment to the growth of people and to building community. All of these characteristics are very important for any leader in today's world of rapid change, but they hold special meaning for the delivery of excellent health services. Commitment to the growth of employees is necessary for the health care leader to obtain the support of all those who deliver health services.

Trompenaars and Voerman (2010) argue that servant leaders have the unique ability to bring people with different points of view together. They allow their people to grow by giving them the room and the opportunity to improve their performance every day. By including everyone in the decision making process, they increase their chances of making the best decision possible for their business and for the employees of the business. This style of leadership also allows for input from the customers, which can also improve the services being offered.

Finally, servant leaders are able to harness the creativity and innovation of each individual to improve the performance of the team—and improving the delivery of most services in health care requires a team approach. Servant leadership may be the answer to the problem of how to make the process of delivering health services more efficient and effective.

EMPLOYEE PARTICIPATION

The delivery of quality health services to a demanding customer requires superb leaders and dedicated, empowered workers operating as a team to deliver excellence on a continuous basis. Servant leadership seems to be the perfect approach to developing, implementing, and consistently improving the self-managed work team in health care delivery. It is not the leaders of health care organizations but rather their employees who deliver excellent services to their customers. This excellence is not a result of the leader's power; it is the by-product of empowerment among those who directly serve patients. It does not happen when employees are told what to do; it results from their knowing what to do and doing it. The administration of the health care facility first needs to realize that every employee must be involved and on the same page if health care delivery is going to be improved. This is where leadership becomes the catalyst in ensuring consistent, high-quality health care delivery. Fottler et al. (2010) assert that only 10 percent of those involved in providing services to others actually love what they do. This is a frightening statistic for those who are managing the delivery of health services and are attempting to empower lower-level employees, and it suggests the need for all health care professionals in the organization to understand the value of hiring the right people, to receive the best training, and to be certain that they are part of the culture of excellent care.

Managers want to hire employees who desire to work and grow at their health care facility. This can only be accomplished through careful recruitment and selection of very special employees who fit into a culture of excellence. To be really effective in the delivery of health services, the leader needs to understand the importance of all the people who work for the organization. Everyone is a critical player in health care delivery, making teamwork, communication, and worker empowerment mandatory in realizing the mission of every employee's providing excellent services every day.

A leader of empowered employees in a health care organization must be truly interested in serving the customers and the greater community that surrounds the health care facility. Such a leader is capable of upholding the vision of the organization while also paying close attention to the development of those who actually produce and deliver health services. This feat is made possible because this servant leader has perfected the ability to listen to both the employees and the customers of the health care facility. This ability to listen is exactly what health care managers need to develop to lead their facility to excellence. It is the ultimate requirement for retaining excellent employees who can consistently deliver high-quality heath care services to their customers, thereby enabling the health care facility to gain and keep a competitive advantage over those who would attempt to take away its customers.

CREATING A VISION OF HEALTH CARE DELIVERY

There needs to be a vision for delivering health care to Americans. This should be a vision that reflects how the patient wants to receive health care, not how providers want to deliver it. Creating such a vision is the most important part of the new world of health care. The leader's vision of how the organization supplies these vital services to customers must be shared among all members of the organization, which is where the ability to listen to employees and customers comes into play. By listening, the leader is able to find out how to improve health care delivery. The customer will tell the leader what is being done right and what can be improved. The employees will tell the leader how to deliver the services the customers want. It only requires the ability to listen.

To respond to this challenge, the leader constantly needs to develop his or her workers, urging them to work as a team in delivering excellent services to all customers all of the time. He or she needs to encourage rather than discourage all members of the health care team to provide help, guidance, and even dissenting views concerning how to deliver high-quality services to customers. The frontline employees know what is working well and where the errors are in the delivery process. These employees are also very aware of what management processes are working and what managerial tasks are actually impeding employee creativity and innovation.

Senge (2006) points out that a shared vision is crucial for the learning organization. This vision provides the focal point of the organization's direction and the energy required for the journey. The organizational vision is capable of bringing everyone together in a quest to make that vision a reality. The question becomes, How do we get the vision to be shared by all members of the health care organization? Health care managers must be able to gain the ability not just to develop a vision but also to get it accepted by every member of the organization. This is also the component of leadership that separates success from failure.

In the pursuit of a shared vision, the leader's primary responsibility becomes articulating the vision to employees in different ways. The vision actually becomes a living, breathing part of the day-to-day activities of every member of the organization. It is not enough to put it in writing for employees when they enter an organization; it has to become a way of life for leaders and followers on a daily basis, and a catalyst for the consistent delivery of excellent health services. The vision needs to include the reduction of medical errors, the improvement of health outcomes, and the delivery of high-quality services by all employees to every customer. This requires placing the customer above everything else in the organization.

Finally, according to Fottler et al. (2010), the vision is a way for the leader to communicate the desired future for the health care organization. It is also a superb means of inspiring and uniting employees in the achievement of a common goal. It is a vehicle for the leader to point the way, encouraging all members to focus their total attention on the customer from the minute they enter the health care facility until they leave. Excellent service becomes the only acceptable measure of performance. It also becomes the center of the culture that is accepted by the vast majority of organizational employees.

EMPOWERMENT AND RESPONSIBILITY

To achieve the vision of excellence in health care delivery, the leader needs the buy-in of all employees because they are the ones delivering the health services to customers. To accomplish this goal, the leader must build a thick culture of trust among all health care employees, thereby empowering them in delivering excellent services to their customers. However, followers may not be ready for empowerment. Health care employees have been conditioned to expect management that uses legitimate, coercive, and occasionally reward power, and they may have a very difficult time understanding transformational leadership and empowerment.

Empowerment involves a whole new way of delivering services without the constraint of direct supervision. According to Blanchard (2009), it entails allowing employees to use their personal power, including their experience, knowledge, and motivation in their position, to achieve the goals of the organization. For the empowerment of employees to happen, the leader needs to be able to devote attention to helping his or her direct reports unleash their personal power. This requires a shift in thinking by the leader; the elimination of the many roadblocks to empowerment, which may include managers who are reluctant to share power; and the training of employees to accept and use their newfound power. Research strongly supports empowerment as the way to achieve goals that were never considered possible (Blanchard).

It should be noted here that the concept of employee empowerment can seem risky for both leaders and followers because it requires mutual trust. Trust has to be earned, and that takes a great deal of time and commitment from everyone involved. The most important reason for the empowerment of health care workers is that leaders cannot achieve excellence in health care delivery without the cooperation of others. For the health care facility to be successful in pursuing its vision, improving health outcomes, and reducing medical errors, the leader must share power with every worker.

IMPROVING HEALTH OUTCOMES

A health care facility, to remain relevant in its delivery of health services over time, needs to spend a great deal of time in the pursuit of improving health outcomes. Fottler et al. (2010) argue that a service-oriented strategy requires the alignment of the organization's mission with all other activities. To improve health outcomes, therefore, health care organizations require a mission statement that is responsive to ever-changing consumer demands. The improvement of health outcomes and the reduction of medical errors are of great importance to all of the major players in health care.

The new focus in health care delivery must become the improvement of health outcomes for all patients entering the health care system. These outcomes for some individuals will not involve curing illness because of the types of medical problems encountered. To sharpen everyone's focus on health outcomes, customers should be able to compare the outcomes achieved by all providers. In other words, there will be complete transparency.

The health care system has consistently concentrated on curing rather than preventing disease. This has resulted in tremendous waste of scarce health care resources, with little attention paid to patients' wants and desires. The recent passage of health care reform legislation is going to force the health care system to change in very dramatic ways. There will be changes in reimbursement, a focus on prevention, and much more attention paid to what the consumer wants in the health care experience.

According to Sultz and Young (2011), medical errors, especially in hospitals, are a well-known problem that commands very little attention by those in power. The Institute of Medicine (IOM, 1999) revealed that forty-four thousand to ninety-eight thousand people die in hospitals each year because of preventable medical errors. Hospital-based errors alone represent the eighth leading cause of death in the United States, ahead of breast cancer, AIDS, and motor vehicle accidents (Altman, Clancy, & Blendon, 2004). Regardless of any debate about these estimates, they remain the standard for describing the scope of the nation's problem with medical errors. The continuance of this epidemic of medical errors within health care facilities is a managerial failure and must not be allowed to continue.

Kenney (2008) also discovered that at least 4 percent of patients suffered injuries that resulted in longer hospital stays, disabilities, and death. The health care manager must begin improving the quality of care in health care facilities by immediately dealing with the problem of medical errors. According to Kenney, these medical errors are a direct result of poor communication between health care managers and their employees. The health care facility must treat every medical error as a failure in its ability to offer quality health services to patients.

According to Brownlee (2007), the most common error in health care delivery involves a mistake in administering drugs to patients. These drug-related errors include administering the wrong drug, giving the wrong dose of the right drug, or prescribing drugs that interact and harm the patient. These drug errors alone add $5,000 to the cost of every hospital admission (IOM, 1999). Looking beyond the cost of drug errors, the needless disability and death following the administration of the wrong drug should command national attention and motivate those in charge of health care to take action.

Too many patients are the victims of preventable medical errors and hospital-acquired infections (Emanuel, 2008). These errors are a result of poorly organized, inconsistent, and dysfunctional health care delivery. Recent research has found that one of the major causes of medical errors is miscommunication among health care professionals (Duhigg, 2012).

It is also becoming clear that a lack of cooperation among the players in the current health care system is behind the epidemic of medical errors (Brownlee, 2007). This is not necessarily to blame individual employees for medical errors, however. In many instances the teams of health care professionals simply do not talk to one another about the care of their patient. Mistakes are often made because of inadequate or incorrect information about a patient, and perhaps because of a lack of incentive to make the system work error free. Many providers are still using paper records with handwriting that is not legible, for example, even though electronic medical records (EMRs) not only are available but also are producing error-free health care delivery in many of this country's hospitals. This provides further evidence of the great value of using EMRs in hospital settings.

Reducing medical errors will require the development of a culture of safety in which teamwork is the norm in regard to delivering health services to patients. Health care teams will be empowered not only to develop their own protocol to prevent errors from occurring but also to deal with an error immediately if it does occur.

The health care system, in other words, must be redesigned such that it is more difficult for mistakes to be made. The system, Brownlee (2007) argues, requires too many people to do everything right every time to arrive at a successful patient outcome. Such a system is perfect for "latent errors," or mistakes that are waiting to happen. Although they are quite often labeled as never events, they are nevertheless occurring too frequently, causing health care costs to rise and patients to be hurt by a system that is supposed to heal them.

This is clearly the case with medical errors, which must be eliminated by dealing with the known flaws embedded in this complicated system. Medical staff must not attempt to work around this problem, but rather must immediately redesign a given process when they uncover problems. To eliminate system flaws it is very helpful to look at other companies that have dealt with—and solved—the problem of workplace errors. See, for example, Chapter One's discussion of Alcoa, whose practice of addressing safety problems in the workplace with a sense of urgency and with an eye toward avoiding such problems in the future is now used by high-velocity organizations.

LEADERSHIP AND CULTURE

The building of a culture of excellence has become one of the most important functions of the health care manager in his or her role as a leader of employees in the delivery of quality health services. The health care manager must work on building culture every day with every employee through establishing trust and improving communication among all employees. The vast majority of employees will respond positively to the process of culture building, as long as they understand the process and the reasons for the effort by health care managers. Bolden, Hawkins, Gosling, and Taylor (2011) define culture as ways of behaving in an organization that are based on values and assumptions shared by members of a group. It is simply "the way we do things around here." We do know that it is dynamic and is usually transmitted to those who belong to specific groups. Kotter and Heskett (1992) argue that the presence of a strong culture can enable a group to become proactive in dealing with the problems confronting it. They also point out that most managers operating within a strong culture usually share with followers a set of relatively consistent values and methods of completing work.

Hickman (1998) argues that a company with a corporate culture that pushes positive change understands the value of the people and the processes that create such change. This company truly believes in its workers and respects its customers, and this shows in the way top managers act in the workplace on a daily basis. The company whose culture fosters enhanced performance takes pride in its workers and customers and strives never to hurt either group. This company takes the extra step needed to produce goods and services with no defects and no negative consequences for its workers in the production process.

Ledlow and Coppola (2011) argue that culture development is a product of a group's learning how to solve problems together successfully. In health care, this development is in part a response to external and internal pressures that require a change in the way the facility does business on a daily basis. It is the leader's responsibility to move beyond power influence to accomplish this change. Exceptional leaders are capable of providing direction and support while empowering followers to move this necessary change to completion.

Schein (2004) defines culture as shared basic assumptions that have been successful in solving problems associated with the external environment and have also worked well in regard to internal integration. Figure 4.4 shows the

Figure 4.4 Levels of Culture
Source: Schein, 2004, p. 26. Reprinted with permission of John Wiley & Sons, Inc.

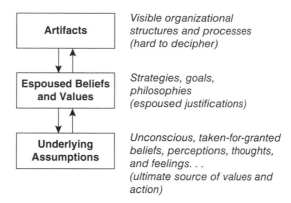

major levels of culture, including artifacts, espoused beliefs and values, and underlying assumptions.

Schein (2004) points out that members of a profession are quite capable of developing a culture of their own. This is a result of their molding into a group as they receive similar education or training. This culture development is very evident among physicians, nurses, and individuals from several other health care professions who share similar attitudes and values in what they do on a daily basis. A few points about culture are important to bear in mind:

- Organizations can have more than one dominant culture and several subcultures.

- If you study any organization long enough you are going to uncover a strong, distinct, and thick culture. There is no right or perfect culture.

- A strong, focused culture usually begins with a compelling vision espoused on a daily basis by the leader. This vision is usually the catalyst for upholding the values of the organization.

The new health care reform legislation is going to usher in tremendous change in the way health care in the United States is delivered (Dolan,

2010). Dolan argues that these changes are going to require health care leaders to have the following skills (p. 6):

- Mastery of change management and change leadership
- Continued quality and patient safety efforts
- Productivity
- Public policy
- Interpersonal skills

It is very difficult if not impossible to find all of these leadership skills in a single leader. However, it is quite possible to find these skills in a group of individuals who have been empowered by a leader and are working together toward a common vision. According to Thompson (2009), excellent leaders develop an instinct that lets them know how to use their emotional energy to push followers toward the attainment of organizational goals. He called these special leaders organizational champions who are capable of using their enthusiasm to unite large numbers of followers with many skills that can be used collaboratively toward the achievement of the common vision.

An organizational champion is capable of energizing his or her followers to embrace new challenges despite any major barriers that could prevent the successful achievement of goals (Thompson, 2009). This leader provides the energy and the inspiration that are so necessary to help others rise to a level of achievement that they never thought was possible. The organizational champion, therefore, becomes an inspirational leader who can unite followers to share their special skills to achieve a common goal.

Lighter (2011) argues that espousing the Baldrige Core Values is necessary for a high-performing organization that is capable of creating and sustaining a results-oriented culture. These values are as follows (pp. 352–353):

- Visionary leadership
- Patient-focused excellence
- Organizational and personal learning

- Valuing work force members and partners

- Agility

- Focus on the future

- Managing for innovation

- Management by fact

- Societal responsibility and community health

- Focus on results and creating value

- Systems perspective

These values are all-important for health care organizations and seem particularly relevant for maintaining a leadership focus in the delivery of health services.

The Baldrige Core Values look very much like Dolan's list of required skills for the health care leader of the twenty-first century. In fact, almost every book or article about leadership of health care organizations written since 2011 argues for the same necessary skills for the new world of health care delivery. It seems like the bureaucratic model still being used in many health care organizations is no longer sufficient to implement the rapid change required to improve the delivery of health services and thus retain patients. The leader has to rely on his or her empowered employees to uphold the core values so necessary to achieve excellence in health care delivery. The rules and regulations found in bureaucratic organizations block necessary change and render innovation and creativity impossible to sustain.

Eliminating the bureaucratic rules and regulations allows the leader to begin the process of inspiring followers by showing them respect, empowering them, and fostering personal development. Successful leaders working in organizations with thick, positive cultures all seem to have one thing in common: they recognize that they will never achieve organizational goals if they are not devoting the vast majority of their time to satisfying their customers' needs and developing their people. These leaders also recognize that to improve the health care experience for customers they require excellent employees who are motivated toward service excellence. Their employees are their greatest resource and their most important responsibility.

You cannot build a thick, positive culture in your work environment if your employees are unhappy and are constantly leaving your company for competitors who better meet their needs. It is a well-known fact that after the compensation package offered by employers, the next most important factor in motivating employees to remain with an employer is the learning and personal development that result from their training and work experiences. When work offers no meaning and no real opportunity for personal growth and development, employees stop being inspired to come to work (Zenger et al., 2009). When this happens they become bored, reduce their effort at work, and usually leave their employer. The leader is now unable to maintain excellent services, thereby losing customers and more employees to competitors that can better motivate their workers.

Zenger et al. (2009) point out that several things happen when individuals are given the opportunity to experience personal growth and development. They want to remain with their employer, their job satisfaction increases, their productivity goes up, and the quality of their work improves dramatically. The leader needs to recognize his or her responsibility for the personal development of employees, and must use this understanding as a starting point for building a culture that delivers opportunities for employees and service excellence for customers.

The question to be answered is, then, What type of culture does a health care leader want to build in a health care facility? In this chapter we have seen the importance of respect for employees and customers, the need for empowered employees, and the demand by all for a vision that is communicated clearly to everyone, every day. We have also learned what a leader must do to build a thick, positive culture that brings everyone together in support of attaining the organizational vision. It seems that the type of culture that would be optimal for most health care organizations has already been designed by Mayo Clinic.

Berry and Seltman (2008) argue that the longevity and continued success and growth of Mayo Clinic are direct results of its core value: "The needs of the patients come first" (p. 20). This one value has become the guiding force and vision for Mayo Clinic's customers, patients, payers, physicians, and other employees. Mayo Clinic's espoused values are the result of collaboration among all those involved in the provision of care (Berry & Seltman).

Mayo Clinic has built a superb, patient-centered culture that brings together all employees in the fulfillment of its mission and values. Management lessons can be gleaned from this clinic that are capable of making a health care organization successful in competing for both customers and employees, but these will require real leadership skills if they are to be implemented in other health care organizations. According to Berry and Seltman (2008), the lessons that come forth from the continuing success of Mayo Clinic include the following (pp. 62–63):

- Act small even if big.
- Encourage boundarylessness.
- Value "how," not just "what."

ADDING VALUE IN HEALTH CARE DELIVERY

To continuously add value in health care delivery we must constantly ask, What does the customer want? What makes a health service valuable to patients? The answer will never be found in the organization because only the customer knows what he or she wants from the health care system. In other words, the consumer of health services determines what does and does not constitute value on an individual basis. The value-adding process does not usually come forth from a bureaucratic organization with a top-down management structure. It is more likely to happen with frontline employees who are close to—and empowered to create value for—each individual customer.

A focus on the customer requires asking customers if their wants are being satisfied by the health care facility (Toussaint, 2010). If their expectations are not being met, the business model needs to be designed to fulfill them, even prioritizing patient demands over organizational needs. There will never be true customer satisfaction in a bureaucratic organization guided by rules and regulations. Toussaint points out that the bureaucratic organization has two major problems: it groups people by function, and it has a top-down command structure. The employees who work for the bureaucratic organization wind up serving their managers rather than their customers.

Because health care delivery is composed of employees offering services to customers, the most important part of the quality equation in health care is those delivering the services, not those who manage that delivery. The health care leader recognizes this fact and spends the vast majority of his or her time aligning the employees to meet the demands of the customer. Sanders (2008) argues that an organization should develop employees to continuously provide optimal services to their customers. This should be the leader's vision for the health care facility. It will require the employees to be empowered to spend all of their time on delivering services rather than worrying about rules, regulations, and time-consuming meetings about quality improvement. These rules, regulations, and meetings do not produce quality; people do.

According to Champy and Greenspun (2010), reengineering health care requires better use of new technology and of the skills and behaviors of the people who actually deliver health services. Fottler et al. (2010) argue that health care managers have devoted their energy to meeting patients' clinical needs. Leaders in health care delivery have realized that although clinical needs are vitally important, health care facilities also must spend a great deal of time and effort meeting other needs of the customer, such as friendly service and on-time appointments. The leader also recognizes that the needs, wants, and expectations of the consumer of health care are met by lower-level employees, not by managers. This means that reengineering efforts must concentrate on technology, processes, and the people who deliver health services.

The delivery of health services has to be organized around the patient rather than around a department or a specific provider of care, such as the physician. To accomplish this goal there needs to be a team approach to adding value to the patient's experience while he or she consumes health services. All health care employees must take responsibility for problem solving, which involves working together to produce continuous quality improvement in health care delivery (Toussaint, 2010). This will usually require a complete reengineering of the care process.

Champy and Greenspun (2010) argue that to facilitate the reengineering of health care delivery, four words are of the greatest importance: *fundamental, radical, dramatic,* and *process*. Health care leaders need to learn how to listen to their employees and their customers (Toussaint, 2010). These leaders need to spend a great deal of time asking their customers how to improve the quality of their health care experience. Leaders then need to seek out the help of their followers in improving the work process of the organization by providing them with training and empowerment.

SUMMARY

There never has been a greater need for leadership in health care delivery then there is in today's turbulent health care environment. Leadership is necessary to improve the quality of the services delivered and the outcomes from those services while also making the best use of health care resources. Health care managers must acquire, develop, and use leadership skills to accomplish the predetermined goals of their health care organization.

The health care manager, to lead others, must be capable of using his or her power in influencing followers to improve the quality of health care delivery. The old forms of power given to the manager include legitimate power, coercive power, and reward power. However, these types of power are no longer sufficient to influence health care employees. The health care manager must learn how to develop personal power, including expert power and referent power (also known as charisma), which have become absolute necessities in the accomplishment of the many goals of health care reform.

There are several theories of leadership that can help health care managers better understand how to influence and empower those actually delivering health services. The theories of transformational leadership and servant leadership seem to offer health care managers the skills necessary to respond to a changing health care environment.

The health care manager must also gain a much better understanding of the role of culture in a health care organization. He or she must learn how to help all employees build a thick, patient-centered culture that will promote constant quality improvement. This requires the manager to empower employees to add value to the health care delivery process.

KEY TERMS

high-performing organizations

inspiration

sustainable momentum

transformational leadership

vision

REVIEW QUESTIONS

1. Why is leadership so important in the improvement of health care delivery? Explain.

2. Compare and contrast the various styles of leadership discussed in this chapter.

3. Explain how health care leaders can empower their workers to deliver excellent services to customers on a daily basis.

4. Why are transformational leadership and servant leadership considered to be the gold standards of leadership where the delivery of services is concerned? Explain.

5

Change, Motivation, and Innovation
Creating a Culture of Excellence

Bernard J. Healey

LEARNING OBJECTIVES

- Understand the major challenges found in responding to changes in our health care system
- Recognize the need for a culture of excellence in health care facilities
- Become aware of the advantages of a proactive approach to health care problems
- Understand the value of innovation in the delivery of health services
- Become aware of the need for disruptive innovation in health care
- Be able to explain how the process of innovation in health care delivery works in health care organizations

This chapter is about the health care manager's role in change management. This role involves motivating employees to attain far-reaching goals and using **innovation** in solving many of our current problems, both of which are necessary to address the tremendous **change** that is occurring in health care delivery. Our country can no longer afford to pay trillions of dollars for a health care system that is not producing good health. Our employers, the government, providers of health services, third-party payers, and consumers are all demanding a health care system that delivers what they want, when they want it, while also offering quality care at a reasonable price.

Health care organizations generally have a bureaucratic structure held together by the legitimate power of those in charge. Managers in a bureaucracy are expected to establish rules and regulations for employees, and these employees are expected to follow these rules and regulations and get the job done. Employees are not empowered to change procedures, and they certainly are not expected to make any recommendations for improving performance. The bureaucratic organization is usually incapable of recognizing environmental change because everyone is too involved in following the rules, even when these rules are outdated. In such an organization the change process only happens when it is forced by outside competition. Unfortunately, this is where health care organizations have resided for many years.

Change is never easy, but it is particularly difficult in bureaucratic organizations that have always been insulated from environmental forces of change. These organizations block the change process through a power structure designed to keep things the same. They fear change because it threatens their base of power. This causes health care managers to fear change, even when they realize that change in health care is of great importance and may not be negative in the long run. It is ironic that nearly everyone in health care delivery in our country is aware of the need for change except for those who control the power. Fortunately, this attitude is breaking down as managers of large health care organizations are gradually allowing a shift to a more decentralized way of delivering care.

Health care involves a large number of services that are evaluated by consumers as they are produced. The vast majority of health care consumers have indicated in recent years that they are not very happy with the services they are receiving. This means that health care organizations must change how they have been doing business. According to Champy and Greenspun

(2010), reengineering health care will require a rethinking and a radical redesign of the process used to deliver these services to consumers. Such a reengineering effort requires managers to seek input from consumers about what changes are necessary and from employees about how best to make these changes. It seems like a complicated process, but it becomes much easier if managers begin to listen to those around them. Because the process of health care delivery has always been bureaucratic, any change that caters to consumer demands will be a vast improvement.

Changes in the health care system will require empowered and motivated employees who are capable of delivering superior services on a daily basis. Lombardi and Schermerhorn (2007) argue that health care managers, by designing change strategies in health care delivery, are able to respond effectively to the evolving health care environment. Managers should empower their staff to exploit the environmental changes to improve their organization and become more competitive. In other words, change does not necessarily have to be negative; it may very well be an opportunity to gain a significant competitive advantage in delivering health care the right way at the right cost.

Health care managers must accept the need for positive change, which would entail better serving patients, not only as a method of improving health care delivery but also as a progressive force within the health care organization (Lombardi, 2001). In the past health care managers were empowered to resist change because organizations feared the potential impact of that change on their long-term profits. That attitude by top health care managers has certainly shifted, however. Now there is a strong mandate both to respond to change and to view it as a positive force for achieving organizational success.

According to Hamel (2007), over the last ten years every business on the planet has been spending most of its precious time attempting to reinvent the process of developing and selling products and services. Businesses have also paid a great deal of attention to their management practices. Health care organizations, too, need to reinvent the process of developing and selling services, and they must similarly cultivate new management techniques.

Hamel (2007) argues that to better understand a business problem you must tackle it at its roots. At the roots of the many problems found in how we deliver health services there is inefficiency in the use of scarce health care resources and poor quality in the health care delivery process. Inefficient delivery of health services is the primary reason for the continuous cost escalation that health care facilities are experiencing. This can only change if the employees delivering the services work as a team to stop wasting resources. The health care manager must play a central role in this effort by helping his or her team design a new work process. This is going to require health care managers to become empowered, to learn how to motivate and empower their staff, and to spend a great deal of time figuring out how to improve the quality of services through innovation. The manager's employees, once empowered, need to buy into the change process and become motivated to make it work. The same employees need to become creative and innovative in developing a new work process that not only eliminates the inefficiency in health care delivery but also improves the quality of services delivered and the outcomes achieved. Once these changes become a reality, they need to be embedded in the new culture of the health care facility.

THE CHANGE PROCESS IN HEALTH CARE DELIVERY

There is no question that health care organizations must not only allow the change process to occur but also seek out change to exploit it before the opportunity is seized by their competition. This continuous change process is going to involve all of the providers of health services as they move from a protected environment into the new world of health care delivery, and it is going to require tremendous leadership. The change leader, to be effective, must actively participate as a learner in the change process (Fullan, 2011). Those who are responsible for making positive change happen must learn to do what matters most. In other words, the starting point for change must be discussions with the customers and employees about what is wrong in the current state of the health care delivery process at the organization.

It takes deliberate practice to discover what really works and what improvements are needed to make positive change happen on a daily basis (Fullan, 2011). Health care managers must start the change process by understanding the necessary change and then helping their employees achieve the goals required for positive change to occur. Employees are watching their managers to see if they are actually involved in improving the services delivered in their respective departments.

Figure 5.1 shows the seven elements that need to be part of the change process, throughout which the change leader must remain resolute, staying the course in the improvement of health care delivery. The outer foundation of the change process should include deliberate practice and sustained "simplexity," which is defined as a complementary relationship between complex and simple. This outer core allows one to double-check or evaluate the success or failure of one's goals. The inner core includes the managerial skills of motivation, collaboration, and learning. This model offers an excellent strategy for health care facilities not only to deal with required change but also to allow employees to actively search out change for exploitation.

Lombardi and Schermerhorn (2007) argue that health care managers have to be alert to the need for change and prepared to assume a leadership role in the change process. This requires the manager to be open to new ideas about how health services should be delivered and to have the requisite skills to support the implementation of new ideas in actual practice. This

---

Figure 5.1   Elements of the Change Process
Source: Fullan, 2011, p. 24. Reprinted with permission of John Wiley & Sons, Inc.

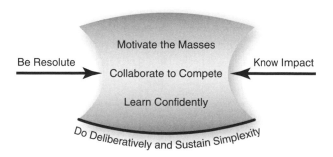

obviously would represent a new way of doing business for the vast majority of health care organizations in our country. Health care management has always involved power that originated in the organization—legitimate power, coercive power, and reward power. Upholding this type of power structure does not entail asking employees how to better respond to change, and it does not involve asking patients what they want and delivering it to them. The attitude has been, "This is the way it is, and we are not going to change." The new world of health care delivery makes this bureaucratic outlook obsolete. Figure 5.2 offers a contrast between change leadership, which implies looking for change to exploit on a daily basis, and status quo management. This figure clearly demonstrates the problems inherent in status quo management and the tremendous opportunities that come from practicing change leadership.

Figure 5.2 shows that we are looking for creativity and innovation from more employees and also from their managers. In fact, thanks to the rapidity of change, if we are not actually creating value and producing new and better products and services, we are not going to be around very long. Status quo managers are threatened by change and spend way too much time waiting for things to happen, and then reacting to the changes instituted by the competition. In fact, if status quo managers would spend as much time preparing for change as they do resisting it, they could eliminate many of

Figure 5.2   Change Leadership Versus Status Quo Management
Source: Lombardi & Schermerhorn, 2007, p. 310. Reprinted with permission of John Wiley & Sons, Inc.

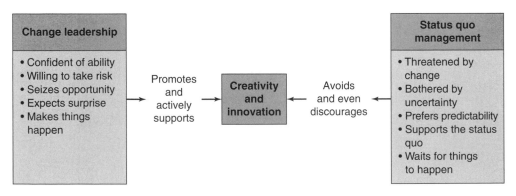

their future problems. It makes a great deal of sense when you know change is coming to become proactive rather than reactive. If you're not prepared with both good management and empowered employees dedicated to the delivery of quality health services to all of your customers, your future is not very bright. By contrast, change leaders seize opportunities because they are proactive in their approach and will be able to take advantage of the many chances for advancement that are usually present when rapid change occurs. Health care organizations have to decide which type of management is necessary in today's very turbulent health care environment. It must be understood that if your organization has decided to focus on change leadership, your managers and employees have to receive serious training on how to deal with change and how to lead the organization through the temporary crisis situation that usually develops when change becomes the norm. The health care manager must also realize that employees and customers can actually help make the change process easier and improve the likelihood that the change will be positive.

The health care manager has to become the facilitator of the change process. Organizations must adapt and adjust to change that comes forth from the external environment (Bennis, 2009). To be successful in these tasks the health care manager must involve and listen to his or her employees. By including all of the employees in the change process, the manager can enable positive change to actually become absorbed into the organization's culture.

The change process in a health care organization requires the health care manager to focus on the most important components of that process. Following the insights from Figure 5.1 is critical for the health care manager in determining how to make understanding change one of the most important managerial responsibilities (Fullan, 2011). As you can see from this illustration, the critical components of managing successful change are learning, motivation, and collaboration. This is why health care managers require a solid grounding in how to motivate health care employees to be proactive when it comes to thriving in a changing external environment. It is also extremely important that it become part of the culture of the health care facility for employees to seek change opportunities.

THE SECRET OF MOTIVATING HEALTH CARE EMPLOYEES

One of the most important skills that must be present in any manager and especially in any health care manager is the ability to motivate his or her employees to offer quality services. This has not been the case in health care because, for the most part, health care consumers have been passive in their demand for quality when entering a health care facility. The consumer has been very happy just to receive the services, and because these were paid for by his or her insurance company the consumer did not think it was appropriate to complain. Today's better-informed consumer, who is also in most cases paying for a portion of health care costs, is now making the same demands in health care that he or she makes when purchasing any other product or service.

To respond to changing consumer demands, those who deliver health services need to become motivated to deliver excellence on a daily basis. It has become the responsibility of the manager to learn how to motivate followers to improve the quality of the services delivered and to achieve any new goals set forth by the administration. For many health care managers motivation is itself a brand-new concept for which they are not properly prepared. This must change if the organization is not only to improve its competitive position but also in some cases to remain in business.

According to Pink (2009), **motivation** is the energizing force that leads us to pursue and ultimately attempt to achieve our personal goals and the goals of our employers. Psychologists and management theorists have put forth numerous theories over the years about what motivates people. The theories of motivation that are discussed in management courses usually involve employee needs, along with intrinsic and extrinsic motivators. It is interesting to note that much of what was believed about what motivates most individuals has been rapidly shifting in recent years due to more intense research and the ever-changing needs of individuals. It is necessary for health care managers to know what motivates their staff if they are to obtain their help in dealing with the turbulent health care environment. These managers are finally realizing just how important motivated staff members are in reducing costs and improving the quality of care as experienced by health care consumers.

One of the major responsibilities of a manager is to motivate workers to achieve organizational goals. Rewards and punishments have always been thought to be very effective motivators for use by managers. Pink (2009) argues, however, that intrinsic motivators become increasingly important as basic needs are met. The starting point for motivation in any organization involves negotiation among employees and managers to decide what each side wants from the process of work. Many of the successful health care organizations have also spent a great deal of time asking customers what they desire from their health care experience. It is so very important to ask this question because more and more health care customers are deciding what they want and who will deliver their health services. Once the customer has decided what he or she wants, it is then up to the operating worker to go about the process of delivering a quality health care experience to that consumer. This means that the quality of health care delivery is actually determined by the customer and the operating worker. It seems that this understanding of quality in health care delivery changes all of the rules that were previously in place in bureaucratic, power-driven health care facilities.

According to Lombardi and Schermerhorn (2007), health care employees and customers need to be placed at the very top of the organizational chart. This is certainly a profound change in how the health care manager must conceive of delivering health services. In effect, everyone working in health care delivery must become a **value-adding worker.** The worker who adds value is an individual who is actually doing something that the customer considers to be valuable. The starting point will always be the determination of what adds value to the consumer's purchasing process. The best way to find the answer to this question is to be very close to the consumers of health services, constantly quizzing them on how their purchasing process can be improved. It seems that in the delivery of health services the most important players are not the health care employees or the managers but rather the consumers who purchase health services and the employees who deliver this care, indicating that the old organizational chart—the business pyramid—should be turned upside down, as shown in Figure 5.3.

Figure 5.3   "Upside-Down Pyramid" View of Today's Organizations
Source: Lombardi & Schermerhorn, 2007, p. 11. Reprinted with permission of John Wiley & Sons, Inc.

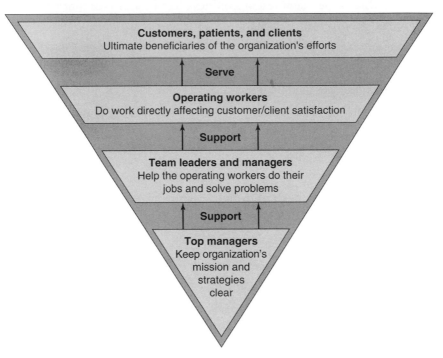

It is evident that health care organizations have to develop a better definition of value for both their employees and their customers, and managers must continually ask questions of members of both groups. Questioning is one of the most important tools to be used by health care managers and their empowered employees. We will discover later in this chapter that questioning is also a mandatory skill for those who are innovating to meet the competition in health care delivery today.

The upside-down pyramid shown in Figure 5.3 makes it very clear that employee skills in delivering health services are critical, teamwork is mandatory, and managers are responsible for guiding the team to deliver quality. This figure supports the notion that today's successful health care managers really have to become coaches, helping and supporting all of their employees to become value-adding workers. Health care managers and their staff have to recognize the beauty of the team approach to delivering health care. As we will discuss later in this chapter, the health care manager also needs to recognize that both customers and employees are critical in the innovation process. Figure 5.3 places top managers at the bottom of the pyramid only to emphasize that their direction needs to come from the customers, who should be dictating what they want to the employees empowered to serve them. This is the only way to remain in business—and prosper—in health care today. Empowered employees who are already close to the customer have a much better opportunity to determine exactly what the health care consumer desires from the health care facility.

To begin motivating those who work in health care delivery, managers should gain a better understanding of the concept of motivation. Unless employees and managers have a degree in business administration, the chances are quite good that they have never really explored any of the theories of human motivation that have evolved over the years. There has been a change in thinking among many researchers concerning the value of money and promotions as motivators over the long term. Recent research has uncovered a very strong link between intrinsic motivation and the long-term motivation of individuals in their place of work. Let us start from the beginning with the development of motivational theory.

As discussed in Chapter Two, the Hawthorne studies that were completed at a Western Electric Company plant in Illinois in 1924 marked the beginning of our interest in motivating employees in the workplace. These studies involved experimentation with various changes in the workplace designed to improve the productivity of a select groups of employees. The study involved such factors as better illumination in the work space and wage incentives to motivate employees toward increased productivity. The experiment uncovered the value of nonmonetary work factors that were capable of improving motivation of workers along with their productivity.

In the 1950s Frederick Herzberg, a management professor, proposed that there are two major groups of factors that motivate individuals in the workplace. The first group is made up of "hygiene factors," such as pay, job security, and working conditions. The second group is made up of motivators that include personal growth, the purpose of the job itself, and a feeling of achievement from work. This theory helped managers understand that satisfaction and dissatisfaction at work arise for various reasons.

Edwin Locke developed the theory that organizational goals can be great motivators if they are well established and properly managed (Locke & Latham, 1984). Presenting goals affords health care managers an opportunity to give direction to employees as well as to empower them to practice behavioral self-management. This theory provides an excellent framework for achieving the goals of eliminating medical errors, improving efficiency, and providing health services of increased quality. For this theory to be properly tested in an organization, managers and the various lower-level team leaders must work together in establishing and managing goals.

The management theorists just outlined were attempting to discover what incentives are necessary to motivate workers to produce more and better products or services. After years of study, psychologists and management theorists seem to be in agreement that motivators can be extrinsic and intrinsic. **Extrinsic** motivation usually comes from outside of the individual and involves such things as salary or benefits. **Intrinsic motivation** usually involves factors that improve an individual's self-concept. This powerful type of motivation comes from within an individual.

Pink (2009) argues that a great deal of what we thought we knew about motivation has been proven not to be completely true. As the standard of living rose in our country, such basic needs as money and security became less important. There's no question that pay and benefits are still very important motivators and are among the primary reasons individuals go to work every day, and there is certainly a minimum level of pay and benefits each employee desires. It seems that after that level has been reached, however, the ability of these lower-level benefits to motivate diminishes rapidly. The real problem lies in that most organizations are still attempting to increase employee motivation using such out-of-date strategies as short-term incentive plans and pay-for-performance schemes that only motivate individuals for a short period of time. According to Pink, much of the current research on motivation has confirmed that human beings are really "intrinsically motivated purpose maximizers and not only extrinsically motivated profit maximizers" (p. 31). This is so very true when dealing with those who primarily deliver services rather than products. I believe that the vast majority of health care professionals, although relying on their work to pay their bills, are also intrinsically motivated to deliver quality services to their patients. According to Pink, a great deal of the recent research concerning motivation has actually uncovered negative results from applying too much extrinsic motivation to certain types of employees, and it seems that intrinsic rewards have become the real source of long-term motivation for many. The companies that have realized this have begun to grant their employees the autonomy to design and develop their own work process, which seems to motivate them to perform at a very high level.

Pink (2009) spends a great deal of time discussing the differences between Type X behavior and Type I behavior. Type X individuals find less satisfaction with the work itself and more with the external rewards to which work activities lead, such as pay and promotions. Pink argues that the major problem with Type X behavior is that it is difficult to sustain. To understand the problems inherent in Type X behavior, we need to pay more attention to the results of new research, which has found that in the long run Type I individuals always outperform Type X employees.

According to Pink (2009), research into individuals demonstrating Type I behavior has shown that they are more motivated by freedom, challenge, and the purpose of the work itself. These individuals have a strong internal desire to control their lives, learn more about their world, and accomplish something that endures. It is interesting to note that these are many of the same qualities found in entrepreneurs. Successful entrepreneurs create wealth for themselves and their community. It is too bad that many health care managers cannot unleash the same entrepreneurial qualities in their staff. Research has further demonstrated that these individuals have higher self-esteem, better interpersonal relationships, and greater overall well-being. These are all qualities that are necessary for employees who deliver health services. As already argued, the responsibility for motivating employees rests with the manager, who must continually question employees about what they want from their current position. By empowering most employees, successful businesses have found that these individuals continue to grow and develop, allowing the services they deliver to continue to improve in quality, with resultant customer satisfaction.

Pink (2009) also points out two assumptions about managing people that are no longer true, especially in the delivery of services. The first is that health care managers, to move forward, need to either reward or punish their employees. The second is that once employees get moving they require direction or they will be unable to complete their task. Pink argues that managers must eliminate the desire to control people and instead try to create a sense of autonomy among their staff, which can become the catalyst for solving many of our health care problems. For example, a work group or team might be allowed the autonomy to make all of the decisions involved in the delivery of a particular service, with the goal of pleasing the consumer.

THE NEED FOR INNOVATION IN HEALTH CARE

Innovation refers to the creation of better or improved products or services. It is important to point out that innovation is not the same as invention, because innovators are usually not creating something new that never existed before. The starting point for innovation is a creative idea that is acted on by an innovator (Gallo, 2011). The process of innovation can result from creativity from anyone in the organization. Innovation does not just happen; it results from a continuous effort on everyone's part to make new things happen that improve the way a process is completed. This is probably what makes innovation in the delivery of services so difficult. Such creativity requires real effort, and innovation is not something that you do once and then stop. Creativity has to become part of the normal way of doing business if an organization is to remain innovative—and competitive—in delivering services over time. Innovation was never an area of particular concern for bureaucratic health care organizations. Most health care facilities and many health care practitioners occupied a monopolistic position, meaning that competition was actually the least of their worries. But this has changed, making innovation of great importance in health care delivery.

Health care organizations, to compete effectively in the turbulent health care environment, must embrace the process of innovation, but first they need to understand how it works. Innovating has become standard practice for successful businesses that operate in the delivery of products or services throughout the world. Unfortunately, this is not the case for health care facilities, which deliver services as they are needed by the customer. This is not to say that creativity and the resulting innovation are not possible in the delivery of health services. The problem has been that this process is typically blocked by rules and regulations enforced within bureaucratic organizations. However, health care reform and competition among health care facilities have moved these firms from a bureaucratic organizational structure to a more decentralized one, making the ability to innovate a sought-after skill.

Many physicians and hospitals are frozen in the old bureaucratic model, whereby change and innovation in the delivery of health services are blocked. The health care manager needs to learn how to foster creativity and innovation in the workplace, making these the norm for all employees in the creation of value for the health care consumer. Innovation has become a necessity for survival in the modern world of business, including in health care organizations in which managers must develop and support the skills associated with innovation as they go about the process of improving health care delivery.

Many companies, such as Apple, Facebook, Google, and Nordstrom, have been very successful in allowing their employees to be creative and innovative in seeking to please consumers. Similar creativity and innovation are being practiced by many health care facilities as consumers become more active in demanding health services. This capability should also be critical for those who truly believe in health care facilities' enormous potential to improve the quality of health services while reducing their cost. This is going to require health care managers to make bold moves that bring tremendous change in how services are delivered. The secret to success for most health care managers who are trying to make change happen seems to revolve around their passion not only to dream but also to spend the vast majority of their waking hours making their dreams come true. The health care manager has to work very hard to motivate employees to buy into the vision and become highly creative in their approach to meeting the large number of consumer demands they face on a daily basis.

Health care workers usually love what they do, or they would have abandoned the health care field many years earlier. The compensation is only moderate, promotions are rare, and frustration is a daily experience. Those who choose this career area do so because they are passionate about trying to improve the health of the population. The problem is not in the passion of the health care employee but quite often in managers' inability to motivate lower-level staff to continually improve the performance of the health care facility.

A combination of passion and aptitude seems necessary for health care organizations to begin improving health outcomes while reducing the cost of health care delivery (Gallo, 2011). Dedicated health care employees must be empowered to use their creativity to find innovative solutions to the complex problems in health care, especially the current epidemic of medical errors. The health care manager needs to build a culture among his or her followers that is dedicated to the vision of quality improvement.

The health care manager needs to spend a great deal of his or her time building on the existing culture within the organization to foster the expansion of creativity and innovation among all employees. This will involve using well-developed communication skills to help all employees to understand their very important role in discovering what value means for their customers and then finding creative ways to deliver it to them. This dedication to customers will not happen in a bureaucratic structure that is held together by rules and regulations. It will only happen when the climate is right for lower-level employees who deal directly with customers to feel empowered as they attempt to create meaningful value for these customers.

Innovation and creativity are required to deal with the challenges we currently face, including escalating costs in health care delivery and widespread poor service quality. A recent statement made by Gary Hamel (2007) rings true for our health care industry: if consumer ignorance is a profit center for you, you're in trouble. Unfortunately for the health care providers, consumers are no longer a passive recipient of health services. Consumers are now paying a greater share of health care costs, and they have become aware of the increasing number of medical errors in many health care facilities. Thanks to technology, consumers are now able to find out a great deal about a product or service before they purchase it. These new active consumers can represent an opportunity for those health care organizations that are attempting to improve value in their delivery of very important health services.

Clayton Christensen, author of *The Innovator's Prescription: A Disruptive Solution for Health Care,* has studied innovation and management for decades. **Disruptive innovation** addresses the question of how complicated and costly products or services can be made simpler at a lower cost for consumers (Hwang & Christensen, 2008). They believe that this concept can be very helpful in improving the quality and reducing the cost of most health services. The three key elements of this type of innovation include a technology enabler, a business model innovation, and the development of a value network.

In regard to the first element of disruptive innovation, technology as an enabler is central to innovation in the field of health care already, but it has not resulted in significant quality improvement and cost reduction in health care delivery. Electronic medical records and telemedicine, for example, provide evidence of technology's role in extending access and potentially containing costs. Adapting other forms of technology for use in the health care system seems plausible and necessary.

The second element of disruptive innovation relates to the business model of the health care organization of the future. The new emphasis on outcomes and on reducing medical errors will call for new ways of thinking in regard to how physicians are paid. The current fee-for-service model rewards the wrong behaviors, both from the health care provider and the consumer. The new business model will require payment for outcomes, which should force providers to adopt a more innovative approach to delivering health services. This new model will pay providers based on the improvement of the health of the individual and of the population served by a given health plan. Although the argument for prevention has been in the health care conversation for a long time, the money has yet to follow.

Because prevention will ultimately improve health outcomes, the new system of health care delivery will provide incentives for prevention efforts by physicians and health care facilities.

Hwang and Christensen (2008) argue that a business model for health care can be divided into these categories: solution shops, value-adding process businesses, and facilitated user networks. These authors define solution shops as units constructed to solve unstructured problems. The value-adding process businesses turn inputs in the production process into outputs that have a value greater than the cost of the inputs. The facilitated user networks also deliver value through effective operation of the network and its user transactions. As you can clearly see, this business model has a very strong emphasis on solving problems and adding value to the process of producing health services.

Christensen, Grossman, and Hwang (2009) point out that the third element of disruptive innovation, developing a value network (the context within which each firm establishes its business model) that is sustainable, is likely to require buy-in from all employees in the health care organization. The health care facility that is attempting to improve the quality of its services while also attempting to reduce the cost of those services must involve employees throughout the entire planning process.

Unleashing these transformational forces has worked well in lowering the cost and increasing the availability of a product or service in the business world (Christensen, Grossman, & Hwang, 2009). In health care, managers and empowered workers, as well as resources, are needed to respond to the opportunities presented by disruptive innovation. All health care managers and employees must support the concept of innovation.

Disruptive innovation allows resources in the production process to be combined in new and innovative ways, which usually means that greater value is produced by the process. This is exactly what is required for our health care system to survive and deliver better-quality services at a lower cost.

Innovation involves the change process and usually results in improved products or services, quite often at a reduced cost for the consumer. This is exactly what is required in our health care industry—better services as defined by the consumer at a lower price. Dyer, Gregersen, and Christensen (2011) argue that successful innovators exhibit the following skills: associating, questioning, observing, networking, and experimenting. In their new book *The Innovator's DNA: Mastering the Five Skills of Disruptive Innovation*, they argue that these skills can be learned, and that businesses that employ individuals who have acquired these skills can make much-needed innovation a standard practice. These five skills are precisely what must be added to the health care manager's recipe for successful innovation in the delivery of health services. The most important of these five skills for use in health care are associating, questioning, and observing how services are delivered to consumers.

There is no question that true innovators think differently than other workers. They do not see the world in the same way that most other people see it. They are able to associate things that are not usually thought to belong together. The process of associating usually involves connecting relevant information from different areas or knowledge bases to produce diverse ideas. This skill will be very useful in bringing together different disciplines to develop new ways of solving current health care problems.

Questioning is probably the most important skill necessary for innovation in health care. By this I mean that health care managers and their employees should constantly question every aspect of the health care delivery process. Such questioning is meant to determine how best to serve the customer as well as to illuminate many of the processes found in health care that do not add value to either the overall production process or the ultimate delivery of services. The questions should be aimed at the various professionals working on a health care team; questioning should also be used to discern the perceived value of each service by the customer. According to Dyer et al. (2011), asking lots of questions allows health care team members to move into disruptive territory as they explore the areas that might lead to the improvement of our health care system.

Innovators usually have a strong, well-developed ability to observe. They can develop this skill to the point where they not only know what works but also have become very aware of what does not work. This is an area in which the health care manager can learn a great deal from the floor nurses who have direct patient contact on a daily basis. Because they actually deliver direct patient care, they will have observed areas for potential innovation in health care delivery to patients. Also, because they have usually gained the trust of their patients, they can help the manager get questions answered concerning what would improve the quality of care and patients' overall health care experience.

Conway and Steward (2009) argue that the organizational climate for innovation requires goal clarity, open discussions between managers and employees, and supervisory support for new ideas that come forth from the team. In recent years such support has become the key to a sustained competitive advantage for an organization. This makes the development of relationships critical in managing health care professionals. If these employees leave the organization, they are able to take their knowledge and creativity with them.

THE EFFECTS OF CULTURE DEVELOPMENT ON MOTIVATION, INNOVATION, AND THE FACILITATION OF CHANGE

The culture of the health care organization is a significant factor to consider when attempting to establish motivation, innovation, and acceptance of change as organizational norms. The exploitation of change through disruptive innovation has to become the norm for successful health care organizations. The health care manager has to learn how to weave change exploitation, intrinsic motivation, and disruptive innovation into the thick culture of the health care facility. It is the organization's culture that will continue to motivate all health care workers to seek out change for exploitation through their creativity and innovation.

According to Cameron and Quinn (2011), a large volume of recent research has shown that one of the major reasons for failure by managers in responding to a changing environment is neglect of the organization's culture. This points out the great value of understanding the culture before embarking on the delicate task of reengineering the work process. Cameron and Quinn also argue that culture can have an enormous effect on the overall performance, both short-term and long-term, of any organization. It can also have an effect on the individual members of the workforce. In many ways correct culture diagnosis, along with facilitating cultural change, is among the most important functions of health care managers as they attempt to respond to environmental change while encouraging innovation from their employees.

Many managers erroneously believe themselves to be responsible for building the culture of the organization. In reality, the culture has already been developed, nurtured, and thickened by the workers. In fact, this culture may have been developed as a reaction to poor management and poor employee relations. Workers have their own way of accomplishing organizational goals, and this worker unity becomes the culture that determines how things are done in the workplace. The best the manager can do is to try to work with the existing culture to accomplish goals. Although the culture already exists, however, it can be developed to encourage motivation, innovation, and change through management's efforts to facilitate such a shift. This is particularly true of those working in health care delivery. These employees enjoy a unique bond, nothing less than a sense of family unity, that draws them to work in health care and convinces them that this is where they want to spend their career. The manager has the responsibility of helping the culture continue to grow by providing employees with the requisite skills, tools, and trust that are needed to continually improve.

Innovators not only think differently but also usually arise from a work environment that is much different from that of those who do not innovate. True innovators will never last long in a bureaucratic organization because it is too structured and does not allow them to think in unique ways. Innovators need to work in an organization without a rigid structure that allows them time to be creative and to make novel associations as they develop new and exciting products and services. Innovation will only happen in organizations that go out of their way to create and sustain a culture that supports diverse thinking among all members.

There are two additional areas that must be addressed in this discussion of health care managers' attempt to integrate change, motivation, and innovation into the thick, positive culture of their organization. These areas include the quality of health services, which has become an overriding issue for the consumers of care, and the value of health care managers' creating touch points, which offer managers a new way of thinking about their new responsibilities. Establishing touch points, according to Conant and Norgaard (2011), involves nothing more than two or more individuals' getting together to deal with an issue with their employees.

In regard to the first area, according to Michelli (2011), "Value can be calculated by combining the perceived quality of the products or services with the perceived quality of the consumer's experience and then subtracting the price charged for those goods and services" (p. 127). This formula works very well for most businesses but runs into difficulty when applied to health services. The major problem with measuring the quality of health services is that the consumer actually pays a very small portion of health care costs. The attitude that consumers of health services are passive because they only pay a small portion of the cost of their care is very rapidly changing, however, as consumers have begun to realize just how much they are spending for health care in terms of nonmonetary costs. Such nonmonetary costs as having to wait for an appointment or having to wait to receive services do reduce consumers' perception of quality in relation to the cost of receiving health care. Other major quality and cost issues for consumers of health services are unnecessary medical care and medical errors.

The Institute of Medicine (2003) gave health care a very workable definition of quality by stating that it is manifested in products and services that are safe, effective, patient centered, timely, efficient, and equitable. To achieve all of these variables the health care facility must count on motivated followers who have become obsessed with providing quality care to their patients. What is more, the health care facility must spend a great deal of time talking to its patients and training employees to deliver quality services to every patient every time. This can be accomplished through better teamwork that includes communication among all team members and the patient who is receiving the care.

Medical errors and hospital-acquired infections cannot be tolerated. But as you can see from the definition, quality services also must be delivered in a timely fashion and at a reasonable cost, and they must be designed to achieve predetermined outcomes. Therefore, paying providers to produce activities rather than quality outcomes is a counterproductive way to do business, and will almost certainly increase medical errors and infections for the patient.

In regard to the second area, Conant and Norgaard (2011) argue that touch points represent crucial opportunities for managers to influence the course of events scheduled in their overall agenda. These touch points occur when two or more people work together to solve a problem or attempt to get something accomplished. Health care managers can use touch points to transform an encounter with staff into a moment to improve their performance. Touch points have three variables: the issue, the other people, and the leader. For example, the issue could be the reduction of medical errors and infections to zero. The other people would include anyone involved in direct patient care, and they would have to understand and be willing to support the new zero-tolerance policy for errors and infections. The leader in this instance would be the health care manager responsible for implementing the new policy.

According to Conant and Norgaard (2011), the manager responsible for implementing change needs "to be both tough-minded on the issue and tender-hearted with people" (p. 19). In the example just given, the health care manager needs to make all staff understand that both the health care organization and the patient are deeply concerned about the problem of medical errors and infections and will not tolerate anything less than full compliance from everyone. At the same time the manager must help his or her staff gain appropriate skills so they all can meet their new goals. The manager must actually work harder than his or her staff to make this new policy part of the culture. Culture is critically important to the innovation process and relies on human relationships to make things happen (Holstein, 2011).

According to Chesbrough (2011), a critical component in accelerating or inhibiting innovation is information technology. Information technology is fast becoming one of the most important factors in improving health levels for the entire population. All health care organizations need to do to exploit this technology use in health care delivery is to understand how and when consumers use this technology for future innovation. Chesbrough also points out that customers, when touch points have been established, will be only too happy to offer an opinion concerning the use of technology in their care process. This is where most health care facilities have had great difficulty because so many consumers are disappointed by the poor quality of the services they receive. What is needed is a culture of candor and transparency.

According to Bennis, Goleman, and O'Toole (2008), to create a culture of candor the organization must become transparent, allowing a free flow of information among all organizational stakeholders. If information flows freely, the organization can better solve its problems, surpass the competition, and innovate to better meet short- and long-term goals. For this transparency to be perceived as genuine, employees must believe that they are allowed to share good and bad news with upper management. In other words, the element of trust must be present among the organization's managers, employees, and customers.

Trust is the most fundamental component of employee engagement (Marciano, 2010). Relationships with people require respect and trust or they will not work. This is especially true for relationships between managers and their staff. Strong relationships between managers and employees usually lead to greater creativity and initiative, which in turn lead to innovation and risk taking by employees. This will ultimately contribute to a thick, positive culture in the workplace. The end result of the exploitation of change through innovation by motivated employees can be the reduction of the costs associated with the delivery of health services, as well as an improvement of these services' quality.

SUMMARY

The health care manager must confront constant change and prepare employees not just to deal with change but also to be proactive in exploiting it as many opportunities become available in our turbulent health care industry. The process of implementing change is difficult for everyone in an organization, especially the employees. Health care managers have to gain a sound understanding of the change process and learn how to assuage the almost certain resistance to change.

Creativity and innovation are needed if health care organizations are to be proactive rather than reactive in the face of health care reform. Reform efforts will also require empowered and motivated employees to deal with change and the conflict that will develop among departments and even teams in the health care workplace. To better assist employees with change, the health care manager has to understand how to keep employee motivation high, which will help employees deal with change and still keep improving the quality of health services.

Gaining a better understanding of what motivates employees will help the health care manager constantly improve performance. Recent research has placed a great deal of value on intrinsic motivation, which comes from within each employee, making it very important for managers to understand the desires of those they supervise. It seems that intrinsic rewards have become the long-term source of motivation for a group of employees that grows ever larger, which means that health care managers must work even harder at discovering what makes health care employees want to come to work. Time and again it seems that the more that you empower your employees and earn their trust, the more likely it is that their motivation will increase.

Health care patients have turned into consumers of health services because they are now paying for a portion of the health care bill. These consumers have also become better informed about their health care and are now demanding to participate in their medical decisions. The health care manager must understand this new world of health care delivery and prepare his or her staff to better deal with a more knowledgeable and demanding health care consumer. The health care manager must also help employees become value-adding workers in the process of health care delivery. All of these changes require a knowledgeable manager, empowered workers, and a real desire to better serve patients.

KEY TERMS

change

disruptive innovation

extrinsic motivation

innovation

intrinsic motivation

motivation

value-adding worker

REVIEW QUESTIONS

1. Name and explain the various reasons why health care organizations are experiencing mammoth change.

2. How should the health care manager best prepare his or her employees for the necessary change process?

3. Please explain fully the process of innovation in the delivery of health services.

4. What role does a motivated employee play in the improvement of our current system of health care delivery? Please explain.

6

Communication
Can You Hear Me Now?

Bernard J. Healey

LEARNING OBJECTIVES

- Understand the major problems found in the communication process in the workplace
- Recognize the need for better communication skills among health care managers
- Become aware of the value of open communication when encouraging new ideas from all members of the organization
- Be able to explain the process of communication

The delivery of health services in the United States has become extremely disorganized. This disorganization has affected the trust of patients, resulted in increased medical errors, reduced the morale and productivity of health care employees, and increased costs while ultimately reducing positive health outcomes. One of the themes running throughout these problem areas is poor communication between those providing health care and the recipients of that care. There is also poor communication among members of the organization attempting to deliver quality health services to their customers.

The health care system in our country delivers almost $3 trillion worth of services to customers on an annual basis. These services are delivered by dedicated employees who, for the most part, have chosen their profession because of a desire to help individuals who have become ill. Most of these employees are not happy with the disorganization in many health care facilities. They realize that industry reform is never easy, and they want to be part of the change process so that they can better serve their patients. Health care managers can play a pivotal role by leading this change process.

To be competitive in today's turbulent health care environment you must keep everyone inside and outside your organization informed. According to Tracy (2010), 95 percent of the problems affecting an organization are a direct result of having a poor communication system, or no communication system at all. Communication with members of the organization, therefore, becomes one of the most important functions of the health care manager. Communication skills can be learned and improved through practice, but first the administration of the health care facility must fully appreciate how valuable a well-developed communication system is to that facility's future success. Those who provide health services require constant communication from those in charge of the health care organization to improve the productivity and quality of the delivery of those services.

Accordingly to Lee and Mongan (2009), the provision of health services can become organized through formal groups of providers, such as physician groups, which can take responsibility for problems that individual providers cannot. These organized groups are also capable of developing and implementing a sophisticated communication system that places the health of the patient as the number one priority. Communication seems to be the missing ingredient required to make health care reform work. Fortunately, new technology is available to improve the communication network in our health care industry, but it will take time and effort. Tracy (2010) argues that health care managers need to understand that for employees to do their work well and make good decisions about how best to deliver services to their patients, they need to be informed about what is expected from them.

The process of communication, if properly undertaken, can facilitate the sharing of information and can provide meaning to the members of an organization. It has become evident from the available research that you cannot be successful as a manager unless you learn how to communicate with others (Lombardi & Schermerhorn, 2007). There is a positive relationship between the effectiveness of a manager and his or her ability to communicate. This ability to communicate has become a crucial part of overseeing the provision of health services, which are delivered by professionals to consumers who are measuring the quality of those services. Quality services cannot be delivered to their recipients unless communication systems in health care organizations are improved.

In the case of health care management, communication involves employees and customers. According to Champy and Greenspun (2010), the vast majority of research on health care management has concluded that one of the most important functions of a manager is communicating to lower-level employees, but the manager must also be able to communicate with customers. The problem is that in most bureaucratic organizations communication begins at the top and filters down the organizational chart to subordinates who usually do not have the ability to communicate to members of the upper-level hierarchy. This style of management works very well in demonstrating power, but it does very little to bring forth new and creative ideas from all employees. Champy and Greenspun point out that in times of rapid change **open communication** is a prerequisite for success.

The most successful companies in America today have one thing in common: rapid communication from the top down and from the bottom up that results in many new and successful innovations. These companies have recognized the value of communication for their future success and for the achievement of their vision. These companies have learned how to listen, and they position themselves such that they are able to hear their employees. This is so very important when an organization is going through rapid change, and all employees need to be on the same page every day to make communication meaningful. Honest and open communication can be the difference between success and failure as an organization responds to the changing health care environment.

There is one fundamental fact concerning the ways in which workers are managed and products or services are sold to consumers: regardless of whether your business is selling computers or providing health services, both your workers and those who buy your products need to be empowered. Thanks to technology and its widespread application, both groups have gained a great deal of power, which needs to be better understood by all health care managers. This is not necessarily a bad thing for managers as long as they can turn this new world of work into an opportunity to increase employee and consumer trust and loyalty, making total control unnecessary. This can only be accomplished through better communication from managers.

Mayo Clinic is an example of an organization that has become extremely successful by keeping the needs of the patient first. Patient needs are at the core of Mayo Clinic's culture. Excellent communication among managers, clinic employees, and their customers is a major part of all decisions made by this premier organization (Berry & Seltman, 2008). The employees make decisions that are always patient focused but also team supported. This team approach to patient care, facilitated by an excellent communication system, always results in superior patient care. Mayo Clinic has decided that clear communication among all stakeholders is necessary to provide excellent patient care.

How we communicate has changed dramatically in recent years. The development and rapid expansion of new methods of communication are resulting in a loss of control by those in power. To many health care managers, losing power is a frightening prospect because it represents tremendous change, but it can also be an opportunity to become innovative in their management style. Li (2010) argues that technology allows us to let go of power and still be in charge, resulting in open leadership. Li goes on to point out that it is all about the development of relationships between managers and followers and managers and customers. These relationships involve trust, which is a by-product of honest communication among all parties.

Demonstrating exceptional communication skills allows a manager to connect with employees. This usually improves relationships, which in turn will improve the manager's ability to influence his or her employees. This connection with employees is crucial in an environment that is rapidly changing. Health care reform in America is forcing every health care organization into such an environment, necessitating faster communication exchanges between managers and employees that are understood and acted on immediately.

COMMUNICATION METHODS AND SKILLS

Communication is a critical component of the management of any organization, but it takes on even greater value in the delivery of health services. As already mentioned, communication is also a major component of building trust between the health care manager and those he or she supervises—and this trust becomes the foundation for the strong, thick, positive culture that is so necessary to deliver quality health services consistently. Unfortunately, the topic of communication has been ignored in many of the health care organizations in our country. This needs to change.

The health care manager has to learn how to improve communication with his or her direct reports and with all of the customers of the health care facility. Figure 6.1 shows the process of **interpersonal communication,** which is essential in the changing health care environment. It is hard to believe that the constant communication process managers undertake on a daily basis involves the many steps depicted in Figure 6.1. It is not surprising that for many managers this process can be very difficult and can cause numerous problems for lower-level employees.

According to Lombardi and Schermerhorn (2007), the process of interpersonal communication involves sending and receiving symbols with messages attached to them. After **encoding** a message to convey a certain meaning, the sender transmits it to a receiver, who then works on **decoding** the message. The process of communication is successful only if the message that is sent and the message that is received are the same. Effective communication between the manager and subordinates has the ability not only to increase trust but also to motivate team members and improve the process of innovation while helping accomplish organizational goals. This is why health care managers have to spend so much time learning how to improve

Figure 6.1   Process of Interpersonal Communication
Source: Lombardi & Schermerhorn, 2007, p. 341. Reprinted with permission of John Wiley & Sons, Inc.

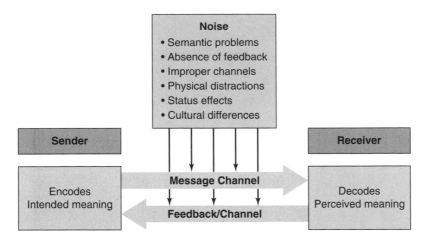

their communication skills for use with the people they manage and all of the customers they serve.

The health care manager, to achieve success with employees and customers, requires a well-developed communication plan for both listening to members of these groups and imparting information to them. This communication process will not work very well in an organization that has a bureaucratic structure because communication usually flows from top to bottom. The bureaucratic structure in many health care organizations is slowly changing to a more organic form, but the changes are not happening fast enough to solve all of the current communication problems in health care. Because the vast majority of health care facilities are still practicing bureaucratic management techniques, there is a very real need to improve the communication process in most health care institutions. It takes very special skills to communicate effectively with all members of the health care team who are attempting to improve performance and beat the competition in the delivery of health services.

What specific types of communication skills are most important for a health care manager today? There are many skills that are required to communicate in today's rapidly changing environment of health care delivery, four of which are listening, evaluating the message being communicated, communicating with passion and enthusiasm, and avoiding overdependence on electronic communication.

Listening

According to Becker and Wortmann (2009), individuals who are excellent communicators can alter the ways in which they communicate to meet the needs of those to whom they are attempting to impart information. This skill takes time to develop and depends on the manager's also spending a great deal of time listening to the individuals in the communication process. It is much easier to do the talking and expect that others will listen to and agree with you. This methodology of not listening to lower-level employees works well in a bureaucratic organization but will fail in the new world of change and rapid communication. This one-way communication can actually be the major reason why an organization loses good employees and valuable customers. The remedy is very simple: health care managers have to learn how to listen.

There is probably no industry in our country that is more dependent on accurate **two-way communication** than the health care industry, in which there is very little room for misunderstanding in any communication involving the delivery of health services. We need to have a well-informed employee delivering the services, and a well-informed consumer receiving these services. This is because employees need to understand the vision of the organization, and the customers need to be able to provide instant feedback to the health care facility on how well the services are being provided.

Health care managers may need to both talk and listen to their employees and customers, but listening does not come easy to individuals who are responsible for the supervision of large numbers of employees in a bureaucratic organization. This lack of two-way communication can then result in the delivery of poor health services.

Both employees and customers are capable of informing managers what is being done right and also what needs to be improved or changed in the delivery of health services. The process of listening gives the health care manager the opportunity to discover what it is the customer wants and how best to deliver services to that customer. Szollose (2011) argues that companies that fail to listen to their employees and their customers are going to find out sooner or later that they are in trouble. What is more, if the customers are ignored they will tell the competition what they want and will probably get it. Similarly, if the employees are not allowed to speak the truth to managers, they will usually withdraw their innovative ideas and eventually go to competitors that will be more than happy to listen to them.

It is a sad commentary on the state of an entire organization when it suffers from fear and distrust that could have been eliminated with simple communication skills. All that is required is the development and expansion of an open communication system. But the most important part of the communication process between manager and follower is for the manager to learn to listen to what the follower has to say, because the follower is much closer to customers and knows better how to serve them. This poses special problems for health care managers in bureaucratic organizations, however, because a top-down communication system virtually eliminates any advice from those who deliver the services and who are usually well aware of the flaws in the delivery of these services.

Health care managers need to realize the value of being open and truthful with their employees, who have the ability to share the real problems that the organization faces. Employees are also capable of helping the health care manager find solutions to current and potential future problems. The manager only needs to be visible during the process of producing and delivering services and to ask and answer questions. There is no shame in asking lower-level employees how to improve the delivery of health services. Those who desire to speak up need to be encouraged to do so because they usually care a great deal about the future of the organization. The problem, however, is that managers tend to forget that it is not *their* organization. The real owners of the health care organization are the employees and the customers, but they are nevertheless very willing to collaborate with management to make the organization work better. For this to happen, the manager needs to talk less and listen more. Most of the recent research strongly suggests that listening is the hardest skill for the health care manager to develop

(Becker & Wortmann, 2009). Managers working in a bureaucratic organization have been used to dictating how tasks should be accomplished because that's the way top-down management works. We must not forget that the bureaucratic form of management has been and continues to be in some organizations the only way to do business. However, we are in a new world of health care delivery in which open communication among managers, workers, and customers is critical. It is also a wonderful opportunity to build employee and patient trust in the services the organization offers and to expand the organizational vision to more closely engage employees and consumers.

The health care manager also needs to encourage feedback from both employees and customers about how he or she is communicating. This is very rarely done in bureaucratic organizations because managers fear that these two groups might tell them that they are not doing a good job. In an open system of communication, feedback is strongly encouraged because it can be very helpful to the manager in making future communication that much better. We should look at such feedback as free advice that has a great chance of improving both the manager's performance and the services being delivered, which is a winning proposition for everyone involved.

It is critical for the health care manager to confront his or her own mistakes and learn from the process. According to Kouzes and Posner (2010), continuous feedback, even if it is negative, will help managers learn about themselves, especially their ability to manage. This is very true when it comes to developing communication skills. Most managers in health care do not like to hear negative things concerning their ability to manage, but constructive feedback from employees can actually help them grow and develop the requisite skills to deal with the changing health care environment. A manager should be very happy that his or her employees care enough about the development of their superior that they would risk confronting this individual with constructive criticism. Receiving feedback is the only way to become a better health care manager.

The health care manager must understand that to facilitate change, he or she needs to understand why individuals behave the way they do. This requires communicating with both employees and consumers to find out as much as possible about their behavior. The manager will never have all the information he or she needs to make sound decisions without first listening to what others have to say.

Evaluating the Message Being Communicated

Health care managers, because they are in a position of power, need to spend a great deal of time fine-tuning a given message to employees or customers before sending it through the channel of communication. Imparting information to these groups becomes much easier if mutual trust has been established, but it still requires the sender of the message to think about what it is he or she is trying to communicate and why this is being communicated in the first place. Such a message generally involves the vision of the organization and how this vision relates to employees and customers. Quite often the message itself is not as important as the way it is communicated. This is where communication skills, especially the ability to think about what it is you're trying to communicate, come into play. Evaluating the message is a vitally important communication skill that managers need to use whenever they are communicating important information to employees that may be confusing. In other words, managers must make a constant effort to be certain that the receivers of the message understand what it is he or she is actually saying. If the receiver does not understand, the message should be changed until it is completely understood.

This skill can be learned, but it will take practice and time. Unfortunately, the vast majority of health care managers have not given mastering this very important skill the priority that it deserves. It is interesting to note that if the organization is practicing open communication, the manager doesn't have to spend as much time evaluating the message because communication will usually flow from the sender to the receiver and vice versa with very little effort or thought.

Communicating with Passion and Enthusiasm

To be successful in the communication process the manager needs to believe in the message, to be open in communicating the message, and to show passion and enthusiasm in the entire process of delivering the message.

According to Zenger, Folkman, and Edinger (2009), the most effective communicators are capable of sending messages with emotion and passion that the receivers perceive to be real, thereby making the communication more meaningful for them. This is not an easy thing for managers to do every time they communicate, but it is essential. Although it requires practice and dedication to the communication process, most managers can eventually improve their ability to communicate with passion and enthusiasm.

Using this communication skill becomes difficult when the manager has to communicate bad news to his or her followers and still show passion and enthusiasm. If staff reductions or changes in responsibilities are necessary for the good of the overall company, then that must be communicated to everyone along with the other reasons for the changes.

The health care manager must believe in the vision of the health care organization to be passionate about sharing it with others. The manager cannot fake enthusiasm because the employees will realize that the message being communicated is disingenuous. Perceived insincerity will negate the value of the entire communication process. The more genuine passion and enthusiasm evident in the communication process, the more likely that the message will be well received by employees and customers.

Avoiding Overdependence on Electronic Communication

The methods of communication have changed dramatically in the last decade. The health care industry has been slow to respond to the information technology revolution, but health care organizations are now seeing the advantages of rapid communication, and some of the best-run health care organizations have been using information technology to improve their competitive position. These organizations believe in open communication and the transparency that this technology can offer them. For example, they are using electronic medical records to improve the quality of health care delivery by improving the accuracy of the information gathered, sharing health information with everyone who needs to know, and bringing transparency to the medical process.

A well-organized information system in health care delivery is capable of improving coordination among tasks (Gittell, 2009). This coordination is a prerequisite for increasing quality in health care delivery. Electronic communication can help alleviate many of the quality issues currently found in our health care system. But electronic communication can also create problems for the health care manager. Face-to-face communication is still necessary to instill passion for the message that is being communicated. According to Gittell, electronic communication needs to be combined with face-to-face communication to maximize the effectiveness of the communication process in health care delivery. The rationale behind this assertion is that dependence on automated communication can result in weakened relationships among workers over time. There are individuals who respond better to face-to-face communication than they do to receiving information from a computer and then having to interpret the sender's frame of reference from a distance.

The ability to share information rapidly is critical in the delivery of health services. Medical errors have become a major problem in our health care system, and this problem can only be resolved through better communication methods that convey accurate and timely information, such as the medical history of an individual with comorbidities or the drug records of each patient. Accuracy and timeliness are both components of successful electronic communication. Unfortunately, improving quality via electronic communication may have the side effect of inadvertently harming the relationships among health care workers by creating distance between them, which in turn may negatively affect the culture throughout the health care facility.

HOW TO BUILD TRUST IN RELATIONSHIPS

The best-run companies in America have one thing in common: their employees trust each other and their managers. Trust is also one of the most important ingredients of successful health care organizations. This trust is found among employees who work for these health care organizations and among the consumers who purchase health services from them. It is built over time and requires a great deal of effort on the part of the health care manager to maintain.

Charlene Li, in *Open Leadership: How Social Technology Can Transform the Way You Lead* (2010), writes the following about establishing trust: "Rather than actually using the word 'transparency,' which implies complete openness and candor, I prefer to describe this skill as making information and processes 'visible'" (p. 193). This is really relationship building, which is accomplished by responding to challenges and providing detailed information in a manner that engenders trust. Building trust can lead to empowerment and better performance, and has the potential to help assimilate the health care manager into the culture of the organization. This requires the manager of the health care facility to share goals, challenges, threats, and opportunities with employees. The manager must constantly give his or her people updates and even options in the process of change.

Communication is a critical component of building trust because people are listening to what the manager says and watching what the manager does. This is how trust develops, taking time, effort, and communication skills. Building trust requires managers to provide timely information to employees that is readily understood and always available. This will tell employees that they are part of a team trying to accomplish the goals of the organization. Managers are then better able to ignite the passion of their employees in the delivery of health services, with their only resource to achieve this feat being their ability to communicate the importance of delivering quality services to every patient every day.

According to Burchell and Robin (2011), the dimensions of a great place to work include credibility, respect, fairness, pride, and camaraderie. Figure 6.2 shows these five dimensions and all of their components. Credibility, respect, and fairness are all shown to be components of trust. It is interesting to note that a great deal of two-way communication is necessary to achieve these ideals. With communication being such a critical part of management—and particularly health care management—it is amazing how little attention most managers pay to this process.

The organizations that foster the immediate sharing of information with their employees are able to increase trust among and between their members. It seems almost self-evident that to build trust between managers and employees there must be continuous communication between these two

Figure 6.2   Dimensions of a Great Place to Work®
Source: Burchell & Robin, 2011, p. 4. Reprinted with permission of John Wiley & Sons, Inc.

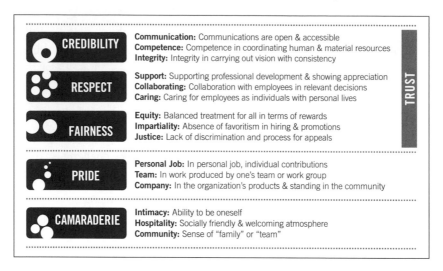

groups. It also becomes very clear that to build a thick, positive culture there has to be trust among all members of the organization. Again, this trust is built step-by-step over time, and it does not happen overnight. The manager has to realize that employees are listening to everything he or she says and watching everything he or she does.

Kouzes and Posner (2010) point out that when managers discuss their intentions with subordinates, many employees will view these intentions as promises. If these promises are not kept, trust will begin to diminish, creating a credibility issue for the manager. In the absence of trust, employees lose motivation, making the accomplishment of goals virtually impossible. This is because the loss of trust among employees destroys the organization's thick culture, causing employees to not want to come to work and to be less driven while at work. This can result in talent leaving the company and joining the competition. It can also result in customers leaving the organization because of poor service from less-than-enthusiastic employees. When it comes to sharing information among all employees, most of the research in recent years is strongly endorsing the development of an **open organization,** in which good and bad news is immediately available. This is a definite departure from the approach to communication in bureaucratic organizations, which resist sharing vital information with anyone except the administration, even though this information ultimately affects all employees.

When information is shared with employees, their sense of ownership of the work process increases, along with the sense of pride they feel from working for an organization that cares about their involvement. Li (2010) argues that open communication entails information sharing and collaborative decision making. As part of open information sharing, information concerning the operations of the company is shared in numerous ways with all employees in a timely fashion. Many of the best workplaces in the United States share everything with their employees, which in turn increases their motivation to be part of something special. Decision making involves using available information to make choices that are optimal for the organization. The best workplaces also involve employees in the decision making process, thereby making rapid change possible. This also increases the creativity and innovative spirit of everyone who works for the organization.

The bureaucratic organization does not share information with employees because the withholding of information gives managers a sense of power. It also is a very direct way of telling employees that they are not trusted, which in turn causes employees not to trust management. The serious mistake of limiting the information shared slows down the organization's response to environmental change. Further, when information is kept secret, employees feel that they are not important, they will lose interest in the goals of the organization, and they will look to change employers.

The bureaucratic organization also does not involve employees in decision making. This shows employees that their expertise is not valued and that they are not trusted to help the organization make decisions affecting its future. This is a very serious problem because the input of all employees is critical to making appropriate and timely decisions in the improvement of the health care system.

Transparency in decision making is a concept intrinsic to building a thick culture that is capable of improving health outcomes and the safety of health care delivery across the United States. All employees have to trust their managers and feel free to speak up when the organization is making mistakes. Culture is the subject of the next section.

COMMUNICATING TO BUILD A THICK CULTURE

A thick, positive workplace culture is mandatory for the continued success of an organization. This type of culture can enable the organization to face all challenges and prevail. According to Schein (2004), work groups that come together require a system of communication that helps them interpret their overall environment, thereby allowing members of an organization to understand what is not important and concentrate on what is important for the future success of the organization.

Szollose (2011) argues that the most creative cultures are most often found in new businesses. This is because these businesses are hungry to win, they push risk taking to the limit, and their small size usually allows for open communication between managers and lower-level employees. One of the disadvantages of growth for a business is the inability to keep sponsoring open communication: the company starts applying rules and regulations, which destroys employee creativity. The companies that continue to act small even when they have grown large are usually the most successful over the long term. Frequent communication with employees can help build strong and long-lasting relationships, even after a business grows larger. These strong relationships are necessary for developing a thick, positive culture over time. The health care manager has to understand the value of a thick culture in the accomplishment of organizational goals. The days of motivating individuals through a bureaucratic model are long gone.

A strong, positive culture is mandatory for long-term survival in the new and rapidly changing business world. The only way to survive the turbulence produced by rapid change is through better and faster communication between the manager and all stakeholders, especially employees and customers. This is especially true in the delivery of health services in our country. Health care organizations have grown in size and have been faced with tremendous change that has made all employees very uneasy about the future. These changes are a real threat to the stability of the employee culture in a given health care organization. The solution to the problem of cultural instability is better and more frequent communication from health care managers to lower-level employees who want to know about potential changes in their working environment.

According to Connors and Smith (2011), the experiences people have in the workplace affect their beliefs about their contribution in the work process, which in turn contribute to their actions at work, which ultimately affect the results the organization sees. It seems logical, then, to assume that the culture that exists in the organization produces that organization's current results. It also seems appropriate to assume that to improve results for the company, the culture will need to change. Connors and Smith also point out that the way to get individuals to change how they behave at work is by getting them to change how they think at work. These authors believe that there is a results pyramid that includes experiences, beliefs, actions, and results. The starting point for achieving improved results is past experiences in the workplace. If these experiences have been bad, usually due to poor management, then the manager must improve employees' ongoing experiences.

This change will take a long time, but it can be facilitated by improved communication throughout the organization. Managers communicate with employees in an attempt to get them to change their beliefs, resulting in a behavioral shift by the employees. This shift in employee behavior toward the achievement of organizational goals will ultimately lead to actions that result in better results. In this case a change in the culture has led to improved results.

Because the beliefs of employees are a major determining factor in their actions in the workplace, the health care manager must understand the role of beliefs in his or her attempt to improve the quality of health care delivery in this country. Being mindful of the beliefs of both employees and customers is key to enhancing the experiences of those receiving and those providing health services.

A belief statement that reflects the employee culture that is communicated to all employees every day can be the driving force for employees

(Connors & Smith, 2011). The development of this statement has to be a joint venture between the administration and the employees of a health care facility. This belief statement has to be the product of two-way communication among everyone involved in the provision of services to customers. Further, the belief statement needs to be modeled by health care managers. Managers also need to understand that they are capable of creating experiences for their employees every day that can build and grow a thick, positive culture of service for the entire organization. Managers are always creating experiences, and employees are observing and living these experiences and developing beliefs about their workplace. If these beliefs are positive and are communicated throughout the organization, the results produced by employees will improve, resulting in favorable consumer attitudes concerning the organization.

COMMUNICATING TO MOTIVATE

One of the most important responsibilities of the manager is to motivate his or her employees. A thick culture filled with mutual trust can lead to a successful organization that consistently produces superior results. Employees of such an organization are naturally motivated to achieve organizational goals because these and their personal goals have become the same. These goals have become one in that the organization and all of its employees exist to serve each other and their customers. Their motivation to produce quality services becomes contagious—almost epidemic—throughout the organization. This type of motivation is absolutely necessary when the organization is delivering services that the customer must have. To produce this type of intrinsic motivation in others it is quite often necessary for managers to use various communication methods to continually reinforce the wonders of working for the organization.

Motivation is a critical component of the production and delivery of superior health services. Motivation to purchase the health services on the part of customers is also critical for success in the world of health care delivery. Because the health care manager does not usually deliver health services directly to customers, he or she is responsible for motivating others to deliver these services. This is probably one of the most difficult responsibilities of the health care manager. It is also a skill that has been neglected in the training most new health care managers receive.

Organizations in the reforming health care system are starting to realize the importance of motivation to those who actually deliver health services to our population. This is going to require the health care manager to communicate a vision of quality to those delivering these services, which is where motivation becomes a critical variable. A vision that is widely shared can help large numbers of individuals become truly committed to group goals because these have become personal (Senge, 2006). The shared vision of what can be is capable of changing the relationships among employees within the organization. It allows all of them to come together with the courage and resolve to do whatever is necessary to achieve their shared vision. The communication skills of the manager become the conduit for bringing this vision to all of the employees. It is one thing for the manager to be enthusiastic about delivering services; it is quite another thing for employees to be motivated to achieve excellence in what they do. Motivating employees in this way requires trust building and the development and maintenance of a thick work culture. It also requires health care managers to gain a solid understanding of how the motivation process works and what role communication plays in motivating lower-level employees to deliver quality services on a daily basis.

According to Becker and Wortmann (2009), the best way to motivate employees is through the use of a motivation matrix. This matrix includes items that individuals are motivated by (ethos, emotions, and logic) and that which they are motivated for (achievement, recognition, and power). The motivation matrix can easily become part of the orientation of every new employee. This matrix is a critical starting point for understanding how to motivate employees to deliver excellent health services for each consumer every time.

Recent research concerning motivation is finding that once employees have satisfied their basic needs with acceptable wages they move toward more intrinsic forms of motivation (Pink, 2009). This is an important revelation for managers: to motivate health care employees they need to pay more attention to employee development and less attention to the compensation package. To be sure, a certain level of compensation is still important, but the worker is also motivated by the job that he or she is performing. This is where better communication between managers and employees in health care delivery becomes critical, in that the manager has to spend a great deal of time communicating the vision of the health care facility and why it is so important, above and beyond making a profit.

One of the most important building blocks of trust consists of interpersonal relationships (Hamm, 2012). These relationships can go a long way toward reducing fear in an organization, which in turn reduces defensive employee behavior. This is one more reason for the organization to support open communication, encouraging complete transparency of all work-related information. Hamm argues that all great businesses encourage a free flow of information in all directions, all the time. This information flow allows employees to concentrate on creativity rather than fear, which builds the culture of trust that is so necessary to achieve greatness. Such trust building by health care managers through open communication is a vital attribute of successful organizations.

Employees are also very interested in being part of something that they consider to be important to both their own lives and their community. They want to feel as if they are growing personally and professionally through the work they do. This is quite often their greatest motivation and needs to be shared with and understood by the health care manager. Nonmonetary motivators are relatively easy to develop and offer to employees. Extrinsic nonmonetary rewards can be something as simple as individual and team recognition by the health care manager for a job well done. This type of motivation works best if it is communicated to all employees at the same time. They only require two-way communication with employees to be discovered.

Employees are more motivated when they believe that they are part of something special in the workplace. This generally means that they feel challenged and respected by the work process, and their managers know what the organization wants to accomplish both in the short term and the long term. Employees desire to work for an organization that has a real understanding of the challenges it faces and has developed a plan to meet those challenges. Excellent organizations have learned how to communicate their vision for their employees, their customers, and their community.

Coherence in the way an organization does business, according to Leinwand and Mainardi (2010), has become a critical advantage. These authors expand the normal definition of coherence to include more than just "having your act together," encompassing an alignment of market position, the organization's most distinctive capabilities, and the products and services that are produced by the organization. This coherence can virtually guarantee success for the organization, and it also provides a motivating environment for employees. The underlying factor that has been found in coherent organizations is an open system of communication, whereby all employees participate in making things work. In fact, the distinctive capabilities of these organizations are produced by their human capital.

According to Leinwand and Mainardi (2010), the secret to success in almost every market involves the organization's reinvesting in its own capabilities. In the delivery of health care the successful companies are the ones that continuously invest in the people they employ. Unfortunately, the vast majority of health care facilities have not developed among their employees a significant capability in the form of constantly and consistently delivering quality services to customers. The health care manager therefore needs to learn how to offer change leadership in the process of shifting the ways in which his or her employees approach the delivery of quality services. Anderson and Anderson (2010) argue that there are three critical focus areas in the production and expansion of change leadership. The health care manager needs to pay particular attention to the content of change, the people in change, and the process of change, as shown in Figure 6.3.

The critical focus areas are all further developed through the communication process. Because health services are usually delivered by groups of people, the communication between managers and health care employees becomes a critical factor in gaining an essential advantage over the organization's competitors. Employees need to know where the organization is attempting to go and the strategy that is being used to get there. They also need to know what part they are expected to play in goal achievement, and

Figure 6.3   Three Critical Focus Areas of Change Leadership
Source: Anderson & Anderson, 2010, p. 25. Reprinted with permission of John Wiley & Sons, Inc.

Content of change
The organizational focus of the change
(structure, strategy, business process,
technology, culture, product, or service)

People in change
Handling the human dynamics of change: people's
mindsets, commitment to change; emotional
reactions, behavior, engagement, relationships, politics;
cultural dynamics impacting the change

Process of change
The way in which change is planned, designed,
and implemented; adjusting to how it unfolds;
its A–Z roadmap, governance, integration
strategy, and course corrections

what type of power the organization has granted them to achieve organizational goals. This is where communication becomes one of the health care manager's most important tools.

COMMUNICATION PROBLEMS AND MEDICAL ERRORS

One in four Medicare patients experiences some form of medical error when hospitalized (Sarver, 2010). How can this be happening in our hospitals, which are equipped with modern technology and well-educated health care professionals? Recent research indicates that these medical errors are quite often a result of poor communication among the members of the health care team.

A major study was released by the Institute of Medicine (IOM, 1999) that revealed that as many as 98,000 of the 33 million individuals hospitalized each year die, and that many more receive hospital-acquired infections because of poor-quality health care while hospitalized. According to Schimpff (2012),

This total is about three times the number of deaths due to car accidents, five times the number of homicides, and sixteen times the number of

U.S. servicemen and women killed in Iraq and Afghanistan since the start of hostilities in 2003 (p. 127).

These medical errors and nosocomial infections, better known as hospital-acquired infections, represent a medical tragedy that continues as a major problem threatening our delivery of health services in the United States. It represents a serious epidemic that must be eliminated, now.

These medical errors typically occur in operating rooms, emergency departments, and intensive care units. There is mounting evidence that entering the health care system at any location increases the risk of adverse drug events, errors in health care delivery, and hospital-acquired infections. Emanuel (2008) points out that the danger associated with acquiring additional infections during a routine hospital stay is very high, reaching as high as 10 percent in many larger hospitals. This translates into two to three million hospital-acquired infections each year, resulting in over twenty-six thousand preventable deaths on an annual basis. This problem is entirely preventable by health care managers enforcing strict hand-washing techniques among all employees who have direct patient care responsibilities. It is nothing more than a breakdown in communication between managers and employees concerning the importance of following standard quality of care procedures.

The major problem with this epidemic of medical errors in our health care facilities is that many who work in the health care field have accepted these horrible statistics as normal. They are not normal, and they do not have to be accepted. An excellent example of how to solve this frightening problem is found in Alcoa's success story concerning accident prevention, as discussed in Chapter One. According to Duhigg (2012), in 1987 the new CEO for Alcoa, Paul O'Neill, declared war on accidents at his company. He determined that the improvement of one of the worst accident records would be the focus of all of his attention—the most important goal of his tenure at the company.

Paul O'Neill told the world at his first news conference that worker safety would be the focus of the entire company and that he would accept nothing but constant improvement in this one factor as he moved the company forward. He used managerial communication skills to change the culture of one of the largest companies in the United States. He told all employees that accidents would be reported to managers when they occurred, and that he would then receive these reports with a cause and a prevention strategy at the same time. He even offered his home phone number to employees to report safety issues directly to him for immediate resolution. This act of communicating the importance of safety by the CEO not only reduced the incidence of accidents but also improved productivity, efficiency, and profits for the company.

Duhigg (2012) argues that the key to getting to the O'Neill goal of zero injuries was to gain a much better understanding of why these workplace accidents occurred in the first place. To eliminate injuries across the organization, each unit of the company had to build a new communication system that allowed for the rapid transferring of information about injury occurrence along with immediate investigation of the injury's cause.

We can also see these same results in the health care industry in regard to medical errors and hospital-acquired infections if we use the power of communication and follow the lead of Paul O'Neill and Alcoa. It will start with health care managers communicating the desire for zero medical errors and hospital-acquired infections to all employees at the same time. This communication needs to followed by immediate reporting of medical errors and infections acquired in the health care facility to the manager assigned to the unit in which the event occurred. This will be followed by an immediate investigation into the cause with one goal in mind—to stop it from ever happening again.

The health care manager must continuously seek out solutions to the problem of medical errors from all employees. Employees need to have trust in their manager and an understanding that all of their ideas concerning how to avoid medical errors will be considered and, if possible, implemented by the entire health care team. Although these discussions are presided over by managers and staff of the health care facility, we want to be certain to avoid groupthink. Groupthink usually occurs when there is more interest in harmony among group members than there is in a realistic evaluation by group members of possible alternatives. The costs associated with the manager's allowing this to happen could include the loss of employee creativity and independent thinking, both of which are necessary for innovation to occur. It is an obvious conclusion that groupthink will be less of a problem in an organization that has truly empowered employees and a culture of trust. In addition, groupthink may also be avoided if the health care manager is perceived as authentic in encouraging employees to openly discuss how to improve the vision of the organization, the process of work, and the organizational status quo.

COMMUNICATING TO INNOVATE

The chaos produced by health care reform, compounded by the fierce competition in the health care industry in recent years, is producing tremendous opportunities for health care organizations. There is a need for change in the way health services are delivered to improve the health care system for all, and to deliver health services in the way that consumers want them to be delivered. Although adapting to make changes demanded by consumers is a source of opportunities, however, this process will also entail a degree of risk.

To exploit these opportunities, health care organizations need creativity and the ability to offer their customers innovative ways to address their medical issues. Such creativity and innovation will not come from health care managers, but from the people they manage. It is the workers who know what innovations are required to improve the services they currently provide and create the new services their patients desire. Innovation in any industry requires workers to experiment with the products or services they deliver to customers (Hamm, 2012). This experimentation in turn requires great risk by the innovator, which necessitates an environment of trust and belief that failure will be accepted by the organization. This acceptance of failure while trying to improve health care delivery needs to be communicated to employees on a daily basis. Employees need to know that their employer truly appreciates their attempts to improve the services they deliver. Giving employees room to innovate and sometimes to fail requires ongoing two-way communication that goes up and down an organization's hierarchy. The atmosphere for innovation is built through constant communication from management to employees that it is okay to take risks and make mistakes, as long as employees learn from these experiences. The more this type of entrepreneurial spirit is communicated to the entire organization, the more likely it is that it will become ingrained in the way business is done. The best providers of health services in recent years have allowed open communication among managers, employees, and customers.

To make the innovation process happen in the delivery of health services requires a great deal of communication among the health care manager and his or her employees. There needs to be an environment in which new ideas about how to better serve the customer come forth on a daily basis. Szollose (2011) argues that the most innovative companies foster the growth of an environment in which outrageous ideas are encouraged and supported. Workers need to be encouraged by managers to take chances and occasionally make mistakes without any type of penalty. To make this type of environment work, the health care manager needs to communicate the reality of this environment to all of the employees every day. An open system of communication in which everyone has value and can tell the truth even if it hurts can be the catalyst for great innovation.

Innovation involves bringing a problem-solving idea into the open for discussion (Conway & Steward, 2009). This process can be better accomplished through the rapid sharing of information among innovators. It is a fact that innovation should be the concern of everyone who works for a business because all employees have a stake in the success of that business. This holds true in our rapidly changing health care system. The competition for health care consumers continues to intensify, and a given health care organization will only survive through creativity and innovation in the delivery of health services.

COMMUNICATING TO ADD VALUE TO HEALTH CARE DELIVERY

The major goal should be to achieve exceptionally high value for the consumer of health services. Value in health care can be defined as the health outcome achieved for each dollar spent (Porter, 2010). The pursuit of high value alone is capable of uniting the consumer, stakeholders, and those involved in the delivery of health services. Communication between managers and their employees is probably the most important facilitator of the value-adding process.

Measuring value in health care delivery is very difficult because of the bureaucratic structure and information flow in most health care organizations (Porter, 2010). Therefore, as the bureaucratic components of health care delivery break down, there must be a commensurate increase in open communication among all members of the organization. Different communication methods are required to get all of the health care employees involved in the quality improvement and value-adding process within the health care facility.

Many successful companies are moving to an open strategy for conducting their business (Li, 2010). This type of strategy for accomplishing business objectives involves learning, dialogue, support, and innovation. The most important component of this strategy for most organizations is learning. Health care managers have to learn what their consumers value when the health care organization is delivering services to them. They then need to share this information immediately with the employees who actually deliver the services to their customers. This process is difficult to implement in a bureaucratic organization in which information is not gathered from customers and is rarely shared with lower-level employees. If you have an open system of communication among managers, employees, and customers, it becomes much easier to make an open strategy work. This is mainly because trust is present, the culture is thick, and everyone involved wants the services produced to be excellent.

There is also a movement in health care delivery to establish shared decision making and informed patient choice with all patients who enter the health care facility. According to Wennberg (2010), this type of change is going to be very difficult because it will require a major transformation in the culture of medicine. It is nothing short of the doctor's beginning to share decision making concerning medical care with his or her patient. This is also going to require a major change in the communication process involving physicians in health care delivery—and this is a shift health care managers must encourage.

Connors and Smith (2011) point out that the organization must be in perfect alignment in regard to the cultural change process that is also necessary to add value to health care delivery. All employees need to be part of the cultural change process to achieve a critical mass of agreement, causing a rapid multiplication of the number of individuals in the organization who support this effort. Numerous distractions may disrupt the cultural change process, which is where constant communication by the health care manager comes into play. The manager needs to communicate to all employees a compelling case for cultural change to improve the results of the health care delivery process. The health care manager must ensure that all employees realize the importance of the change in the way things are done by members of the organization.

According to Leinwand and Mainardi (2010), successful companies have a very clear understanding of what makes them different in regard to how they add value for the customer. This is the chosen way that the organization does business, and it produces a sense of direction for all employees of the organization. This is a constant choice that can lead the organization for years. It becomes the way things are done, what gives meaning to those who work for the organization, and why the organization remains in business. The employees become absorbed into this culture through constant communication between managers and employees.

SUMMARY

Ninety-nine percent of problems in the workplace are a direct result of poor or inadequate communication between managers and employees (Tracy, 2010). This is certainly the case across the U.S. health care system. The success of health care organizations is dependent on rapid communication among managers, employees, and customers. Better communication systems are an absolute necessity if we are serious about improving health care delivery in this country.

In an organization with bright people who communicate with each other in pursuit of a shared vision, anything is possible (Szollose, 2011). Managers who establish a system of open communication that dispenses up-to-date information to all employees of the organization at the same time change everything for the better. In the delivery of health services, information has become the most important component in improving the health of the population. Information is not to be hidden from employees or patients because then it becomes useless. Information instead needs to be shared immediately with everyone who needs to know. This makes the ability to communicate one of the most important skills that a manager can develop to improve everyone's performance in health care delivery.

The starting point for improving communication in a health care facility is recognizing that there is a communication problem. Then the health care organization must spend a great deal of time helping its managers understand the importance of communication, and managers must then make an effort to improve their communication skills. It seems that improved communication in health care delivery may very well be the most important component in responding successfully to the need for health care reform.

Without better communication among health care professionals, it becomes very difficult if not impossible to improve the quality of health care delivery. The problem with bureaucratic organizations like those found in the health care industry is that communication usually flows only one way: from top to bottom. Health care organizations are slowly moving away from a bureaucratic structure to a more organic structure that is conducive to productive communication.

KEY TERMS

decoding

encoding

interpersonal communication

open communication

open organization

two-way communication

REVIEW QUESTIONS

1. Please offer a complete explanation of the process of interpersonal communication, and discuss how it can be applied to the delivery of health services.

2. Explain the value of the motivation matrix and how communication skills can be used to improve lower-level employees' motivation to produce and deliver quality health services to consumers.

3. How does the communication process help in building trust and increasing innovation in the health care organization?

4. Please explain the value of an open organization in regard to retaining talented employees.

7

Physician Management

Dan F. Kopen

LEARNING OBJECTIVES

- Understand the multiple dimensions of managing physicians that exist and will need to be addressed in the future

- Recognize the need for a greater awareness of what motivates physician behaviors

- Comprehend the values associated with better management of physicians

- Become aware of physicians' ability to create their own demand

- Be able to explain the importance of preparing physicians for a managerial position in health care delivery

The physician should be one of the key players in any serious effort to improve the way we deliver health services in this country. As the private practice model of physician practice declines, effective management of physicians as employees becomes an increasingly important dimension of successful health care delivery. In addition, physicians need to be considered for key managerial positions across the full spectrum of health care facilities. According to Leatt (1994), physicians bring important understandings to such positions, including problem-solving, analytic, and ethical decision-making skills.

Physician management has become an increasingly disconcerting topic of investigation as the medical landscape has undergone tremendous change over the past few decades. Of particular note, the leadership role of physicians, both at the bedside and at policymaking levels, has eroded significantly. The reasons for the deterioration of physicians' influence are many, and the result is a confusing mixture of physician management strategies currently being applied, ranging from increasingly popular command-and-control regulatory and ownership models to disappearing, hands-off, and hope-for-the-best observational approaches.

Starting from an overarching viewpoint, the management of physicians is generally viewed from two perspectives: that of those who manage and that of those who are managed. On the one hand, management and its associated considerations are a practical concern for those who do the managing, whether they are nonphysicians, physicians, or a combination thereof. On the other hand, for those who are the objects of managerial decisions, management is a field of administrative overlay that has a broad spectrum of increasingly profound impacts on practicing physicians' attitudes and behaviors.

Depending on one's viewpoint, what seem to be similar concepts in the abstract may be viewed quite differently in terms of actual effects. Interpretations of the impacts of management on the interests of the involved party or parties can vary widely along a spectrum from beneficial to harmful according to one's perspective. Complicating the process of evaluating the divide between those who manage and those who are managed is the fact that there are individuals and groups occupying overlapping positions on both sides of the management divide.

An additional panoramic consideration that adds a dimension of complexity to this topic is the source of power of the managing entity. Federal and state government sources of oversight and control are growing in influence, both directly and indirectly. Both nonprofit and for-profit private enterprise origins of power, largely founded on financial concerns subjected to overarching legal and regulatory agendas, are the second major source of management overlay. With regard to the private practice realm, large corporate practice models are fast replacing individual and small-enterprise managing entities in health care.

Given the diversity of perceptions of management and the various impacts of management on the participants in a management system, it is necessary to understand and address several dimensions of management methodologies ranging from design and intent to practice and outcomes. A brief historical review provides a foundation for better understanding various approaches to the current issues involved in physician management.

A half century ago nearly all physicians were self-employed. The large majority were supportive members of their respective county, state, and national medical societies. Those societies were effective in addressing most key political and economic issues facing physicians, and they were influential in determining public policy concerning the practice of medicine. In addition, those societies served as gateways to establishing successful community practices, especially in urban and suburban settings. In many instances, active membership in county medical societies was a prerequisite for obtaining staff privileges at community hospitals. Hospital staff membership afforded welcome participation in a group that held sway over the policies driving that organization as it sought to achieve the nonprofit mission of providing health services to the community. Physicians, through membership on hospital staffs and in their county and state societies, provided leadership both at the bedside and at diverse policymaking levels in the delivery of health services.

Out-of-hospital physician management and behaviors were essentially the sole priority of the private practitioner. Office management was minimally burdened with bureaucratic and regulatory overlay. Decisions were made on an ad hoc basis, and these generally focused on patient care and financial concerns, with virtually no imposition of third-party pressures.

The major source of management concerns were unofficial "good-old-boys" networks of private physicians, whose extent and influence varied across a nation that was largely underserved by physician manpower, with the exception of certain urban settings. These entrenched power bases were often firmly invested in preserving the interests of existing participants and resisting change at almost all costs. Even clear change for the better was often seen as a threat to the comfort zones of practitioners, who held sway over local health care referral networks and community hospitals. Furthermore, physician cohorts were almost exclusively male in composition.

In addition, in those bygone days most community hospitals were run by the male medical chief of staff in association with the female head nurse. Their collaborative decisions were effected through the offices of a CEO, who had little influence or control over policy formation or implementation. Community hospital CEOs earned salaries far lower than the incomes of hospital physician staff members. This hospital leadership model was clearly there to serve community needs and not to reap financial rewards.

Externally there were minimal levels of regulatory overlay, and threats of legal action against the institution and its practitioners were not of major concern. The total health care economy constituted roughly 5 percent of gross domestic product, and the medical arena was not high on the list of areas targeted as potential sources of major financial reward by most service and manufacturing industry leaders. Medicine was a profession left largely unto itself.

The major exception to this community-based model was the academic medical center. At such an institution there were more layers of administrative input, with attendant influences placed on physicians as they sought to care for patients while also meeting educational and research obligations. Even in academic institutions, however, outside pressures from private third parties and government sources were modest. Physicians based in an academic institution were free to concentrate on their primary agendas of medical care, education, and research with little day-to-day interference from sources of institutional financial management or government regulation.

In regard to community hospitals, a look at the simple metric of hospital square footage devoted to direct patient care versus administrative activities reveals that a few decades ago the vast majority of space was used primarily for direct patient care. In today's hospitals, by contrast, the percentage of space devoted to administrative and other activities not related to direct patient care often exceeds 50 percent of building square footage. Clearly a major shift has taken place, with direct patient care concerns being challenged and in many cases superseded by administrative and management priorities. The reasons for this change are numerous and include increasing government and regulatory overlay, burgeoning private bureaucratic machineries, and altered priorities. Depending on one's agenda, the categorization of space based on its use can vary considerably and thereby bring this commonsense observation into dispute. For example, those who seek to provide the public with reassurance of the mission of the hospital will often include space that is only indirectly related to patient care as constituting patient care square footage. However, for those who have worked in hospitals during the past half century, the huge shift in the allotment of institutional square footage from direct patient care provision to other concerns is both real and apparent. What is more, the associated redirection of operating expenses and total costs is compelling evidence of shifts in the top priorities of management.

CHANGING ENVIRONMENT FOR PHYSICIANS

Physicians have always held tremendous power in health care delivery. Because of their advanced education in medicine they are usually the ones who determine the testing and medical procedures that are ordered, and they oversee hospital admittance and discharge. According to Feldstein (2012), the physician has become the supplier of both advice and services; and because the doctor gets paid for supplying a substantial part of those services, the advice he or she provides could be biased. This power has in many cases allowed the doctor to be able to create his or her own demand. Managed care organizations in various forms, now including the emerging class of accountable care organizations, are attempting to take this power away from physicians. Depending on the particulars of individual patient circumstances, physician control over the advice given and the acceptance of service provision can have negative or positive connotations for the patient.

Changing political, legal, and economic environments have served to erode physician hegemony across the health care landscape and render physicians and their general societies largely ineffective in advocating both for their patients and for their own interests. Community hospitals are fast decreasing in number, with the attendant growth of large corporate practice models of institutional ownership. With the exception of a small number of physicians who occupy positions of power within institutions (who are often viewed by physicians in private practice as politically connected ingratiates), hospital staff membership has devolved significantly. What was once a position of meaningful influence has become one of mere physical presence at a required percentage of scheduled meetings per year—meetings in which administrative staff members make decisions aimed largely at satisfying imposed legislative and accrediting body procedural mandates, in ultimate service to institutional financial concerns. Most physician staff members are afforded very little opportunity to influence institutional policies concerning the delivery of care. The minutes of meetings often fail to reflect the input of practicing physicians, and as a result fewer physicians choose to make comments on the issues raised, most of which reflect agendas that are predetermined by bottom-line financial concerns, or even to attend more than the minimum number of required meetings per year.

There is no question that the physician is one of the most important players in the delivery of health services. He or she is part of a team of health care professionals who are all needed to deliver quality health services to their patients. The most successful health care organizations in our country have spent a great deal of time developing better working relationships with their physicians. According to Lombardi (2001), extra effort needs to be made in making the physician believe that he or she is an important part of the team.

That medical care must be delivered in a team environment is an area of particular emphasis in regard to health care reform. Gone are the days of the individual practitioner holding a singular, authoritative, paternalistic position in patient care decision making. Today it is widely recognized that medical care decisions have become increasingly complex across a broad spectrum of patient concerns, and that the ultimate legal right to make such decisions rests with the patient or the patient's legal surrogate. The principle of patient autonomy has been recognized for over a century, but it has emerged in fuller force over the past few decades. As a consequence of increasing medical complexity and legal patient autonomy, the team approach to medical decision making has gained favor. This approach offers input into patient decisions from a variety of pertinent sources and thereby often takes into consideration a broader range of concerns in making individual diagnoses. Today's medical care team includes not only a group of appropriate physician specialists and generalists but also nurses, therapists, and social workers.

On a national scale, the growing presence of special interest power brokers over the past half century has radically changed the entire landscape of health care. Beginning with the huge influx of taxpayer dollars with the introduction of Medicare and Medicaid in 1965, we have witnessed exponential growth and radical changes in the medical economy. On the positive side, there have been tremendous advances in diagnostic and treatment modalities as a result of the increased availability of financial resources. On the negative side, however, general medical societies' ability to effectively advocate for their membership has eroded, given the concurrent and disproportionate growth of nonprovider administrative and business cohort influence in the health care arena. Ever-increasing pressures applied to practicing physicians by changing political and legal climates have transformed the spectrum of physician management issues and the ability of physicians and their societies to address those concerns. As a result of these seismic changes, physician organizational allegiances and physician management strategies have shifted substantially.

Although there used to be a safe and secure future for the vast majority of those who entered the medical profession as private physicians, private practice has become an undertaking characterized by increasing risk, debt loads, and uncertainty. The business dimension of the medical economy has mushroomed, while the hands-on patient care dimension has stultified in most areas of medical treatment. Exceptions to this observation include the growth in certain emerging areas of largely behaviorally induced illnesses, such as mental dysfunctions, obesity, and some clearly preventable chronic diseases.

An interesting report from the American Medical Association in 2011 demonstrated that in a large and growing number of physician practices administrative employees now outnumber clinical staff. This is further evidence of the increasing focus on the business aspects of medical care and the increasing costs to practitioners. Physicians must factor these rapidly increasing business costs into their decisions when choosing which practice model to pursue.

An overarching reality facing the medical profession is the unspoken national political and economic agenda of decreasing aggregate physician reimbursement for covered medical services. That is, services recognized and categorized as being "medically necessary" and therefore falling under the umbrella of federal, state, and private sector insurance coverage are targeted for reimbursement reduction by those who control the purse strings. As a result, divide-and-conquer strategies have become a part of the professional medical management environment, and have been applied from both external and internal sources. The external motivation to divide and conquer is the desire to capture increasing percentages of the medical economic pie at the expense of practicing physicians by weakening the physician base of influence. Such external sources include the Patient Protection and Affordable Care Act (PPACA) and its Independent Payment Advisory Board, which will, if allowed to become a reality, gain control over physician reimbursement independent of physicians, physician societies, and our federal and state governments. The internal force driving this strategy derives from understanding that the slice of pie earmarked for the provision of medical and surgical services is growing proportionately smaller, and that each specialty must therefore struggle to capture as large a bite of this shrinking slice as possible for its stakeholders. As a result, some of the most consequential rifts that weaken the influence of physicians across the health care landscape come from within the medical profession itself.

Our nation's medical economy is experiencing what amounts to a national strategy of redistribution of health care dollars away from the providers of services to legions of middlemen who serve diverse political, economic, and legal agendas. There is some merit to the flow of dollars into the pockets of those who are not actually providing care, given that we have witnessed some remarkable advances in technology, enhanced medical knowledge, and an increasing amount of resources available to drug and device manufacturers and research entities. The problem as seen from the physician perspective is that this redirected flow of reimbursement comes largely as a result of financial redistribution rather than wealth creation strategies.

As an example, one of the major topics of technological advancement is in the area of health information technology and electronic medical records (EMRs). This is an area with tremendous upside potential for improvement in health care delivery, but it also harbors significant downside risks, many of which have not been recognized or addressed in the current mandated rush to adopt these technologies. Managers need to understand that these computerized forms of information gathering and exchange were largely developed for primary care practice settings, and that there have been significant, expensive failure rates of incorporation of these technologies ranging from about 40 percent in primary care practice settings to as high as 80 percent in specialty practice settings. The advantages are real for improved patient care where there are information highways that are secure from unauthorized access and allow the easy exchange of safely encrypted information among multiple authorized medical venues, each using different EMR vendors. Most practices using EMRs have had to hire additional staff to ensure the functionality of the hardware and software, and some have employed "scribes" to allow the practicing physicians to continue their hands-on patient care delivery in an efficient manner. When using EMRs there exists the very real danger of HIPAA violations resulting from both intentional and inadvertent access to patient information by unauthorized parties. It was reported in 2011 that over ten million patient records were subjected to unauthorized access over a two-year reporting period, and that number continues to rise. Managers need to recognize these problems and the attendant costs and liability risks, which can far exceed the government subsidies targeted for EMR adoption. Good management will entail addressing these problems prior to signing purchase agreements for these services for use in private practice, in larger private practice groups, and for institutional purposes.

Today there are too few areas in which membership in general medical societies and hospital staffs affords physicians the opportunity to contribute effectively to policy-related decision making, either at the bedside or at administrative levels of health care provision. As a result, the bulk of practicing physicians have shifted their allegiances from local hospital staffs and general medical societies to other entities that offer the promise of advocating more effectively for what amount to changed priorities resulting from the redistribution strategies among an increasingly diverse physician population.

Also of importance is that during the past few years our nation has witnessed a landmark change in the professional status of physicians—a change that signals major evolutionary alterations in physician management strategies. For the first time in our nation's history there are more physicians who are employees of larger entities than there are in private practice. This has been the result of many external and internal forces placing pressure on members of the medical profession. Government regulatory pressures have significantly reduced allowable resident work hours and have altered attendant professional behaviors that are part of the residency experience, and time commitment expectations have changed. It is clearly the case that for many residents in surgical and medical domains the reduction in allowable weekly work hours and daily time slots has relegated patient care to a secondary status in many instances in which time allotments run out while a patient's care needs are significant and often expanding. Managers are forced to remove the residents from their work position to comply with regulations or face penalties. Residents are deprived of a continuous care learning experience.

In addition, unionization of residents has appeared on the scene, and the expected market participation and postresidency job-related time commitments of physicians have altered considerably. Widely promulgated and imposed requirements for the adoption of electronic medical records have altered the physician-patient interface and the relationship between the institution and the physician at many levels. Taken together, these types of structural changes in the education, training, and professional commitments of physicians have significantly changed the aggregate composition of the parties to physician management strategies. The end result is a need to examine the multidimensional aspects of physician practice patterns to better appreciate the moving target that is the aim of physician management programs.

PHYSICIAN MANAGEMENT CONCERNS

Several dimensions of physician practice contribute to the effectiveness of management strategies employed in the health care provider arena. What once amounted to the rather simple, blanket application of a fundamentally hands-off strategy for managing physicians is now a multidimensional quilt that takes into consideration not only manifold practice concerns but also the changing nature of the profession vis-à-vis increasingly burdensome legal, regulatory, and administrative overlay. We will examine some of the categories of concern that help define the multiform physician cohorts and that therefore are the focus of management strategies.

Practice Specialty

One of the most obvious divisions among physicians pertains to their field of practice. This division represents a major barrier to managers' successful adoption of a blanket physician management strategy. An approach to management that might appear to make sense from the perspective of a primary care physician or primary care group can represent an abuse of logic if it is applied to certain specialty physicians or specialty groups. Similarly, management issues of major concern to certain practice specialists may be of little or no concern to other specialists or generalists.

A few generations ago professional medical specialization was an exception; today it is the norm. The forces that have led to specialization are many. The expansive growth in both medical information and available treatment options continues to present the profession with an overwhelming range of medical knowledge and therapeutic modalities. Taken in combination with the fact that physicians are human and thus limited in their ability to learn and apply knowledge and techniques across the entire medical spectrum, this growth in understanding and treatment methodologies has been a significant factor in leading many physicians to limit the scope of their practice to a specialty or subspecialty. The attendant shrinking ability of generalists to fully understand and apply practice guidelines and standards of care across the expansive diagnostic spectrum has lessened the attraction of general fields of practice for those who desire not only to diagnose but also to treat patients effectively.

Another factor playing a role in the move toward specialization has been the differential reimbursement for time spent in the delivery of care between specialists and generalists. This differential evolved in large part from the increased number of years of training required to attain specialty certification and the attendant opportunity costs of specialty training. Although there are ongoing efforts to decrease these differential reimbursement rates, the differences in training times and opportunity costs cannot be totally erased. There is also a supply-and-demand dimension that factors into the increased reimbursement rates for specialists. The numbers of specialty physicians in a given field are usually limited in most geographic regions. Patients are becoming more knowledgeable and demanding of care by specialists. Of additional concern to medical school graduates are the tremendous debt loads they carry upon graduation, often in excess of $200,000, and their future ability to pay down those loans—a worry that makes specialization more attractive in most instances.

Issues of major concern that have a behavioral impact on practicing physicians will often vary widely, not only between generalists and specialists but also among specialty physicians and their respective societies. A regulatory demand that affects a narrow range of patient care issues and physician behaviors can justifiably be viewed as a major interest by one specialty, while being effectively of no concern to generalists or other specialty groups. Similarly, an issue of health care for a specific patient cohort may be central to one specialty group, but marginal or even nonexistent to other provider groups.

Taken together, the factors encouraging specialization also serve to divide physicians into opposing camps with regard to the prioritization of concerns. The diversity of specialization renders a blanket physician management approach difficult in many respects. However, concomitant with specialization are several other categories of concern, outlined in the paragraphs that follow, that must be taken into account in an effort to arrive at effective physician management strategies.

Practice Model

A confounding factor in categorizing physician cohorts aligned along the spectrum of medical specialty fields is the practice model in which they work. In some instances practice model will trump practice specialty in terms of identifying effective management strategies.

Private practice is the traditional model of professional physician practice. Until the past few years this was the archetype that had to be understood in an effort to engage physicians in any management strategy. Each private physician's **value** set combined with his or her selected areas of practice largely determine the concerns inherent in managing that physician. Such individual concerns are often at odds with those pertaining to other parties across the value set and specialty landscape. Successful managers take these often conflicting aspects into consideration to arrive at effective management strategies. These multifaceted and often contravening concerns have made management of physicians in this environment a difficult if not impossible endeavor. An example of a private physician management conundrum emerges from hospital management's application of federal laws concerning the provision of emergency services and the availability of practitioners in the emergency setting. Such availability can seriously interfere with other patients' needs and practice concerns while placing practitioners at serious risk for malpractice lawsuits. Many physicians have been forced to withdraw from active hospital staff participation to avoid the resulting emergency coverage requirements, placing their private practice concerns above the imposed requirements. The hospital is often a loser in this situation with regard to the use of its resources and exposure to liability risks resulting from the emergency coverage rules and regulations. In the recent past, the common refrain among management scholars was that attempting to manage physicians was analogous to trying to herd cats. The private practice model still represents a significant cohort, but it is losing enlistment and struggling to maintain enrollment as the political, legal, and economic environments in health care have evolved to favor elimination of this model, especially the procedural-based specialists. The cost of starting and maintaining a solo medical practice under this model has become unacceptable in many areas and across many specialties. The disappearance of private practice will serve to remove many of the barriers attached to this model of physician management over the next decade.

Corporate practice models have grown significantly over the past decade as the challenges facing physicians who would otherwise enter the private practice sphere have increased in size and scope. Regulatory and economic overlays have made corporate practice models much more inviting. Physicians entering this environment are a step removed from burdensome start-up costs and voluminous regulatory decrees. In return for a guaranteed salary, physicians relinquish certain degrees of freedom in their decision making, both at the bedside and at business practice levels. The indirect, and sometimes direct, imposition of institutional financial concerns can weigh heavily on some practitioners, especially those who have embraced the "patient first and foremost" value set. Practice patterns are subjected to modifications in service to the corporate financial bottom line in conjunction with overriding provider financial concerns, and as a result physician management is more easily established and maintained. Managers operating within this type of model usually enforce compliance with efficiency measures that encourage lesser aggregate resource allocation per patient case. There are both beneficial and harmful dimensions to this strategy on a case-by-case basis. In the majority of cases the results have been neutral in regard to patient outcomes. Aggregate data that are self-reported by the organization are used to promote the management model. To date, many corporate practice models are in their first-generational stages, with a resultant high turnover of employed physicians. High turnover rates are a clear indicator of dissatisfaction among employed physicians that is usually hidden from public view as well as regulatory overview. A healthy bottom line is the internal metric most often used to measure the success of the organization, and it is increasingly attained at the expense of individual physicians' judgment and in many cases even patient satisfaction. Compliance with procedural mandates rather than outcome quality measures is more easily demonstrated and acceptable to external accrediting bodies and commissions facilitating government oversight. The corporate practice model is on the rise, and management strategies geared toward corporate concerns will become prevalent in the near future. Many managers in the corporate realm have come to view physicians as replaceable providers and patients as numerical clients in a strategy to meet bottom-line, short-term financial objectives.

Academic practice models offer a management standard that is more than a century old and that often serves to combine the best value-adding dimensions of the private practice and corporate practice models while minimizing their downsides. Management in the academic environment keeps patient care, education, and research at the head of the value set while maintaining appropriate respect for financial concerns. Physician commitment and organizational values are usually more in sync in this type of model than in corporate environments for the majority of practitioners. Management strategies need to embrace a wider spectrum of issues than in the other models, but managers' ability to work with practitioners rather than being at odds with them is enhanced. Management offers a buffer for practitioners between regulatory overlay and practice-level issues, and does not simply subordinate practitioner concerns. Academic practice models are more amenable to physician interests, and the complexities of integrating research, teaching, and patient care do not lead to widespread deference to financial matters. An emphasis on long-term success over short-term profits reflects the overarching time metric employed in academic practice models. For example, whether a cohort of medical students has been successfully educated will take more than a decade to establish. The success of some research initiatives and objectives may take multiple decades to determine. Powerful corporations have come to recognize the value of an academic practice model in health care and are reaching into the academic sphere in attempts to gain access to this clearly superior health care management arena. As money matters grow to trump almost all other concerns across the spectrum of health care reform, even in some academic institutions, powerful corporate entities are likely to emerge victorious in their desire to take over academic bases with which to legitimize their own health care management strategies in the minds of the public and of political leaders.

Many of the physicians within the **government practice** models are largely employed in the VA hospital system. There are also opportunities for military and state government employment, often in prisons and other institutional settings, as well as opportunities in the Indian Health Services federal program. A federally employed physician is in a position of significant safety, and is protected from market pressures and malpractice liability concerns. Even in the most litigious jurisdictions, VA physicians are protected under the Federal Tort Claims Act. This act renders bringing a malpractice action against a provider much more difficult than it is under most state laws. What is more, the institution of electronic medical records has been extensive and fairly well accepted in this atmosphere of relatively lower productivity and lessened growth expectations. The financial bottom line is an almost nonexistent worry for practicing government physicians and managers, as taxpayers always pick up the tab and upper managers have the force of the federal government behind their interactions with drug and device manufacturers and suppliers. On the downside, administrative overlay is immense, and physician initiatives at all levels are submerged under heavy layers of bureaucracy. Managers are similarly subjected to cumbersome layers of administrative burdens, which render most change initiatives difficult to effect. Government careers for physicians are often electively shorter, with the prospect of greater retirement benefits than in other models of practice.

Although these work model categories are fairly distinct from one another, it is important to understand that many physicians occupy positions in which their practice can overlap with more than one model category. Some private practitioners hold academic positions as well as VA hospital staff assignments, usually on a part-time basis. Further, there are some corporate practice models that incorporate aspects of private and academic practice as well as VA part-time membership. Private practice features appear in the form of productivity bonuses in corporate settings and fee-for-service or salary arrangements in VA settings. Physicians seek academic appointments to enhance public respect. Also, many private practitioners form allegiances with academic and corporate entities to better access services for their patients and also to provide a layer of insulation from exposure to personal risk. These combinations and permutations are driven largely by both reimbursement and service provision concerns.

All of these practice model combinations will continue to change with time as our nation's fixed-asset medical landscape is undergoing rapid ownership transformation. There is no one-size-fits-all approach to managerial decision making that will serve all practice models and combinations well. Decisions that are attractive to one cohort may be deal breakers for another. When attempting to make managerial decisions, the different concerns that are associated with the different models along with the complexities that come with overlapping models must be taken into account.

PHYSICIAN REIMBURSEMENT ISSUES

One evolving force that lends strength to the position of managers of physicians is our societal shift away from more traditional professional values toward an overriding attention to and concern for financial reward. This evolution has enticed all cohorts of citizens, including professionals of all types, to pursue monetary success as a primary goal rather than to consider financial gain as a secondary effect of providing professional services. The more thoroughly financial rewards replace patient care as the top priority in the value sets of physicians, the easier the imposition of successful management strategies. Traditional professional values, such as placing patient care at the top of one's value set as well as not creating demand by engaging in direct-to-consumer advertising, subsequently present less of a barrier to the imposition of successful management strategies. As physicians have experienced growing debt burdens and have continued to more highly prioritize monetary compensation, the reimbursement model of a given organization has become the primary determining factor in effective management strategies.

The three major categories of reimbursement models are fee-for-service, capitation, and salary. Each has nuanced subcategories, and each can be employed in any of the four practice models just discussed. The degree to which a physician's income is defined by any one or any combination of the reimbursement models will play a large part in determining which management strategies will be successful in supervising and directing physician behaviors.

Fee-for-service has long been the dominant reimbursement model across U.S. professional sectors. The definition of a fee-for-service model is rather straightforward: a provider of care receives a specified payment for a specific, individual service provided, which is characterized in terms of either a defined time period or a defined unit of work. The more work done, the more money received. This remains the accepted method of payment for services among most professions. However, because the costs associated with health care have grown disproportionately when compared with median family incomes and gross domestic product over the past few decades, this model has come under increased scrutiny. The fee-for-service model has good and bad aspects. Feldstein (2012) argues that patients have their highest confidence in physicians who receive payment in this form as opposed to capitation and salary forms. There is also the benefit of the provider's increased willingness to work harder and for longer hours to meet patient expectations, including making after-hours and weekend visits to render care. Arguments can also be made that this model encourages provider-induced demand for services, and there is truth to this claim. The result is often the provision of unnecessary services. The practice of defensive medicine lies in synergy with this model, as provider protection from lawsuits and provider income often increase hand in hand. However, many persons in policymaking positions fail to realize that physician provision of services is not the major driver of increased health care costs, and they therefore attribute more weight than is warranted to this payment model as a cause for our nation's skyrocketing health expenses. The result of the combination of factors outlined has led this model of physician payment to fall into disfavor among political and corporate leaders as well as managers. The changing behaviors and value sets of physicians are also leading to less ardent aggregate physician support for this payment model. However, fee-for-service still remains one of the major reimbursement methodologies, and it must be understood and addressed by management personnel.

Capitation was introduced on a national scale with the federal-government-incentivized push for HMOs as a means to reduce spending on patient care. According to Barsukiewicz, Raffel, and Raffel (2010), under capitation rules a physician receives a set amount of money for each patient in a group to which he or she is assigned to provide defined services, regardless of the services provided. In some cases, physicians may make additional money for providing fewer services during specified periods of time, usually in the form of year-end bonuses for having expended fewer dollars in aggregate patient care for the patients covered. The clear message in this reimbursement strategy is that the less work done, either in terms of units of work provided or time spent in patient care, the more money received per unit of work or hour of service provision. This reality is not lost on patients, many of whom question the commitment and availability of physicians who work under this system of reimbursement. Physicians who are morally driven to provide the most comprehensive patient services in what amounts to a large grey zone of "necessary care" often find themselves penalized for the expenses incurred as a result of their decisions. The penalties can be direct in the form of nonrenewal of contracts, or indirect in the form of a lack of access to bonuses paid to colleagues who expend less in the care of their covered patients. Under this form of payment, management has a significantly stronger leverage base to control provider behaviors than under fee-for-service arrangements. However, under this model provider productivity often diminishes, and patient satisfaction often suffers.

Salary reimbursement models are the fastest growing of the three model categories, as physicians are increasingly attracted to corporate employment. For the reasons outlined elsewhere in this chapter, the external and internal forces acting on the medical landscape are driving physicians away from private practice and into positions as employees of larger entities. A salary reimbursement model is the easiest under which to manage because agreements that physician behaviors will be subject to corporate regulation can be established up front in the contractual language of employment contracts. Contracts are growing in extent to cover far more than simple agreements to pay a stipulated salary in return for a defined time commitment from physicians. The wording of the contract can be massaged to capture many dimensions of physician behavior, beyond the provision of time in service to the organization. In addition to the corporate requirements, imposed federal and state behavioral mandates enter the equation and render physician autonomy a relic of the past. Just as an example, the contractual agreement in combination with attendant regulatory compliance demands can set requirements for vaccinations, disease testing, behavioral norms, and obedience to process regulations over which the physician has no say or control, unless he or she decides to break the contract. Salary reimbursement models have both good and bad aspects for the managed and the manager. On the positive side, the salaried physician is relieved of the growing burden of external regulatory overlay, startup costs, and the uncertainties of attempting to capture an effective market share. The manager is freed from the necessity of focusing undue energy on the multidimensional aspects of provider concerns outlined throughout this chapter. On the negative side, employed physicians will have their hands tied concerning many dimensions of practice behaviors. The manager often will not enjoy the cooperation of a fully committed provider cohort, as managed physicians understand that more effort will most often result in little or no increase in salary. Incentive and bonus clauses written into the contract may offset some of the loss of potential productivity, but many physicians entering this model are geared toward a lower productivity goal in return for more time to commit to concerns outside of their medical career. On balance, a salary reimbursement model offers the best opportunities to engage in effective physician management strategies, especially where there is buy-in by the managed physician.

An often overlooked physician management concern is the compatibility of value sets of both the targeted physician and the managing entity. Values alone are not predictive of behaviors. Rather, it is value sets—the prioritized inventories of values held—that determine human behaviors. The difference between individual, held values and inculcated value sets can be enormous in terms of their effect on behavior patterns in response to management strategies. Understanding this difference is essential to successful management.

For instance, a practicing physician and a managing party can both hold values that include high-quality patient care and institutional financial well-being. When those values are in good alignment, the parties will be very satisfied in their management relationship. However, when the same values are held in differing alignments, the result can spell disaster. If a physician places the quality of patient care above all other concerns, major problems can arise. For example, the desire to provide the best possible care to a patient may result in the transfer of a well-insured or wealthy self-pay patient from one hospital to another institution that offers better-quality services to address the problem confronting the patient. The transfer decision, which will result in lost revenues, can meet with serious disfavor among the management team as well as other physician staff members. The management outcome can create huge barriers to that physician's ability to practice in the institution that places institutional reputation and financial concerns above individual patients' well-being. Alternatively, for the indigent uninsured or poorly insured patient whose ongoing presence represents a drain on institutional finances, just the opposite scenario will often play out along the physician management spectrum. Transfer of the nonpaying or little-paying patient out of the facility to avoid further financial drain is an accepted management strategy, even if the transfer is to a venue of lower-quality care.

In summary, value sets determine attitudes and behaviors. In the case of practicing physicians, the individual physician's value set defines his or her prioritization of such matters as patient care concerns, personal and family issues, and organizational allegiances. It is also important for management to understand that although value sets are the main determinants of physician responses to administrative input, these arrangements of values, some conscious and some subconscious, are subject to change over time.

PATIENT QUALITY OF CARE CONCERNS

Among managers of physicians in corporate and institutional practices, one of the most disliked value sets is that of the time-honored physician whose top three priorities are (1) patient care, (2) patient care, and (3) patient care. That type of physician will not be welcome in the majority of institutional, especially corporate, settings, in which organizational financial strength is no lower than a close second in priority on the value set ladder, and is often the unspoken top priority. There are too many grey zones of decision making along the patient care continuum, all of which have significant associated cost differentials, to accede to the judgment of a physician who always places quality patient outcomes as the top priority with less regard for the financial impacts on the institution of patient care decisions.

Management also must understand that a physician's placing a top value on the quality of patient care has nuanced meanings that can significantly influence behavioral responses from both the manager and that physician. Although the majority of physicians will state that they place patient well-being at the top of their value set, they will have diverging views of what constitutes the best philosophical approach to achieving that goal. These differing approaches will often force managers to alter how they attempt to control physician behaviors. The major classifications of approaches to patient care priorities include physician paternalism and patient autonomy, each with subcategories that include beneficence, nonmaleficence, and justice.

Historically, physician **paternalism** was the norm. The physician was the sole proprietor of the decision-making process regarding individual patient health care choices. This paradigm was based on assumptions of a huge asymmetry of medical knowledge between the physician and the patient; full faith in the ability of the physician to understand the patient's needs and desires; and trust in the ability and willingness of the physician to comprehend and employ medical knowledge and treatments effectively while above all else doing no harm. This model has fallen into disfavor over the past half century as a result of wider availability of medical knowledge, legal precedents, third-party payer pressures, and devolution of the individual physician-patient relationship. Concomitant with the decline of physician paternalism, there has been growth in institutional and government paternalism. These emerging alternative types of paternalism are often established under the appearance of primary concern for patient well-being, most often in the form of promulgated standards of care requiring providers to adhere to a set patient care process.

The concept of **patient autonomy** has emerged and prevailed as the accepted approach to medical decision making. The law recognizes that an adult of sound mind and body has the ability and the right to decide whether to accept or reject health care recommendations made by those providing health care. The burden lies with the provider to offer, in an accessible form, the information necessary to allow a patient, or the patient's legal surrogate, to make a reasonable decision concerning health care choices. This falls under the concept of informed consent and is a major issue that managers must deal with effectively. Although the definition of reasonable informed consent varies from jurisdiction to jurisdiction, the ultimate arbiter of this concern is a lay jury. In addition to the many risk-benefit issues that must be spelled out, along with associated cost-benefit concerns that are often left unspoken, increasingly present cultural and language barriers must be accounted for in management strategies concerning informed consent to recommendations for patient care. One government requirement is to provide interpreters to meet this challenge. What had traditionally been a need to provide a translator for a patient who is not fluent in English has evolved into a multilane language highway that includes the need to supply a translator to compensate for some physicians' own English language shortcomings when caring for English-speaking patients. Cultural differences present an even more challenging barrier to effective informed consent that falls in the realm of managerial responsibilities.

Patient autonomy is being challenged by standard of care mandates that emerge from regulatory and accrediting bodies. Standardization, which has beneficial as well as harmful dimensions, has begun to replace physician judgment at the physician-patient interface. The result is likely to be less patient autonomy in medical decision making as we move forward with institutional and government paternalism, which includes rationing of care, especially to the elderly. Standard of care mandates will probably lessen the problems associated with cultural and language diversity because there will be less latitude for decision making among patients.

Both physician paternalism and patient autonomy have philosophical subcategories that add differing definitional perspectives. **Beneficence** offers the perspective that medical decisions should be geared toward offering the patient help in attaining either an optimal or at least an improved physiological and psychological health status, with the understanding that all actions as well as inactions carry risks and benefits. **Nonmaleficence** is understood as the obligation, above all else, to do no harm, either intentionally or unintentionally through actions or inaction. **Justice** takes into consideration such elements as equity, needs, merit, and the rights and responsibilities of the parties to medical decision-making. Whereas the beneficence and nonmaleficence subcategories are easily applicable on an individual, case-by-case basis, the justice subcategory calls aggregate population concerns more fully into play, and may find more resistance at the bedside than it would in the administrative office when providers and patients are making decisions about personal medical care. Put another way, there is a difference between rendering recommendations to real patients as opposed to statistical patients. The justice perspective is most easily applied to population statistics, whereas beneficence and nonmaleficence are more readily transferred to the bedside and acceptable to real patients and families.

The impacts of these principles' complex interactions on physician behavior are far reaching. For a manager it is important to understand that the often unstated and at best poorly articulated moral philosophy of patient care that guides individual physicians in their decision making can make it difficult for practitioners to comply with managerial decisions, regardless of the apparent reasonableness of those decisions from a managerial perspective at the corporate office level. A manager should have in his or her arsenal of understanding a basic knowledge of these multiple philosophical dimensions and their influence on physician behavior. These can be brought to the table in a way that diffuses disagreements between managers and managed physicians and increases physician willingness to comply with managerial decisions. Absent an understanding of these principles, managers are often at a loss to address the behavior of noncompliant providers effectively. In addition, an understanding of these issues can elevate the quality of management deliberations in service to patient care while remaining true to corporate well-being.

PHYSICIAN CONCERNS

Just a couple of generations ago the priority standard inculcated in the medical student population was that of professionalism, with patient care concerns placed above all else. Although not always adopted by practicing physicians, this was the top priority for the majority who entered the profession. These physicians often neglected personal and family concerns to meet this professional medical standard. The costs were often severe for many in regard to their personal and family lives. Today this prioritization scheme does not prevail to the overwhelming degree it did in medical training. For those physicians who still place their concern for patients above their personal and family issues, it should be expected that patient concerns will also trump institutional priorities.

Personal and Family Concerns

Growing numbers of physicians are replacing the old model of professionalism with one that places top priority on personal and family concerns. These concerns are also likely to prevail over those of the institution to the extent that institutional ownership and control of physicians do not explicitly allow practitioners to give sufficient attention to their own personal matters. The private practitioner is, somewhat ironically, best positioned to serve both personal and family agendas as well as patient-first agendas before corporate concerns. For the employed physician, when these priorities clash the result is often a parting of ways, with resultant high turnover rates among physician employees. Successful management strategies must afford leeway to physicians in addressing personal and family concerns, and contractual agreements should respect these issues.

The types of concerns that will fall under personal agendas include compensation, length of work days, time on call, vacation time, sick days, scope of practice, freedom to make patient care decisions, coverage arrangements, and ability to identify and address manifold other issues as they arise. Family concerns will, in addition to health and well-being, include the financial situation of the physician, with emphasis placed on current and anticipated debt loads, practice costs, accrued savings, planning for retirement, and net worth considerations. These subjects of personal and family concern will be approachable in different ways, depending on the physician's practice model and specialty. In addition, reimbursement models will have a heavy impact on these issues.

In terms of the family status of the practitioner, physicians who are married with children will most likely have this area of attention at the top of their value set. Unmarried and uncommitted physicians without children or other family obligations, such as caring for elderly parents or covering alimony and child support costs, will often place other values higher on their prioritization schedule. Managers need to take these multiple dimensions of outside-of-practice concerns into consideration to differing degrees, with the understanding that changes should be expected over time. The shift from the old model of professionalism toward new models, especially those focusing on financial concerns, does make intervention into physician behaviors by management more acceptable across the physician landscape.

A review of Abraham Maslow's hierarchy of needs (discussed briefly in Chapter Two) can enhance managers' understanding of the work-life balance issues embodied in this chapter's review. This standard teaching in managerial and marketing courses points out a series of requisite needs that must be satisfied to achieve personal fulfillment through self-actualization, the highest level of realized potential.

At each of Maslow's five levels there are appropriate management interventions that can help physicians achieve their needs. These interventions include working to facilitate satisfactory reimbursement; safety in the work environment; meaningful interpersonal relationships; appropriate, positive evaluations; and the delegation of reasonably achievable, value-adding goals. Although Maslow's theory is neither universally applicable nor unequivocally accepted, in our culture of individualism it adds an important perspective to management oversight. In collectivist cultures it is less useful.

Practice maturity represents another dimension of personal concern that factors heavily into the equation of acceptance of managerial decisions. Practices that are in the infancy or start-up phase confront significant costs and uncertainties that offer managing entities more latitude in forming associations with the young physician or physician group. Start-up physicians may demonstrate a willingness to sacrifice never-experienced behavioral freedoms to reduce risks and ensure incomes. Healthy practices in their more mature phases that are running smoothly and meeting expectations are more resistant to change. It is more difficult to gain a position of effective management leverage when a physician has a mature practice if the medical environment is stable. However, with the huge waves of uncertainty fomented by the onslaught of legislative and regulatory initiatives introduced in and emanating from the PPACA since 2010, there exist opportunities for larger entities to capture these locally and regionally lucrative practices. Many of these practitioners have assumed financial commitments based on assumptions of stability that place them at risk in the rapidly changing medical economic environment. For practices that have attained seniority status in which the energy and enthusiasm of the practitioners are winding down, managing entities may find a more willing acceptance of subservience to management oversight in return for assurances of what amount to comfort measures that protect the practitioners from competition, ensure more personal time, and provide for a steady income in return for acquired market share by the managing organization.

In summary, personal and family concerns have grown to majority status in the minds of most young physicians who are emerging from altered education and training atmospheres and entering a highly regulated and increasingly uncertain medical economic environment. Managers should be aware of these shifts in priorities and the reasons underlying the changes over time.

Organizational Concerns

Physicians across all generalist and specialist divisions and practice models deal both personally and professionally with a maze of organizations, both directly and indirectly. Depending on the extent of their organizational associations this concern can vary widely across the value sets of physicians both within an institution and across multiple organizations. It is at the organization-physician interface that the rubber meets the road regarding many management strategies.

A plethora of organizations are involved in physician management. These include third-party payers, corporate health care entities, regulatory bodies, accrediting organizations, community hospitals, academic health centers, volunteer organizations, service suppliers, drug and device manufacturers and suppliers, and professional societies. All have interests in physician management for widely varying reasons. Some of these entities have direct physician management interests and responsibilities; others have indirect or peripheral approaches to physician management. Many of these managing sources overlap the same physician or physician group, and their respective perspectives on physician behaviors are often in conflict concerning their respective organizational goals.

The category of third-party payers includes government, for-profit, nonprofit, and quasi-government entities. Management from one perspective can include concerns similar to those of other sources of reimbursement, but these differing sources of management oversight can also be at odds. Certain third-party payers have much more control over physician behaviors. Other payers are subject to fraud and abuse at higher rates. Certain payers will gain the respect and allegiance of physicians and physician groups; others will be sources of disdain and avoidance. For managers, the approach to physicians will vary widely among these third-party payers, and this needs to be understood by those who enter the physician management field. The third-party payer with the most powerful influence is Medicare. Medicare decisions concerning both reimbursement schedules and compliance with increasingly burdensome standards of care spill over into the strategies of many other third-party payers in dealing with physicians. The Medicare Sustainable Growth Rate reimbursement formula is the major existing financial threat to providers of covered services. Under the PPACA, the Independent Payment Advisory Board represents a major source of contention for practicing physicians, particularly in regard to its further government-imposed price controls on physician reimbursement. The political and economic course we are on as a nation suggests to many observers that we are headed for a single-payer system over the next couple of decades, with the possible emergence of an alternative market of private providers to serve private payers. In addition, the medical tourism industry is rapidly emerging in response to the huge costs that regulatory overlay and profiteering are imposing on our health care economy. The number of patients traveling offshore to receive surgical services is growing rapidly on a yearly basis as the costs associated with similar services are multiples less offshore than they are in the United States, largely as a result of provider freedom from regulatory burdens and legal risks outside of this country.

Corporate entities are a fast-growing segment of our health care landscape. Large intrastate and multistate hospital owners, representing powerful special interests driving legislative and regulatory agendas, are growing in influence. Smaller corporate entities are subject to acquisition strategies by larger corporations. Managers in these smaller organizations must realize the uncertain future that awaits them, as their ability to influence physician behaviors may be irrelevant among the higher-ups in the expansive and growing conglomerates. Management behaviors that are effective on smaller scales may be of no interest to larger and more controlling organizations. Physicians are experiencing similar uncertainty concerning their future ability to render care in their customary fashion. These corporate entities believe that they can profit handsomely by inserting themselves between payers and providers of services in the health care field. The result for physicians and for some of those who manage physician practices is a shrinking slice of the health care economic pie as a consequence of administrative, bureaucratic, and shareholder overlay.

Regulatory bodies have burgeoned under recent federal and state legislative initiatives. Virtually every aspect of health care delivery in any model is subject to heavy regulatory oversight. Regulatory organizations are often held in disrespect but also in fearful regard by most parties in the health care economy, including not only physician providers of care but also corporate entities, insurers, and community hospitals. A few parties are benefiting from the heavy overload of regulatory decrees, including large, growing corporations seeking to acquire smaller entities that are buckling under the pressures of government oversight and control. In addition, increasing classes of nonphysician providers of care (including nurse practitioners, physician assistants, pharmacologists, optometrists, and so on) are benefiting through the acquisition of expanded patient care roles as a result of physician manpower shortages, which are growing in part due to the increasingly burdensome regulatory climate. Managers at all levels of physician activity, including managers working on behalf of these regulatory organizations, need to be aware of this emerging trend. Physicians for the most part stand in opposition to these entities and the increasing pressures they exert on the physician-patient health care interface. Depending on which side of the regulatory divide a manager sits, physician management in this environment will require different approaches based on differing goals and expectations.

Accrediting organizations have emerged as a growth industry that fills a void between health care entities and government regulatory bodies. Much in the same way that middlemen insinuate themselves between hands-on providers of care and payers, accrediting organizations have found a rewarding niche between health care entities (including physician providers, insurers, institutions, and drug and device manufacturers, to name a few) and regulators at all levels. Most observers view these accrediting entities as non-value-adding parties within the health care field. All physicians are subjected to their oversight and evaluations. Most physicians are averse to the mostly indirect management pressures these organizations apply to their behaviors. Managers of physicians need to understand this hidden organizational reality because it affects physicians' attitudes and behaviors and can heavily influence success or failure in practice outcomes.

Community hospitals are disappearing across our nation's health care landscape. These organizations once were held in fairly high esteem by practicing physicians, as they provided venues for patient care delivery that were not reasonable or possible in an office or outpatient setting. The physicians held sway over community hospital administrative decisions, and they experienced little management imposition on their hospital practices. Today's medical regulatory and economic environment has resulted in many community hospitals either closing their doors or selling out to larger entities. The result is fewer but larger inpatient entities for which practicing physicians often hold little or no respect in regard to the organizational mission, which is most often viewed as being primarily in service to bottom-line profitability. What had constituted friendly management arrangements between small community hospitals and most physicians have devolved into adversarial relationships between many physician providers and administrators of large corporate entities that control access to dwindling numbers of inpatient facilities. This change has been the product of multiple forces outlined in this chapter, and it is a growing concern for private physicians and private physician groups. For physicians employed in a corporate practice model the adversarial nature of the relationships between providers and administrators is less apparent. We have entered a second round of hospital acquisition of physician practices. The first round, which occurred in the 1980s and 1990s, was a resounding failure from the vantage points of both hospitals and physicians, as productivity and patient and provider satisfaction declined significantly along with the acquiring facilities' financial bottom line. The ongoing second round involves larger and more powerful institutions facing far fewer competitive pressures and a more corporate-minded and financially strapped young physician cohort. Corporate managers whose strategies resulted in financial disasters during the previous round of practice buyouts are now better positioned to succeed because of the climatic changes in the health care economy and altered physician training regimens.

Academic health centers have represented an exception to the general rules and practice concerns just outlined. These institutions have maintained a high degree of respect among the physician population for their mission of improving the health care of our nation's inhabitants. Many physicians have sought to be associated with these centers for the dual purposes of giving their patients greater access to higher-quality care and also enhancing their own reputation in the communities they serve. Management issues are less offensive to private physicians and physician groups in this arms-length association. For physicians employed by the academic health center, management concerns are usually more in sync with those of the practitioners than they are in the nonacademic realm. Both managers and the managed understand that they are there to uphold missions of education, research, and patient care. The academic health center itself is usually under the auspices of a larger university with a centuries-old mission that again serves agendas concerning education, research, and the public good. With these multifaceted top priorities, financial gain has been relegated to a lower tier on the organizational ladder of values. The unpleasant reality of increasing regulatory overlay and powerful special interests across the health care economic landscape has meant that even academic health centers are beginning to bow to pressures that divert focus and attention away from education, research, and patient care and toward monetary issues. Corporate entities are actively seeking and accessing greater influence and control over these institutions. Managers of physicians, including physicians in managerial positions, need to be cognizant of this dimension of the health care environment, as it has both direct and indirect impacts on physicians practicing at all levels.

Volunteer organizations have traditionally represented one of the purest work environments concerning service to the mission of providing care to patients in need. The attraction of such organizations for physicians has been their ability to pursue a medical mission without needing to take into account the multiple confounding factors that play a role in successful medical business management. However, what was once an area free from the burdensome oversight of most other practice management concerns has become one of increasing complexity. For instance, medical malpractice carriers often justifiably dissuade their covered private physicians from engaging in such voluntary activities because of the attendant exposure to malpractice liability, which is intensified by the typical absence of an established doctor-patient relationship and the lack of serial, well-documented patient records. One result of this metamorphosis from the pure and simple donation of services to increasing **liability exposure** has been a move by physicians to volunteer their services overseas. At foreign venues in underdeveloped countries, volunteer providers of care are insulated from liability exposure and are free to offer their services essentially without fear of legal risk. A couple of generations ago medical students and residents were taught to expect that about 15 percent of their work would go to the needy without compensation. This understanding was acknowledged and accepted by most physicians in training and carried over into their professional practices.

However, intense efforts are continuously expended across our nation to hold physicians fully liable under medical malpractice tort law for donated services, and this is a strong dissuader of physician volunteerism on American soil. Managers in the medical malpractice insurance industry are well aware of this issue. Medical managers in office and institutional settings need to be cognizant of the risks attached to volunteer work in the United States and the heavy costs that may accrue as a result.

Service suppliers are a source of growing input into all physician practices as well as institutional settings. The spectrum of outsourced services is vast. Legal and accounting issues are pushing many large institutions toward outsourcing traditional in-house services. These entities are having an increasingly significant impact on physicians at all levels of practice, representing influences on direct and indirect patient care as well as substantial and growing costs. Managers are continually challenged by this cohort of service suppliers, and practicing physicians for the most part want to avoid spending time dealing with the issues pertaining to the provision of services that are perceived as being either too costly or suboptimal. Areas that provide outsourced management input on physician behaviors include health information technology providers of hardware, software, and support services. With the $20 billion earmarked in the PPACA of 2010 for what amounts to premature, widespread adoption of electronic medical records there has been explosive growth in entities that provide and manage information technology. Health information technology service suppliers to date have provided high-cost products that have had marginal effectiveness in meeting "meaningful use" standards toward which health care reform legislation is aimed. These vendors are having a substantial impact on physicians across the spectrum of practice models and specialties, as they are on health care organizations. This is an area of management expertise that has ample room for growth and development, as it is currently in a formative stage with huge sums of money earmarked for access by special interests. Other suppliers with which physicians often come into daily contact offer day-to-day, routine services, such as maintenance, room service, and groundskeeping. There are growing cohorts of evaluation entities that will oversee regulatory compliance measures, such as those required by HIPAA, across all venues and practice settings. Managers must also interface with communication, legal, taxation, and retirement investment organizations to cover the full range of physician interests. A practice manager in a single-physician solo practice should be versed in all of these service supplier areas. Some of these supplier organizations will be held in high regard by physicians, others will be viewed with disdain, and many will be disregarded almost entirely. Depending on where each organization sits on the physician's scale of interest and regard, management will be challenged to a greater or lesser degree. Even in large-group and institutional corporate practice models these concerns will come into play from time to time.

Drug and device manufacturers and suppliers continue to exert major influence over physician behaviors, even though regulations have significantly curtailed their ability to directly compensate practicing physicians for their time and attention to distributing their products. Although pharmaceutical and technological advances have added significant value to patient care, these organizations are adept at targeting both patients and health care providers at all levels with strategies that result in the increased use of their products, often at vastly inflated prices. Managers need to protect their physicians from entrapment in behaviors that have been deemed unacceptable by regulatory decrees. At higher administrative levels in large organizations the ability of these business corporations to influence bulk purchases of their products is impressive. Some of these parties have even played significant roles in funding studies and ghostwriting articles that show the advantages of using their products, resulting in increased marketability and profits. Thoughtful managers of physicians in large organizations should be aware of these strategies and encourage physicians to avoid any unnecessary use of such products, thereby reducing patient care costs and helping the organizational bottom line. Unfortunately, some of these manufacturers are so surreptitious and effective in influencing physicians, managers, and organizations, even at national standard of care mandate setting levels, that they have prevailed over common sense and proper disclosure and peer review requirements. If engaged in appropriately, this manager-physician interface concerning relationships with drug and device manufacturers provides another dimension of physician management that can have salutary effects not only on patient care but also on the health care organizational balance sheet.

Professional societies represent a broad array of opportunities for organizational memberships and participatory roles that attract each physician's allegiance to varying degrees based on his or her value set. As already mentioned, physicians have turned away from general societies, which have proven relatively ineffective in advocating for the best interests of both patients and members. This inability to address membership concerns is a result of structural barriers to flexible and effective advocacy, such as rapid turnover of elected leadership as well as bureaucratic entrenchment. Yearly societal elections, with their requisite change of officers, result in a lack of both spokesperson continuity and a consistently articulated agenda. Administrative expansion over time adds an unspoken element of self-perpetuation to the societal mission, and this often supersedes willingness to effectively address specific concerns of membership. The result has been a loss of physician allegiance to long-established general societies, such as the American Medical Association, and state medical societies, with concurrent increased attention to more recently chartered specialty societies. Specialty societies tend to be more conversant with and more responsive to membership concerns across the spectrum, from providing timely political advocacy concerning legislative and regulatory issues, to advancing specialty knowledge and offering continuing education credits that apply to specialty practices. Physician management plays a role both from within each societal structure as well as from the position of the practicing physician who is contemplating which societal affiliations will best serve his or her concerns. Management needs to account for physician interest in professional societal membership and participation.

PROFESSIONAL ETHICAL CONCERNS

What was once a profession marked by the public perception of an overarching commitment to the Hippocratic Oath, and in particular to "above all do no harm," has become a profession of confusing and often confounding medical ethical concerns. Managers should have at least a minimal working familiarity with the Hippocratic Oath and its modern iterations. The original oath held physicians to several responsibilities that are increasingly at odds with modern standards of care, including avoiding the performance of surgery, which was the province of "barbers"; giving preferential consideration to children of doctors in regard to medical education; refusing to participate in abortions; and refusing to participate in euthanasia and legal executions. Today there are multiple more modern versions of the oath that are more compatible with societal norms, and most medical schools administer a form of the oath to students. Patient well-being based on professional responsibility lies at the core of the oath's modern renditions.

The American Medical Association has a detailed *Code of Medical Ethics*. This code makes passing reference to the Hippocratic Oath and its modern iterations. The code book runs to almost five hundred pages of text, with many hundreds of medical and legal references addressing over two hundred areas of concern related to medical practice. The code is published every two years, and new opinions are issued every six months. This text actually finds its way into courts of law when certain physician behaviors are brought under legal scrutiny. Of significance, and in contradistinction to corporate mandated physician behaviors, the book states that "ethical obligations typically exceed legal duties," and further that in exceptional circumstances "ethical responsibilities should supersede legal obligations" (Council on Ethical and Judicial Affairs, 2008, p. 1). These clearly stated ethical mandates are often lost on institutional and regulatory managers, but they are inherent in the attitudes of most practicing physicians. The result often manifests itself in the form of physician opposition to legislative oversight, with managers caught between regulatory mandates and physician behaviors.

The continuing evolution of our medical landscape along the path of expanding legal influence, ranging from general government oversight to individual malpractice cases, plays a large role in the changing definition and application of medical ethics. This will become an area of growing concern for managers as our nation's population and physician cohorts culturally diversify, as health care costs continue to skyrocket, as financial concerns come to trump ethical considerations at all levels of physician and management behavior, and as political processes and the law capture growing and eventually majority status in health care decision making.

An area of increasingly significant influence on some physicians' beliefs and behaviors is religious background. Traditionally our nation has been one in which the ethical obligations of the medical profession have been in sync with the religious beliefs of the vast majority of physicians, patients, and managers. Increasing diversity of religious beliefs challenges the former status quo. In many respects this issue dovetails with ethical concerns. To varying degrees religious affiliation will play a role in a physician's decision making and behaviors. The influence of religious beliefs on a case-by-case basis can range from nonexistent, to minimal, to major, sometimes even resulting in a physician's refusal to render services in response to a patient's desire to receive a medically acceptable intervention. The more religiously diverse our nation becomes, the more likely it is that personal religious beliefs will influence both professional and patient behaviors. Traditionally most physicians have subordinated personal religious beliefs to medical concerns, including most dimensions of patient care, legal overlay, and medical ethics. This approach to patient care is likely to continue among the majority of physician providers of care. However, some physicians place religious concerns at a higher level in their value set and are willing to override other medical and legal concerns. Managers must take this dimension of each physician into account. At the physician-patient interface physicians appear to be more willing to suppress their religious convictions to serve the best interests of their patients. However, the religious beliefs of a physician can be a major factor in determining his or her responses at the physician-management interface. Laws directed at the interface of religion with patient care decisions are subject to change with each election cycle. Federal legislation to date has attempted to address this issue, currently having a limited impact on medical decision making and the delivery of patient care. The scope of legal interjection into the religious realm of medical care will expand as we move forward. Although this is sometimes an area in which people fear to tread in discussions among parties to a decision, managers at all levels of involvement need to understand and account for the religious dimension of each practitioner.

POLITICAL AND LEGAL AFFILIATIONS AND CONCERNS

Political party affiliations represent another dimension of physician management that appears to be gaining prominence. Historically physicians have remained relatively quiet concerning political favoritism. Politics was a field of activity that did not find favor among most medical professionals because it added little to their ability to address patient concerns, and because little if any good would come from patient or public awareness of a provider's affiliation with a political party. There is no question that the role of government across the health care landscape has grown significantly over recent decades. This scenario will continue to evolve and will affect physician behaviors at all levels, from bedside physician-patient interactions and case-by-case decision making to more global medical concerns. Although the major political parties appear to share some aspects of their respective medical-political agendas, they are in conflict over other agenda items. At the divide between political parties concerning control over physician behaviors there are differences that attract individual physicians to particular party affiliations. This is a dimension of physician attitudes and behaviors of which managers should be aware and that they should be willing to address. With the acrimonious political debates over health care reform that have emerged in the past few years there is a growing dissatisfaction among physicians with regard to political processes in general as they apply to the delivery of health services. At the management level, anticipating and preparing for political interventions and mandates are essential to success. The political affiliation dimension of physician management can be a difficult divide to bridge. Convincing physicians and physician groups either to acquiesce or to buy into strategies that provide political protection while accommodating and promoting organizational growth is an important factor in managers' effectiveness in corporate and academic practice settings.

There exists a wide variety of medical-legal issues that require management's attention. All aspects of the health care landscape are subject to legal oversight. Although entire textbooks are devoted to this subject, just a few specific legal issues that have an impact on the physician-management interface and do not appear routinely in most management texts will be briefly examined here.

A major dimension of successful management of physicians is the ability to transfer liability exposure for personal injury from the managing entity or institution to the practicing physician. Quality improvement programs teach that approximately 80 to 85 percent of medical errors are due to system failure rather than individual provider error. Add to this the increasingly intrusive impact of government entities and accrediting bodies on the patient care process and the result is that the organization's management must account for the growing risk of liability exposure in relation to the organizational bottom line. This presents a problem given the associated, increasingly heavy-handed organizational strategy of imposing behaviors on practitioners through the implementation of standards of care while seeking to avoid responsibility for practitioner decisions and service provision. A successful strategy that remains hidden from the physician's awareness, that of both the employee and the private practitioner, is requiring practitioners to sign on to "hold harmless" and in some cases "indemnification" clauses as a condition when accessing institutional electronic medical records and databases. The shrouded insertion of such language into electronic agreements has served vendors of EMRs well and has provided a layer of protection for institutions. It is a fact that adherence to standards of care will not result in universally beneficial outcomes, and in some cases it will result in harmful effects. Successful physician management involves the managing entity's ability to avoid liability exposure for system failures as well as institutionally imposed standardization of approaches to patient care. The use of hold harmless and indemnification clauses has become a widespread and effective management tool for avoiding liability exposure to the practicing physicians in relation to imposed patient care behaviors, system failures, and EMR hardware and software shortcomings that result in harm to patients.

An additional, a hidden medical-legal dimension of physician practice is the cohort of doctors who strongly support the current tort system of medical malpractice. A significant number of practicing physicians derive a substantial part, and in some cases a large majority, of their income from participation in the medical malpractice arena. This cohort includes those who occupy administrative positions in the malpractice industry, those who secretly instigate malpractice cases, and those who provide testimony as expert witnesses. Payment in return for expert opinions represents a form of reimbursement not addressed in the earlier section on reimbursement models. For these physicians, it is important to perform a minimal number of procedures on an ongoing basis in a given specialty to qualify as an expert witness, but their drive to provide services is severely restrained. The payment they receive from the attorneys representing the parties to a malpractice action, in addition to covered expenses, can be well in excess of $1,000 per hour. This far surpasses almost all fee-for-service, capitation, and salary reimbursement models for physician services. A manager of physicians should be wary of this growing number of practicing physicians, some of whom may serve as surreptitious identifiers and instigators of malpractice cases against providers and institutions in return for various forms of compensation. In addition, these hidden sources of reimbursement can have a significant impact on these physician behaviors in response to managerial decisions that would otherwise appear rational and acceptable.

Medical staff bylaws allow managing entities to gain greater control over the behaviors of both institutionally employed and nonemployed physicians. This area of physician agreements in hospital settings had traditionally been left to physician staff members to design and deploy. Over the past couple of decades, however, the drafting of these bylaw documents has come under increasing organizational scrutiny and control as reducing liability exposure, being in compliance with regulatory measures, and increasing organizational net income have emerged as high priorities on managers' radar screens. Bylaw documents have become an effective means of increasing institutional control over physician behaviors. In the past these documents would often remain virtually unchanged over many years or even a decade or more. Currently it is not unusual to see yearly updates and amendments to these agreements as the legal and economic dimensions of hospital management are subjected to constantly changing pressures. Institutional control over the content of these documents is more easily accomplished as the ratio of employed to independent physicians on the hospital staff increases. A hospital's control over a physician's reimbursement can have profound effects on the physician's willingness to accede to certain changes in bylaws. The legal wording of bylaw documents can have profound effects on the hospital's ability to define acceptable physician behaviors, covering topics ranging from interactions with patients, staff, and the administration to compliance with education, documentation, meeting attendance, and reporting requirements, as well as on-call service responsibilities. Bylaws that make reference to physician behaviors have an impact on the hospital's ability to comply with federal and state rules and regulations, including such items as HIPAA and EMTALA. Such concerns as physician discipline and discharge from medical staffs are greatly affected to the advantage of the hospital by physicians' agreeing to and signing the medical staff bylaws. Managers, both those working for the institution and those representing the interests of physicians, should be conversant with the items contained in bylaw documents.

PHYSICIAN MANAGEMENT MODELS

There are multiple ways to classify management strategies for overseeing physicians. The following paragraphs list four management options that allow reflection and introspection on the part of managers with regard to their approach to their duties and their involvement at the physician-management interface. It should be understood that no one option is fully descriptive of any manager's total behavioral package. Also, an effective manager will occasionally feel the need to shift his or her position between the models to achieve optimal outcomes.

Power management models are growing in favor and application. This represents the ability to dictate rather than negotiate managerial decisions. In past times, when most physicians were independent private practitioners with multiple hospital affiliation options, these models were marginally effective. Today, with a fast-growing majority of physicians occupying employee positions and with far fewer hospital affiliation options available, this approach to administrative decision making is gaining applicability. There are circumstances in which a need for urgent or emergent decision making may be best served by this type of model. In addition, some managers have been able to convert otherwise elective decision-making concerns into apparently urgent or emergent conditions to justify this approach to management in certain situations. However, even among physicians who acquiesce to a power management model, usually because of financial dependence based on their employee status, this approach to management is largely disfavored by those who are being managed. Once physicians have been exposed to such dictates by managers, an attitude of disrespect may be fostered that will impair future physician-management relations.

Powerless management models have been traditionally used in the past. These represent a largely hands-off attitude that was more appropriate when management faced far fewer regulatory, financial, and liability exposure concerns. In addition, when nearly all physicians were self-employed, and thus essentially not manageable as a group when it came to their hospital and institutional affiliations, there was far less latitude for managers to engage successfully in any other management model. Even today some who occupy managerial positions view their specific period of tenure as a lame-duck term in which they need not impose pressures on themselves to act on issues, which will simply be passed on to future occupants of their position. Also, although it may be true that some problems, if ignored, will dissolve, the majority of existing and emerging concerns call for attention and a willingness to apply effort to improve the work environment. This approach to physician management may find favor among physicians, but for the most part this represents an abdication of managerial responsibilities.

Principled management models are the most ethical and effective over the long term. In health care the three cardinal ethical principles of behavior are truthfulness, trustworthiness, and integrity. Applying these ethical constructs to all physician-management relationships over time will result in a state of synergy involving honorable providers of care, long-term improvement in regard to institutional effectiveness, and success in service to the mission. Truthfulness calls for the truth, the whole truth, and nothing but the truth in combination with full transparency. Trustworthiness calls for the ability and willingness to meet or exceed the expectations raised and promises made at all levels of interaction. Integrity calls for a keen sense of knowing right from wrong; the willingness to speak to the difference, even when such speech is unpopular; the willingness to act on the difference, even at personal cost; and the fulfillment of these elements day in and day out, year in and year out, without exception. These are principles of human behavior that nurture strong relationships and successful organizational structures over the long term. However, these principles are too often viewed as unnecessary barriers to short-term goal achievement, and most managers will fail to apply them consistently. These principles are also subject to abuse by dishonorable parties engaged in physician-management relationships. This type of model works best when both sides of the management-managed divide adhere to these principles. The more powerful of the parties in a physician-management relationship is more responsible for the model's application.

Pragmatic management is the model most commonly employed across our health care landscape. It is essentially one of deal making, or quid pro quo status, between parties to an agreement. On the surface this appears to make sense, but as the deals made accumulate, the latitude for effectively responding to future problems becomes constrained. Managers who have long-standing deals with numerous managed parties or entities are less flexible in their range of approaches to future issues as a result of the need to avoid breaking bargains made with others, which can and will result in the loss of support from and confidence of past parties to agreements. Rather than making decisions on the basis of what appears to be the right approach, the manager's operative strategy ends up being to offend as few important stakeholders with whom deals have been struck as possible. Although the pragmatic model may at times represent an easier approach to the many problems at hand, the long-term result is often worsened relationships that interfere with organizational success. The overarching approach by very top management is often to dismiss those in managerial positions who have accumulated a heavy web of quid pro quo restraints. These repetitive dismissals serve as a means of diffusing adverse sentiments among the targets of management while maintaining the advantages of the deals made. Boards of directors are placed in the position of finding replacements on a regular basis for pragmatic CEOs and top institutional managers.

Today's rapidly changing health care environment has resulted in most managers' assuming the position of a **pragmatic chameleon** who shifts from one to another of these four models as circumstances change. Depending on the perceived value and strength of a party to an agreement, a manager can choose any of the models to craft a relationship. With those viewed as weak and of little or no significance, a power management model is often effective, provided that the party has been correctly assessed and remains inconsequential. With more powerful and intransigent parties, a powerless approach may prevail, as any resistance may come at significant expense to the manager and the organization. Occasionally a principled approach to issues that are of little relevance but that are high in public profile will bolster an organization's reputation in a way that pays immediate dividends in terms of public perception. The fact is that the infrequently employed principled approach to concerns is the most ethically correct and best serves the long-term interests of both the managed and the managers. Unfortunately, short-term measures of success are the norm, and as a result pragmatic and power management models are the approaches most often employed by health care managers in today's rapidly changing and increasingly challenging health care environment.

PHYSICIANS AS MANAGERS

The world of medicine is changing at an unbelievable pace for both the patient and his or her provider of care, the physician. According to Lee and Mongan (2009), physicians are also suffering from the disorganization and fragmentation found in our current system of health care delivery. The current trend is that the doctor is no longer the sole provider of care, instead being part of a team responsible for health care delivery. Lee and Mongan argue that no solo physician is capable of delivering quality health care to complex patients. The quality of the care that the physician and his or her team delivers can largely now be measured. This situation requires the physician either to be managed or to become the manager of the team.

Physicians and managers have generally worked at different parts of the hospital, using different skills and having different responsibilities (Huff, 2010). Because of the health care system's focus on reducing costs while at the same time improving quality, this relationship is undergoing profound change. Physicians are moving into managerial positions at a rapid rate. In fact, one of the fastest-growing cohorts of managers in the health care field is made up of physicians as managers, a phenomenon that results in no small measure from the fundamental understanding by top management that managers are usually most effective when they possess a hands-on, working knowledge of the processes they are continuously asked to address. This includes familiarity with the attitudes and beliefs of the physicians and other providers of care whom they manage.

Managerial positions are also becoming increasingly attractive to practicing physicians who seek to exchange the mounting pressures that attend the clinical provision of care for a position that often offers more financial reward on an hourly basis, more time off to devote to personal and family concerns, and the prospect of future advancement up the organization's administrative ladder. Physicians are welcomed at almost all levels of management, with the exception of top positions at large, for-profit, corporate health care entities. According to Falcone and Satiani (2008), there has never been a better time for physicians to move back, although under a different title, to a leadership role in health care delivery. The appropriate training of these physician managers will be one of our greatest challenges as we respond to the many changes brought on by health care reform.

Areas of promotion within individual institutions are effectively off-limits to physicians in private practice, and are restricted in scope for employed physicians. These promotional barriers are in part explained by the time demands on management personnel, be they physicians or non-physicians. The time required to address administrative issues is significant, thereby reducing the time available for the provision of clinical services. These barriers are also partly explained by an institutional reluctance to invite outsiders—that is, nonemployees—into the inner sanctum of management. An increasing number of private practitioners are finding institutional managerial positions attractive enough to forgo direct patient care, leave private practice, and join the organization's managerial ranks. More and more opportunities for physicians to enter the field of health care managerial ranks are appearing across the health care landscape. In smaller corporate and nonprofit institutions the prospect of achieving CEO status exists. In larger corporations the highest offices are usually reserved for professional businesspeople rather than physicians. Even in these larger entities, however, there exist many layers of middle and upper-middle management positions that can be filled by physicians. For models at every level of practice, from the office of the self-employed, solo private physician to the largest national health care entities, business management plays a large and expanding role, and physicians are increasingly joining health care management circles.

The solo private practitioner, who a generation or two ago performed, occasionally with the help of an office nurse, all administrative functions in his or her office, can no longer do so under most circumstances. Substantial time, information, and energy are needed to address and comply with the enormity of administrative concerns, including monumental volumes of federal, state, county, and local municipality mandates; employee payroll, withholding, and retirement account issues; dozens of third-party payer contracts and yearly updates and reviews; accounts receivable and accounts payable concerns; staffing issues; coding updates across varied billing venues; multiple vendor relationships; utility and maintenance issues; information technology installation and hardware and software upgrades; rental agreements; scheduling of physician meetings and ensuring required attendance; continuing education and maintenance of certification issues; and legal counsel affiliations that overlap almost all of the aforementioned areas of management oversight. At the solo private practice level, managerial concerns are profuse and require an office manager to allow the solo practitioner the time necessary to attend to patient care. The solo practitioner will not usually seek to hire a physician as his or her manager, but will work in conjunction with a nonphysician office manager.

According to Champy and Greenspun (2010), physicians need to take back their rightful role in the redesign of health care delivery in this country. This redesign is going to require a complete examination of the work that physicians do and how they do it. Whether the physician is the manager or the managed, he or she must be totally involved in the health care reform effort. Because physicians are the most important component of patient diagnosis and treatment, their expertise cannot be ignored if we truly want to improve the quality of health services.

At all levels of the health care provider practice model above that of the solo practitioner, the idea of physicians as managers takes on increased feasibility. The larger the number of physicians in a group, the more attractive the concept of the group's employing a physician as its manager. This manager need not act as the sole provider of all managerial services, but across the spectrum of interpersonal, information-providing, and decision-making roles there are organizational advantages to assigning managerial responsibilities to a physician. This physician as manager need not be a full-time administrator. In many circumstances this person will devote part of his or her time to patient care and part to management. The physician as manager will effectively act as an intermediary between nonphysician managers and physician colleagues. The daily drudgery of attending to administrative details will be left to nonphysician administrative personnel, and the physician manager will identify issues in need of corporate attention, interpret for colleagues the multidimensional issues, and seek input from colleagues to arrive at decisions in regard to these concerns.

As health care organizations grow there will be more opportunities for physicians seeking full-time managerial positions. The smaller the proportional contribution of a practicing physician to an organization's gross income, the less negative the financial impact of having a practitioner assume a full-time managerial role. The benefits to the organization in terms of monetary value added to the bottom line will often be larger than the revenues lost as a result of the physician's change in status. In regard to patient care concerns, there are opportunities for physicians as managers to markedly improve the overall quality of care. Physicians as managers bring to the administrative table a wealth of understanding of the processes involved in providing patient care that can significantly affect health outcomes for the better. With improved patient care outcomes, the organization should see improved long-term performance.

Taking a more panoramic view of the medical management environment, what is happening across our nation is a wave of acquisitions of successful group and private practices by large and growing corporate organizations in response to the economic changes brought on by the recently passed PPACA in 2010. This creates a strong drive for group practices to improve short-term paper profitability, thereby allowing them to sell out to larger entities at profit multiples that result in greater payouts to stakeholders. This strategy should be understood by managers on both sides of the buyout divide. Managers in the organizations up for sale need to protect their position as best they can because elimination of many of these positions will be on the acquiring entities' agenda. For physician managers the option to fall back on patient care provision as a default position once acquired by the larger entity provides a level of security. Nonphysician managers are less protected and at greater risk of unemployment.

Medical schools are increasingly aware of the need to include business and management courses in their curriculum. Whereas just a couple decades ago such courses were viewed by most medical educators as either unnecessary intrusions on students' time or as running contrary to certain dimensions of medical ethics, the business realities facing medical school graduates today are such that failure to provide these educational components can result in less effective physician practices and ultimately poorer patient care. In addition to inclusion of these topics in the medical school curriculum, the increasing accessibility of dual MD/MBA and MD/JD degrees will result in more physicians' being prepared for entry into the large spectrum of managerial positions across the medical economic landscape.

SUMMARY

It has become impossible to discuss health care management without considering the potential role of the physician in the management of health care organizations. This reality is overshadowed by the fact that the influence of the physician in health care delivery has diminished in recent years due to increasing costs and complexities in health care delivery. This is unfortunate because we desperately need the cooperation of the physician cohort as health care organizations change in response to health care reform efforts.

One of the major problems for physicians in becoming health care managers is the need to unlearn many of their previously acquired assumptions about managed-manager behaviors. In the new world of health care delivery there is less of a need for traditional, bureaucratic managerial skills than there is for the interpersonal skills that foster management expertise in the medical arena. Obviously physicians understand health care, but most have very little if any exposure to management education and training. There is no reason why physicians cannot learn how to manage, but not all will be willing to devote the time and energy needed to develop the necessary knowledge and skills. In some instances such a transition may include a willingness to give up their position of power with regard to patient interactions to work with employees to improve health care delivery.

Practicing physicians have been losing their power base in health care for many years, and their future role in health care decision making is constantly under review. That in many cases the physician is both the demander and the supplier of health services becomes problematic. Managed care organizations as well as the accountable care organization cohorts are under tremendous pressure to reduce health care costs. As a result, these organizations have increasingly been taking away a great deal of the physician's power. This too is unfortunate because the physician's medical expertise is an absolute necessity for quality health care delivery in our country.

According to Avakian (2011), physicians need to unlearn autocratic behaviors and learn the best ways to improve the results of those individuals who report to them. Schwartz, Pogge, Gilles, and Halsinger (2000) argue that top-performing organizations develop great team leaders who embrace change for the better. Unfortunately, this has not been the case with most organizations that deliver health services in our country. The vast majority of leaders in health care networks are confined to specific disciplines and work in silos that insulate them from other departments in health care organizations. There is a clear need to transition from isolated pockets of health care delivery knowledge to an integrated understanding of patient needs and expectations if we hope to attain better-quality health care access.

The clear trend is toward health services' being delivered by a team. That team is usually supervised by a health care manager who is not routinely a physician. As this team-based model of patient health care delivery becomes increasingly common, health care organizations are struggling with what role the physician should play. To be a productive member of this team, the physician will need to acquire many new skills, including expertise in the areas of technology use and management.

Whereas the nonphysician health care manager needs to spend a great deal of time learning how to work successfully with the physician who is better educated and more knowledgeable with regard to diagnosis, the physician health care manager is usually much better positioned in regard to the knowledge associated with the patient care decision-making processes. Part of bridging this knowledge divide will have to do with the type of physician manager—whether he or she is a generalist or a specialist, and his or her medical background. Managers must also pay a great deal of attention to medical ethics when attempting to influence medical decision making. The reimbursement of physicians is also of great importance to the health care manager as health care organizations respond to health care reform. What is more, patient quality concerns need to be considered when managing physicians as well as other individuals who are concerned with the broad spectrum of medical errors, usually the result of system failure. Finally, the role of the physician as a team member and team leader needs to receive great attention as we move into the new world of health care delivery.

KEY TERMS

academic practice

beneficence

capitation

corporate practice

fee-for-service

government practice

justice

liability exposure

nonmaleficence

paternalism

patient autonomy

pragmatic chameleon

private practice

salary

value set

REVIEW QUESTIONS

1. List the major factors directly relating to the management of physician behaviors.

2. Explain how the methods of physician reimbursement can become a critical variable in health care delivery.

3. Describe the models of physician practice as they pertain to managing physicians.

4. Illustrate how the physician-as-manager should be involved in the redesign of health care delivery in the United States.

5. What strategies should physicians pursue to become an effective component of the reengineering of health care delivery?

6. What management model best serves long-term organizational success?

PART 4

Creating a High-Performance Workplace

Part Four of our book discusses ways for health care managers and their employees to create a high-performance workplace in which high-quality services can be delivered to customers on a daily basis. It consists of three chapters designed not only to demonstrate to health care managers the importance of helping health care employees achieve excellence in the delivery of services with scarce resources but also to demonstrate how they might do so.

This section of this text devotes full attention to human resources management, staffing, recruitment, and selection—and the pursuit of quality health care delivery. These are probably the most important functions to be performed by health care managers in these turbulent days of health care reform.

The first topic discussed in Part Four is human resources management and the health care workforce (Chapter Eight). A great deal of attention is paid to the role of the human resources department in a health care organization. This chapter also considers the rights of employees and employers as they work toward the improvement of health services for the population

This topic is followed by a thorough discussion of staffing, with attention paid to the recruitment and selection of employees (Chapter Nine). Components of the staffing process, including several alternatives to hiring full-time staff, are presented to the reader. This is followed by an explanation of internal and external recruiting along with how to evaluate the recruiting function. Successful recruitment leading to well-trained and then empowered employees can go a long way toward improving the outcomes of health care delivery. The last area of discussion in Chapter Nine is the employee selection process, including commonly used selection methods.

The last chapter in Part Four of this book addresses employee performance improvement and the pursuit of quality in health care delivery (Chapter Ten). The starting point for improving employee performance in health care is shown to be employee orientation and mentoring. The discussion then moves to employee training, and finally employee performance appraisal.

8

Human Resources Management and Health Care

Marc C. Marchese

LEARNING OBJECTIVES

- Understand the labor market for health care jobs
- Be aware of the challenges for health care employers in maintaining an effective workforce
- Be knowledgeable concerning the role human resources management plays in creating and sustaining productive employees
- Be cognizant of the numerous employee relations issues an organization must prepare for in managing its employees
- Acknowledge the role unions play in affecting the management of human resources in a health care organization
- Be able to identify the key metrics commonly used to assess workforce productivity

One of the most common messages in management texts today is the importance of quality. It does not matter if the industry is in manufacturing or service. Quality is critical for success in today's marketplace. The health care industry is especially concerned with the issue of quality of care. Health care is provided by a wide array of health care workers, whether they are physicians, nurses, medical technicians, and so on, and it follows that a health care organization's workforce is a primary driver of quality. Health care organizations need to attract, motivate, and retain talented employees to flourish in a highly competitive and ever-changing industry.

Human resources management is the process by which an organization manages its employees. In the past, *personnel,* rather than *human resources,* was the term used. A personnel approach to management viewed workers as a company's largest expense. Employees were a cost to be minimized, with the goal of maximizing profits. This approach to management resulted in a disengaged workforce with only a limited commitment to the company and weak concern for quality. A human resources approach to management views employees as talented contributors to organizational success. Employees are a resource that if managed correctly can provide a competitive advantage in the marketplace. This approach is necessary in any health care organization for which the quality of care is of the utmost importance.

The most significant challenge for health care organizations in creating and sustaining a productive workforce is attracting and retaining top talent. The U.S. Department of Labor (DOL) provides an excellent resource with information on jobs in all industries: O*NET (http://online.onetcenter.org). The section on health care lists 87 health care jobs. Of the 87 jobs, 63 have a bright employment outlook, indicating that job growth is much faster than average for these areas. For example, this Web site indicates that there were over 660,000 general practitioners in 2008, and the DOL is projecting over 260,000 job openings for general practitioners by 2018. An even more startling finding involves registered nurses. In 2008 the DOL estimated that there were over 2.6 million registered nurses in the United States. By 2018 there will be over 1 million job openings for this occupation! You can find similar results for pharmacists, physical therapists, physician assistants, and others. With so many job openings in so many health care occupations, talented employees have considerable discretion before accepting any job offer, and they know they can switch companies relatively easily even when the economy is not thriving. Employers need to have a well-thought-out plan to obtain and retain these workers. Human resources management plays a key role in accomplishing this goal.

In addition to the high demand for qualified health care professionals in many areas, a second and related challenge for health care organizations is the increase in patient demand for health services. We are abundantly aware that the U.S. population is getting older. According to the U.S. Census Bureau (2011), about 10 percent of our population is over age sixty-five, and within the next twenty years this percentage will almost double. Moreover, the population of citizens eighty-five and older is expected to triple by 2050 to about nineteen million people! It is not surprising that an older population is associated with a greater need for health services. Thus the demand for quality health care workers will last for the foreseeable future.

THE ROLE OF HUMAN RESOURCES PROFESSIONALS IN ORGANIZATIONS

Human resources professionals have significant responsibilities that will influence how successful the organization is in meeting the aforementioned challenges. To begin with, the human resources department will oversee the analysis and design of jobs in an organization. This process includes defining the tasks, duties, and responsibilities (TDRs) for each position in the organization. Furthermore, once the TDRs for a given job are defined, the knowledge, skills, abilities, and other characteristics required to perform those TDRs will be identified as well. There are many approaches to collecting and compiling this information. The common methods of job analysis include conducting interviews and surveys, making observations, and examining work products to produce accurate job descriptions. The use of this information is especially important for health care organizations as health care jobs become more and more specialized. For example, within the nursing profession there are acute care nurses, critical care nurses, advanced practice psychiatric nurses, licensed practical nurses, registered nurses, nurse anesthetists, nurse midwives, nurse practitioners, and others. Clearly and accurately defining these jobs is essential to identify the top talent for each position as well as to eliminate redundancy in the organization.

Human resources professionals will also explore various ways to design jobs to make them more effective for the organization and the employees that hold them. For example, one commonly used approach to job design is ergonomics, which is the study of the person-machine interface in the workplace. Is there a way to reduce the physical demands of a job on the employee, which in turn could reduce absenteeism, sick days, worker's compensation claims, and fatigue? Ergonomic initiatives cut across a wide array of jobs. For example, there might be ergonomically designed desk chairs for greater back support, soft wooden floors to reduce strain on workers' feet, and lift assist equipment to reduce the physical demands of getting patients in and out of hospital beds. A second approach to job design is industrial engineering, which entails searching for ways to reduce wasted time and motions in the workplace. For example, in a typical nursing shift, a nurse may walk over four miles in performing his or her duties (Welton, Decker, Adam, & Zone-Smith, 2006). Industrial engineering, through the use of time and motion studies, involves looking for ways to arrange the workplace to reduce the amount of required travel for an employee. Thus an employee is more productive for the employer, and both sides benefit. Alternatively, technology can be implemented to improve efficiency. For example, research has shown that nurses found using electronic medical records to improve their organization and efficiency (Kossman & Scheidenhelm, 2008). Reexamining an employee's job description by reassigning certain tasks to other employees can also improve workplace efficiency. For example, a registered nurse's task of recording a patient's vital signs might be assigned to a licensed practical nurse. A third approach to job design is enrichment. Enrichment programs attempt to improve the attractiveness of the employee's job, which in turn aids employee motivation and retention. Enrichment initiatives include job enlargement (giving employees more variety in their work), vertical integration (giving employees more challenging and meaningful tasks), employee empowerment (giving employees more control over how their work gets done), and implementing team-based programs (allowing employees to work together). A fourth and final approach to job design is alternative work schedules. Employees today expect their employer to accommodate their personal needs. Alternative work schedules have been found to be effective in attracting and retaining employees. A common alternative work schedule in health care is the compressed workweek. Instead of having to work five eight-hour days, employees are offered longer shifts, reducing the number of workdays they need to be at work. This enables them to have extra days off during the week to meet their personal needs (such as reduced day care, long weekend getaways, and time to run errands). The most common compressed workweek across industries is the 4/40, which is four ten-hour workdays. Other alternative work schedules include flextime (allowing employees flexibility as to when the workday begins and ends), telecommuting (allowing employees to work from home for part of the week), and job sharing (splitting a full-time job among two employees who prefer part-time work). Overall, effective job design initiatives introduced by human resources professionals can help the employer acquire and retain talented workers.

Human resources professionals play a large role in staffing the organization as well, a process that contains many critical components. To begin with, planning is essential to determine how many employees will be needed, what types of employees are needed, and when they will be needed. From there recruitment strategies are devised to help create a large pool of qualified applicants. After creating the applicant pool, human resources professionals can assist in the selection process to help the organization determine the best fit for a given job opening. This staffing process will be discussed in length in Chapter Nine.

After the staffing process is complete, the human resources department also has responsibilities in regard to managing the performance of the organization's workforce. After an employee is hired, human resources professionals typically provide orientation and training as needed. Due to our dependence on technology and the fact that technology is always changing, all employees will receive training in how to handle technological advances. Moreover, compensation and benefits play a major role in influencing employee performance. Human resources professionals work closely with department heads and management to devise a compensation and benefits package that will help maximize employee motivation. Furthermore, employee performance needs to be monitored and recorded for a variety of purposes, and human resources professionals will assist in devising a performance appraisal system to accomplish this objective. Performance management will be discussed in much more detail in Chapter Ten.

The final role of human resources professionals has to do with general employee relations, a topic that covers a broad spectrum of employment issues, such as employee discipline, worker attitudes, and employee rights. Employee relations are greatly affected, among other factors, by union relations. This chapter will explore many of the significant employee relations and union relations issues for health care organizations, with an emphasis on the role of human resources management as these issues are addressed. Overall, the human resources department plays a major role in helping companies cultivate a talented workforce, and thus helps promote high-quality health care.

RIGHTS OF EMPLOYEES AND EMPLOYERS

To develop an organization's human capital, the employer must be cognizant of employee rights in relation to employer rights. A successful human resources department will educate and counsel managers in these areas to make sure decisions are made that maximize benefits for both parties. Employee rights can be broken down into three main categories: statutory, contractual, and implied. Statutory rights for employees are rights that are grounded in the law. For example, according to the Equal Pay Act of 1963, employees have the right to "equal pay for equal work." The intent of this law was to reduce pay disparities based on gender. In 2009 this right was strengthened further by the Lilly Ledbetter Fair Pay Act, which expands the statute of limitations for filing a claim of pay discrimination on the basis of any protected characteristic. Because of these two laws, employers need to monitor differences in pay for males and females in jobs that require comparable skills, responsibilities, and levels of effort, and that have similar working conditions. An employee has a right to question pay disparities if he or she suspects this difference is based on gender as opposed to legitimate factors, such as seniority, productivity, or qualifications. Another example of statutory rights is based on the Fair Labor Standards Act of 1938, which states that if an employee's job is classified as nonexempt, that employee is entitled to overtime pay (at least equal to time and a half) for all work hours that exceed forty hours in a given workweek. Due to the 24/7 demands of many health care positions, the health care industry can base overtime on a two-week, eighty-hour time frame. Regardless of the time frame, however, health care employers need to be careful in designating jobs as exempt or nonexempt. Certain types of workers, such as registered nurses and physician assistants, are generally considered exempt, but nurses' aides, licensed practical nurses, and workers in any position that pays less than $455 per week are considered nonexempt. For example, long-term care organizations often employ workers in nonexempt positions. Due to the 24/7 nature of this business, these employers need to particularly careful in their compensation practices to comply with this regulation (Lyncheski & Garrett, 2006). The Department of Labor will impose severe financial penalties for misclassifying a nonexempt job as exempt.

Statutory rights can also vary from state to state. For example, in Pennsylvania a relatively new law has banned mandatory overtime for nurses (Toland, 2009). The next chapter will describe employment legislation in much greater detail, but for the purposes of this chapter it's worth noting that there are numerous statutory regulations affecting human resources management in an organization. These regulations address the majority of human resources functions, including but not limited to recruiting applicants, selecting new hires, making pay decisions, training personnel, managing performance, administering benefits, pursuing safety in the workplace, and monitoring union activity.

Contractual rights are based on written agreements between the employer and the employee. The most common type of written agreement is an employment contract in which the employer agrees to provide compensation (such as a base salary, incentives, and pay increases) and benefits (such as health insurance, a retirement plan, and paid time off) for a specified time. The employment contract also specifies the conditions of employment, such as circumstances under which the contract may be terminated, the employee's right to work for another employer, and any materials and resources to be provided by the employer or the employee. In health care organizations employment contracts can be used to secure long-term commitments from workers in certain specialty areas that are in short supply. In a recent article forecasting a severe shortage of physicians over the next fifteen years, Strode and Beith (2009) advocate the use of employment contracts to help health care organizations stabilize their workforce. As indicated earlier in this chapter, there are several health care areas in which a great demand for qualified personnel is expected. It would not be surprising to see employment contracts become more popular as health care organizations attempt to manage this human resources challenge. In addition to employment contracts, other written expressions of contractual rights include noncompete agreements, which may or may not be included in an employment contract. These restrictive covenants are used to prevent former employees from competing directly with the organization. In drafting these noncompete agreements, it's important to make sure they are not overly restrictive on the former employee in terms of where he or she can work and how long the agreement will last. For example, a relatively recent court ruling in New Jersey upheld a noncompete agreement that prevented a neurosurgeon from practicing for two years within thirty miles of his former employer (Lewis & Dambeck, 2005). If this noncompete agreement had been much longer (for example, five years), or if it had covered a much large area (for example, a hundred miles), then the outcome of this case would probably have been reversed.

Employees also have implied rights, which can be affected by implied contracts. Implied contracts are agreements that can be considered contractual in nature, even though their terms are not as clearly specified as they would be in an employment contract. For example, promising a new hire lifetime employment in the job interview may be legally actionable if that employee is later laid off to reduce business expenses. Furthermore, an employer that does not consistently follow the policies and procedures in the employee handbook can be vulnerable to a lawsuit as well. Employee handbooks often contain a disclaimer that the handbook is not a contract. However, employees do have an expectation that the policies and procedures outlined in the handbook, although they can be changed at any time by the employer, will be followed in a consistent manner. An employer disregarding the handbook can be viewed as a violation of an employee's rights.

So far this section has focused on the statutory, contractual, and implied rights of employees. However, there are several areas in which the rights of employees and employers intersect. One such critical area pertains to the concept of **employment-at-will,** whereby an employee has the right to quit at any time for any reason or no reason at all. Comparably, an employer can terminate the employee at any time for any reason or no reason at all (Steingold, 2007). For the employee and the employer to have this right, an employment contract that specifies the length of employment cannot be in effect between the parties. Employees often take advantage of this right and leave companies for a wide variety of reasons that can be quite questionable (for example, they are bored, feel like a change, or don't care for the boss). Employers, however, need to be very careful in exercising this right. If the employee believes that he or she was fired for the wrong reasons, the former employee may sue for **wrongful discharge** (also known as wrongful termination). There are many circumstances that would constitute wrongful discharge. The next chapter will address numerous equal employment opportunity (EEO) laws that apply to termination as well as hiring. For now, suffice it to say that if an employer terminates an employee because of his or her race, color, religion, sex, or national origin, then the employer has violated Title VII of the Civil Rights Act of 1964.

There are many other restrictions on the employment-at-will right of employers beyond those imposed by EEO laws. A few years ago an assisted living facility in Indiana was ordered by the state's department of health to furnish the personnel files of six of its nurses. A payroll clerk for the employer obtained the files and noticed that a couple of these nurses had received discipline notices for stealing patient medications. The clerk alerted the administrator of the facility of these notices. The administrator ordered the clerk to remove them from the personnel files. The clerk refused to comply with this request and was later terminated. The former employee sued for wrongful termination and was successful. The court ruled that the employment-at-will doctrine does not permit an employer to punish an employee for refusing to commit an illegal act ("Wrongful Discharge," 2009). This case is an example of the public policy exception to employment-at-will. A more common example of the public policy exception would apply to an employer that terminates an employee for performing jury duty.

Another case involved a nurse who hurt her wrist on the job. She collected worker's compensation while recovering from her injury. When she returned to work she violated a company policy by giving her keys to the medicine cabinet to a coworker so that person could do the narcotics count instead of her. The employer found out about this violation and terminated her immediately. The nurse filed a wrongful discharge case against her former employer. The court ruled in favor of the former nurse, because the court believed that the motive for the firing was that the nurse filed a worker's compensation claim, not that she had violated a policy (Moushon & Asher, 2007). In this case the employment-at-will right of the employer was superseded by an employee's right to be free of retaliation for collecting worker's compensation. In addition, this case also showed the value of an implied contract based on the company's policies and the enforcement of those policies. If the company had consistently enforced the policy concerning the keys to the medicine cabinet, it would have had a stronger defense in this case. Overall, employers do have the right to exercise employment-at-will with their employees; however, due to the numerous exceptions to this concept (such as those involving public policy, EEO protection, and implied contracts), employers have to be cautious in terminating employees.

There is another concept related to wrongful discharge of which employers need to be aware. Due to concerns over terminating an employee, sometimes an employer may go too far in trying to encourage an employee to quit. If the former employee is able to show that he or she was subjected to extreme conduct that made it virtually impossible to remain on the job, the former employee may sue his or her former employer for constructive discharge. Examples of constructive discharge may include harassment that the employer intentionally ignores, an employee's demotion to a degrading position, unreasonable work hours or demands, and threats to the employee.

Employees have the right to be free of intolerable working conditions (Steingold, 2007).

Another area in which the rights of employers and employees intersect has to do with freedom of speech. Do employees have the right to speak freely about their employer to a third party? Does the employer have the right to terminate an employee for inappropriate or unwelcome communication that may harm the reputation of the organization? These rights have been tested under the concept of **whistleblowing.** Whistleblowing is a topic that receives media attention, but exactly what constitutes whistleblowing is subject to debate. Generally speaking, whistleblowing occurs when an employee discloses an employer's wrongdoing (defined as an illegal or immoral activity) to a third party and the employee is disciplined for this disclosure (Drew & Garrahan, 2005). In the health care industry there have been numerous examples of employees' reporting perceived legal and ethical violations and then being terminated for this disloyalty. Laws protecting employees from retaliation for whistleblowing vary from state to state. At the federal level there is the Whistleblower Protection Act of 2007, which only covers federal employees who disclose government fraud, abuse, and waste (Hill, 2010). There is also the False Claims Act (amended in 1986), which protects whistleblowers who reveal the inappropriate use of federal funds related to health care (Drew & Garrahan).

The challenge with whistleblower cases is determining whether or not the perceived violation is significant enough to warrant protection from retaliation. For example, in California a director of staff development for a convalescent home complained to the director of nursing that a recently hired nurse did not have a valid nursing license or a social security number. This person also complained about unsanitary conditions that were present at her facility. Three days later she was fired, and subsequently she sued for wrongful termination under California whistleblower protection. In this case the California court was on her side, and she received a large settlement from her previous employer ("Whistleblower: Terminated," 2008). In New York a nursing manager complained to management that the surgical instruments were not being sterilized correctly in the operating rooms. The nursing manager was fired, and similar to the previous case sued her former employer. The New York court, however, ruled in favor of the employer because the former employee could not point to a specific law related to sterilizing surgical instruments that had been violated ("Whistleblower Lawsuit Dismissed," 2008). In Pennsylvania a neurologist was fired after reporting the absence of a supervising neurosurgeon when depth electrodes were placed over the brains of epileptic patients. One patient died, and another patient became comatose as a result of these procedures. The Pennsylvania court's ruling was similar to that of the New York court from the preceding example. No specific law or policy was violated, and thus her termination was not covered by Pennsylvania whistleblower protection (Drew & Garrahan, 2005). As you can see from these examples, an employee's right to complain about perceived wrongdoing in his or her organization is legally debatable. Whistleblower laws vary from state to state, thus giving employers the right to discipline an employee for undesired behaviors under many circumstances.

One final area of intersecting employer and employee rights that will be addressed in this chapter deals with the right to privacy at work. What privacy rights do employees have in the workplace? Do employers have the right to monitor employees at work? This topic can include a wide array of issues. For example, does an employer have the right to go through an employee's desk or his or her office? Can an employer monitor an employee's phone conversations? If yes, then does this right extend to e-mail and Internet usage? What about video surveillance or some other form of electronic monitoring in the workplace? The courts have often sided with employers in dealing with these issues. Employers should be able to demonstrate "reasonableness" in their policies and practices concerning privacy. Further, employers should be able to demonstrate a compelling interest behind their monitoring of employee behavior (Cozzetto & Pedeliski, 1997). Employers should draft policies that address the aforementioned issues, and they should also clearly communicate those policies to their employees. Employees need to be made aware of what is and is not an acceptable use of technology in the workplace as well as the grounds necessary for an inspection of an employee workstation or office. Consistent application and documentation should also be practiced.

This section of the chapter has addressed numerous rights of employees and, by default, rights of employers. As part of managing a company's human resources, these rights need to be considered in creating and implementing employee policies and procedures. A failure to understand these rights may place the organization in a legally tenuous situation. As important as the legal ramifications of employee rights are, it should also be noted that denying employees their rights can also damage the relationship between employees and their employer. The next section will address several important employee attitudes, which are affected in part by the degree to which a company respects the rights of its workforce.

CRITICAL EMPLOYEE ATTITUDES TOWARD WORK

One of the goals of human resources management is to create a workforce that is committed to achieving the organization's short- and long-term objectives. To achieve this goal the company has to cultivate an organizational culture that motivates employees to do their best, emphasizes and rewards providing quality patient care, and encourages employees to develop their skills for an ever-changing workplace. For this to happen, the company needs a workforce with not only the talent to achieve this goal but also the desire to make it possible. As you know, employee motivation was the subject of Chapter Five in this text. This section of this chapter will highlight the key employee attitudes that organizations should consider in developing a culture that leads to a highly effective workplace.

In the field of human resources management there is an important concept that has an impact on employee attitudes. This concept is referred to as the **psychological contract,** which is formed based on the perceived, unwritten expectations held by the employee and the employer concerning employment (Bohlander & Snell, 2010). An employee learns on the job what the company expects from its workers and the consequences of various actions, and over time the employee develops this psychological contract with his or her employer based on what he or she sees in the workplace.

This psychological contract can vary along a continuum from transactional to relational (Muchinsky, 2009).

A transactional psychological contract indicates that the employee understands his or her job as basically a simple transaction. The employee provides a service to the employer, and in return the employer provides compensation and benefits to the employee. The employee therefore has the attitude that he or she will do what he or she is paid to do: nothing more, nothing less. In this type of contract, the employee perceives that the employer has no type of attachment to the employee and thus the employee should have no attachment to the employer. The expectation is that this employment will continue as long as both parties view the transaction as mutually beneficial.

A relational psychological contract indicates that the employee has a long-term expectation to remain with his or her employer. The employee perceives that the employer is committed to the employee, and in turn the employee is committed to the employer. The employee wants to stay in the organization and do whatever is necessary to help the company succeed. The employee and the employer are building a long-term relationship in which both parties will benefit.

The importance of the psychological contract has to do with its relationship to valued employee behaviors. Employees who have a relational psychological contract are more likely to engage in organizational citizenship behaviors (OCB) are actions in the workplace that go above and beyond an employee's basic job duties. Empirical research has identified five key OCB: courtesy (being nice to others in the workplace); sportsmanship (not gossiping, not spreading rumors, and not complaining); altruism (helping others out without any benefit to oneself); civic virtue (volunteering for additional tasks or participating in optional activities); and conscientiousness (following the rules, doing things right) (Muchinsky, 2009). As you reflect on OCB, it should become clear that a successful organization would want employees to have a relational psychological contract. Employees with the attitudes associated with a relational psychological contract are essential to providing quality care and high productivity. Table 8.1 provides an overview and application of the issue of psychological contracts.

Table 8.1   Types of Psychological Contracts Applied to a Health Care Setting

Type of Psychological Contract	Employee Attitude Associated with This Type	Impact of This Type on an Organizational Citizenship Behaviors
Transactional	"I do only what I get paid to do."	"I decline an offer to join the company's United Way drive because it's not part of my job" (low civic virtue).
Relational	"I care about the success of this company, and the company cares about my success."	"I lend a hand to a licensed practical nurse who is struggling moving a patient from her bed to her wheelchair" (high altruism).

Often when we think of employee attitudes the first attitude that pops into our mind is **job satisfaction.** Job satisfaction refers to the extent to which employees derive pleasure from their job (Muchinsky, 2009). Not surprisingly, job satisfaction has been associated with relational psychological contracts and with OCB. Unfortunately, numerous reports have indicated that job satisfaction in the United States is at its lowest levels in years (Aversa, 2010). The growing dissatisfaction has been attributed to many factors, such as pay raises' not keeping up with inflation, significantly higher health care costs, unfulfilling jobs, and a lack of growth opportunities. In health care the findings concerning job satisfaction are comparable. For example, there are numerous studies on physicians' job satisfaction. This research suggests that a physician's job satisfaction is influenced by such factors as low reimbursement rates, time pressures, work family stress, and the confinement of working in a managed care environment (Linzer et al., 2000). This poor job satisfaction has been linked to frustration, feelings of powerlessness, and disenchantment with the profession (Cohn, Bethancourt, & Simington, 2009).

Employers in all industries should take the initiative to assess the job satisfaction of their workforce. Across industries the most popular job satisfaction instrument is the Job Descriptive Index (JDI) (Noe, Hollenbeck, Gerhart, & Wright, 2004). The JDI assesses five facets of job satisfaction: pay and benefits, coworkers, supervisors, the job itself, and opportunities for advancement. There are also job satisfaction instruments specially designed for health care positions. For example, in one study of physician job satisfaction an instrument was created that hit on such topics as autonomy, personal time, relationships with patients, patient care issues, relationships with colleagues, relationships with staff, relationships with the community, satisfaction in one's specialty, and income (Linzer et al., 2000). Regardless of the instrument used, job satisfaction should be assessed regularly.

Measuring job satisfaction alone is not sufficient, however. If a company finds job satisfaction is declining, then the causes of the decline must be identified and action steps relevant to those factors need to be created and implemented. As an example, a large medical center in Arizona attributed its high physician turnover to poor job satisfaction and burnout. To address this situation the medical center created an on-boarding program. The program is similar to a mentoring system except that the mentoring of a new hire is conducted by several participants rather than a single mentor for each new hire. In the first year of implementation the on-boarding system was credited with reducing physician turnover from 10 percent to 0 percent (Cohn et al., 2009).

Another employee attitude that warrants attention in the workplace is **organizational commitment.** This term refers to the extent to which an employee feels a sense of allegiance to his or her employer (Muchinsky, 2009). Organizational commitment has been empirically associated with job satisfaction and turnover (Wagner, 2007). There are many forms of organizational commitment.

Research has identified three major types of organizational commitment. Affective commitment refers to the degree to which the employee is committed to the organization because he or she really likes this company. An employee with a high level of affective commitment has a strong sense of attachment or identification with her employer. Affective commitment is the form of commitment that most of us think about when we hear that an employee is committed to a company. However, there are other reasons why an employee may be committed to the employer. Continuance commitment refers to the extent to which employees have a desire to remain with an employer based on their perception of how difficult it would be to find comparable employment elsewhere. An employee may have a high level of continuance commitment because he believes that he is unlikely to find another job that offers a similar salary and benefits package. This employee may have low affective commitment, which suggests he doesn't like working for this company, but due to economic realities he may be highly committed to staying from a continuance perspective. Finally, normative commitment refers to the extent to which the employee is committed to the company out of a sense of loyalty. An employee may not want to stay with her employer because she no longer identifies with what the company stands for (low affective commitment), and she knows that she can find a better job elsewhere (low continuance commitment), but she remains with her employer out of a sense of obligation. The sense of duty or obligation may be the result of the company's demonstrating its loyalty to this employee at an earlier time (for example, accommodating her special needs during a rough period in her life), or it may be due to a promise this person made to the company when she took this job (for example, "I will make sure the merger is completed") (Muchinsky, 2009). Table 8.2 presents an overview of these three types of organizational commitment, all of which are important and indicate very different attitudes.

Table 8.2   Types of Organizational Commitment

Type of Organizational Commitment	"I Am Committed to Staying Employed at My Company Because . . . "
Affective	"I really like this organization and how it treats me."
Continuance	"I don't like my chances of finding another job."
Normative	"I promised my boss I would be here for at least three years."

Similar to how an employer might address job satisfaction and the psychological contract, once the employer assesses these important employee attitudes concerning organizational commitment the next step is figuring out the reasons behind them. For example, one study examined the impact of generational differences on organizational commitment among nurses. Younger nurses' desire for flexibility in work schedules was noteworthy. The authors presented alternatives for health care organizations to manage the generations differently to enhance organizational commitment (Carver & Candela, 2008).

The value of addressing the employee attitudes that influence important employee behaviors is self-evident. The challenge for employers from a human resources view is, What we should do to enhance employees' job satisfaction and affective organizational commitment, with the ultimate goal of establishing a relational psychological contract with them? The answer to this question is that there are many alternatives to consider, depending on the values of the company and the factors contributing to employee attitudes. For example, our company could examine its reward system in terms of its impact on employee attitudes. Based on how we award pay raises or bonuses, what message are we sending to our employees? (For example, do we reward them based on performance or seniority?) We could also examine our job design process. Do we think about ways in which jobs can be enhanced and thus be made more meaningful and interesting to employees? Do we consider alternative work arrangements, such as flexible scheduling and telecommuting? Another factor that influences employee attitudes is balancing work and family. Are our time demands on our employees reasonable? Do we have policies or benefits that accommodate the personal needs of our workforce, such as offering day care or eldercare assistance? Moreover, we may examine the opportunities for growth in our company. Do we offer training and development programs to prepare our employees for new challenges? Do we have a successful career planning system to provide realistic plans for upward mobility? Finally, how we treat employees will undoubtedly affect employee attitudes. Do we treat employees fairly? Do we communicate regularly with employees and give them a chance to voice their opinions? Do we make sure our managers and department heads are properly trained to supervise their staff? As you can see, these questions can provide guidance to improve employee attitudes and relations in an organization. Failure to take the necessary steps to improve employee attitudes may lead to the next topic in this chapter.

UNIONS AND THE HEALTH CARE INDUSTRY

A unionized workforce in any industry presents significant challenges for an organization in managing its human resources. A collective bargaining agreement for the unionized workforce can have an impact on most aspects of human resources management. It is therefore critical to understand the key laws related to labor relations, how a company's workforce can become unionized, the collective bargaining process, and the unique labor relations issues for the health care industry.

According to the Bureau of Labor Statistics (2011), less than 12 percent of the U.S. workforce is unionized, which is the lowest percentage in over fifty years. Further, the percentage of private sector employees who are unionized is just under 7 percent. More than half of the unionized workforce is made up of public sector employees. Local government workers have the highest rate of unionization (42.3 percent). The private sector industries with the highest unionization rates are transportation and utilities (about 22 percent), whereas agriculture and finance have the lowest (about 2 percent). The health care industry falls in the middle of these extremes.

Unionization in the United States became much more popular as a result of the National Labor Relations Act (NLRA) of 1935. Prior to this law's taking effect only around three million workers were unionized. Within a few years the number of unionized workers tripled (Noe et al., 2004). This law gave employees the "right to form, join, decertify, or assist a labor organization, and to bargain collectively through representatives of their own choosing, or to refrain from such activities," as well as to "join together to improve terms and conditions of employment" with or without a union (National Labor Relations Board [NLRB], 2011b). This law also indicated activities in which employers may not engage, which are considered unfair labor practices. For example, employers may not do any of the following (NLRB, 2011a):

- Threaten employees with loss of jobs or benefits if they join or vote for a union or engage in protected concerted activity

- Threaten to close the plant if employees select a union to represent them

- Question employees about their union sympathies or activities in circumstances that tend to interfere with, restrain, or coerce employees in the exercise of their rights under the Act

- Promise benefits to employees to discourage their union support

- Transfer, lay off, terminate, assign employees more difficult work tasks, or otherwise punish employees because they engaged in union or protected concerted activity

- Transfer, lay off, terminate, assign employees more difficult work tasks, or otherwise punish employees because they filed unfair labor practice charges

After the NLRA was passed, the law clearly had a pro-union impact on our workforce. However, abuses of power by unions led to subsequent legislation that restricted certain union activities, which were also categorized as unfair labor practices. The two key laws restricting union activities are the Taft-Hartley Act of 1947 and the Landrum-Griffin Act of 1959. Following are some examples of unfair labor practices by unions that these laws identified (NLRB, 2011a):

- Threats to employees that they will lose their jobs unless they support the union

- Seeking the suspension, discharge, or other punishment of an employee for not being a union member even if the employee has paid or offered to pay a lawful initiation fee and periodic fees thereafter

- Refusing to process a grievance because an employee has criticized union officials or because an employee is not a member of the union in states where union security clauses are not permitted

- Fining employees who have validly resigned from the union for engaging in protected concerted activities following their resignation or for crossing an unlawful picket line

- Engaging in picket line misconduct, such as threatening, assaulting, or barring non-strikers from the employer's premises

In addition to establishing employee rights in regard to unionization and delineating the unfair labor practices just specified, the NLRA also led to the creation of the National Labor Relations Board (NLRB). The NLRB is an independent federal government agency that enforces the NLRA as well as the other labor laws. This agency conducts union certification elections, investigates claims of unfair labor practices, and assists in the resolution of conflicts between unions and employers (NLRB, 2011c). The NLRB consists of a five-member panel appointed by the president of the United States. The members serve a five-year term. In addition, the NLRB has a general counsel whose members are also appointed by the president. Moreover, there are fifty-one regional NLRB offices spread throughout the United States (NLRB, 2011d).

It is not surprising that most employers try to avoid having a unionized workforce. The main question to ask, then, is Why do employees seek unionization? There are many answers to this question, but the overarching response would be a perceived lack of respect by management, and the feeling among employees that the organization does not value them. They are not considered human resources, but rather a cost to be minimized. This perception may be reinforced by below-market wages and benefits, top-down communication, severe penalties for minor workplace infractions, the inconsistent application of work rules, or hostile working conditions. Employers that do not care about employee attitudes and do not perceive the workforce as a valuable resource to gain a competitive advantage in the marketplace are vulnerable to unionization.

The process by which a company's workforce may become unionized is rather straightforward. First, either an employee contacts a union or a union contacts an employee. As a result of this initial contact, support within the organization is explored. The union, along with the interested employees, will attempt to solicit backing from other workers. To prevent the spread of

rumors concerning unionization, some employers will enforce a no-solicitation policy in the workplace. Companies do have the right to prohibit
solicitation on their premises; however, this policy must be clearly spelled
out and consistently enforced. For example, employees at Promedica Health
Systems were disciplined for passing out union literature in areas of the
hospital not designated for patient care. The hospital claimed these employees were violating the no-solicitation policy. The NLRB represented the
disciplined employees and charged the hospital with an unfair labor practice.
The court sided with the NLRB because there was evidence that the employer
allowed employees to sell Girl Scout cookies, advertise Tupperware parties,
and sell Avon cosmetics and other merchandise. Enforcing this solicitation
policy selectively for union activity was therefore deemed a violation of the
NLRA ("No-Solicitation Rule," 2006). If an employer does properly follow
a no-solicitation policy, however, employees will be required to solicit union
support outside of work.

In the next step in the unionization process, interested employees fill out
authorization cards. These cards indicate key employee information (contact
information, company name, job title) and a statement that the employee
is supportive of a union or supportive of a certification election. If at least
30 percent of the workers who would become eligible union members sign
these cards, then an NLRB petition form is completed that requests a certification election to be held. The petition form and the authorization cards
are sent to the regional NLRB office.

At the regional office, the NLRB reviews the petition and examines the
authorization cards to determine which employees would be classified as
"bargaining unit" employees. Bargaining unit employees are employees that
will be able to vote in the certification election and would be bound by the
results of this election. In health care settings many health care professionals
are classified as being part of the management team and are thus ineligible
to be unionized, particularly if their job requires them to exercise independent judgment and oversee other workers. In one case registered nurses and
licensed practical nurses in a nursing home were found to be supervisors
based on the degree of autonomy and authority they had in the workplace
("Labor Law," 2006), rendering them ineligible to be unionized. Once the

NLRB verifies the bargaining unit employees and determines that at least 30 percent of these employees have properly filled out the authorization cards, then an election will be held.

The NLRB will conduct the certification election. All bargaining unit employees will be notified of the time and place of the election. The outcome of the election will be based on a majority vote. It does not matter how many employees show up for the election. For example, if there are five hundred bargaining unit employees and only two hundred of these employees vote, the majority vote will affect all five hundred employees regardless of whether or not they voted or what they voted for ("union" or "no union"). If the union receives a majority of votes, it will be certified as the exclusive bargaining representative of these employees. If the union loses the election, the employees will have to wait at least one year before filing another petition for an election.

Collective bargaining begins after the union is certified by the NLRB as the exclusive bargaining representative for the bargaining unit employees. A union representative will meet with a management representative to negotiate a collective bargaining agreement, which is also known as the union contract. These negotiations are often adversarial, but they can be collaborative as well.

Negotiations cover a wide range of topics. The topics that often receive the most media attention are those pertaining to wages and benefits, which include such issues as starting salaries, pay increases, cost-of-living adjustments, health insurance, pension plans, and paid time off. In addition to covering wages and benefits, these negotiations will also address union security issues, one of which is the length of the contract. From the union perspective, the longer the contract is in effect, the more likely it is that employees will become accustomed to being in a union and thus the less likely it is that they will seek to remove the union from the workplace through decertification. The other key issue with union security is the type of shop clause. A union shop clause in the union contract means that all bargaining unit employees must join the union and pay union dues. In right-to-work states (mostly in the South and the Midwest) union shop clauses are not permitted. In these states unions negotiate for an agency shop clause, which requires all bargaining unit employees to pay union dues but gives them the option to join or not join the union. An open shop clause weakens the security of the union because it allows bargaining unit employees the freedom to choose whether or not they want to join the union and pay dues. This clause provides an opportunity for employers to reward union and nonunion employees similarly, thereby making union employees question the value of paying union dues and thus remaining in the union. Not surprisingly, unions will negotiate strongly for a union or agency shop clause in the union contract.

Collective bargaining will also address the rights of management. Included in this part of the contract will be issues of job security. The freedom management has to terminate or lay off employees will be included in this section. In addition, such issues as changing job descriptions, mandatory overtime, workplace safety, and even modifications to work hours fall within this area. Scheduling and overtime are two critical concerns for many health care organizations (Flynn, Mathis, & Jackson, 2007).

A final, significant part of negotiations in collective bargaining will be to agree on a grievance process. The typical union contract is quite lengthy and covers dozens of workplace issues. Disputes over interpreting and applying the policies included the contract are common in unionized workplaces. Essential to resolving such disputes is a clearly defined grievance process, which necessitates designating a shop steward (a fellow bargaining unit employee) to help the employees involved in the grievance present their side of the story to management. Also, mediation or arbitration will often be included in the grievance process, as a neutral third party that may be able to resolve the dispute.

Once the negotiations on the aforementioned issues have been completed, the bargaining unit employees vote on the collective bargaining contract. Once approved by a majority vote, this contract is in effect for the length of the contract unless provisions are included to alter the agreement. Both management and the union are then bound by the terms and conditions of the contract.

Before leaving this section on labor relations, it is important to note that the health care industry was not covered by the NLRA until 1974 due to concerns over public safety. In 1974 Congress repealed the exemption for the health care industry, but did include a few provisions that are specific to this industry. One of these provisions is that unions representing health care workers must give a ten-day notice of their intent to strike for the strikers to be legally protected from retaliation by their employer. In addition, the Federal Mediation and Conciliation Service (FMCS) must be contacted at least ninety days prior to the scheduled date on which the current collective bargaining contract ends. The FMCS will assign a mediator to the organization to assist with the impending negotiations and resolve any impasses. Finally, if a strike seems imminent, the FMCS director has the right to appoint a board of inquiry to investigate and attempt to resolve this dispute. Moreover, the current contract will be extended for another thirty days as well to delay the possibility of a strike (Flynn et al., 2007).

In conclusion, unions can have a dramatic impact on a company's workforce. Organizations need to understand the implications of labor relations for the management of their employees and their ultimate success in accomplishing organizational goals.

EVALUATING THE MANAGEMENT OF HUMAN RESOURCES

There are many ways to assess the effectiveness of an organization's workforce and in part evaluate the effectiveness of a company's human resources management processes. The productivity of a company's workforce can be considered, to some extent, a reflection of the company's human resources practices. The overall goal of a human resources department should be to develop the human capital of the firm. To develop this human capital the company needs to be effective at acquiring talent through the staffing process. In addition, the talent of the workforce should be cultivated appropriately through well-designed training programs and a well-thought-out performance management system. Moreover, employee policies should be implemented in such a way as to motivate and retain top talent. Thus compensation management and benefits administration should be strategically designed to reward excellence and provide incentives to stay. Furthermore, the company should monitor the critical employee attitudes addressed earlier in this chapter. If these human resources management practices are properly undertaken, the productivity of the workforce should increase. The question is, How do you know how productive a company's workforce is for a given time period?

Although there are many alternatives for evaluating the productivity of a company's workforce, four of these approaches will be addressed here to give you an idea of the variety of ways you can answer this question. A relatively simple way to measure the productivity of the workforce is to determine "labor cost as a percentage of revenue." In this assessment you divide the "total cost of employee compensation and benefits" by the "organization's revenue for the year." This value will indicate the percentage of revenue that is used to cover labor expenses. If the company's human resources management practices are becoming more effective, then the percentage should decrease over time (see Table 8.3 as an illustration of this metric). Keep in mind that labor costs generally increase over time due to pay raises and higher benefits costs. Hopefully these labor cost increases are offset by higher revenue from a talented and motivated workforce.

The next two indices of workforce productivity are closely related. The first one is "revenue per employee," whereas the second one is "profit per employee." To calculate both of these measures the company must first determine the number of full-time equivalent employees, or the FTE, at midyear. The FTE is determined based on the number of full-time employees, with part-time employees added in to some extent. The idea behind this metric is that part-time employees need to be factored into the size of the company's workforce, but that they should not be equal to full-time

Table 8.3 Labor Cost as a Percentage of Revenue

	2009	2010	2011
Labor cost (in millions)	$600	$630	$660
Revenue (in millions)	$800	$900	$1,000
Labor cost as a percentage of revenue	75 percent	70 percent	66 percent

employees. A simple way of counting part-time employees is to multiply the total number of part-time employees by a half. Thus if a company employees 600 full-time employees and 400 part-time employees, the FTE of this organization would be 800 (600 + 200). Alternately, companies may determine the FTE of their part-time workforce by totaling up the number of part-time hours worked for a given year and dividing this number by the typical number of hours worked by a full-time employee, which is approximately 2,000 (40 hours per week × 50 weeks per year, assuming 2 weeks paid time off). Once the FTE is determined, both "revenue per employee" and "profit per employee" can be calculated either by taking the revenue for the year and dividing it by the FTE or by taking the company's profits for the year and dividing that amount by the FTE. As a company's workforce becomes more productive, you would expect to see both of these metrics reveal an improvement over time. Of course, the "profit per employee" metric assumes the organization did not make any major decisions that would greatly influence the profits for the given year. For example, if a company decides to undergo a major expansion, the profits for that year may be significantly lower or nonexistent because expenses greatly increased to cover the cost of the expansion. In contrast, the "revenue per employee" would still be a valuable metric because the FTE and revenue would increase as a result of an expansion. An illustration of these metrics is presented in Table 8.4.

The final metric to assess the overall productivity of a company's workforce is the most complicated to calculate, but also the most useful indication of workforce productivity. This one is called "human capital ROI." The formula for this metric is as follows:

Table 8.4 Revenue per Employee and Profit per Employee

Revenue (in Millions)	Expenses (in Millions)	FTE	Revenue per Employee	Profit per Employee
$500	$450	1,000	**$500,000** ($500M/1,000)	**$50,000** ([$500M–$450M]/1,000)

Human capital ROI = (Revenue − [Total expenses − Labor costs]) / Labor costs

In this formula you can see that key factors from the previous metrics are included. The result of this calculation shows the company how much adjusted revenue was generated over a given time period for every dollar spent on the workforce. Table 8.5 presents an example of this calculation. This formula has the added benefit of including other expenses (for example, supplies, distribution costs, and utilities) in examining worker productivity. Ideally, the human capital ROI should be significantly higher than 1. As with the other indices, tracking this over time will illustrate the extent to which the company's workforce is becoming more or less productive.

The risk of using any of the four measures of worker productivity just mentioned is that they can be greatly influenced by external forces that do not reflect worker productivity. As you are aware, the revenue and expenses of an organization can be substantially influenced by environmental changes, such as a downturn in the economy, inflation or deflation, a change in competitor practices, government intervention, technological advances, and so on. When reviewing these measures, therefore, it is imperative to consider to what extent external influences may be artificially inflating or deflating them. Thus organizations should be cautious before assigning too much credit or blame when reviewing these findings. These metrics are valuable, but overreliance on a single statistic can be misleading.

A broader perspective on evaluating the workforce would go beyond a productivity measure or two. When examining the human resources of a company, another key dimension that should be factored into this analysis

Table 8.5 Human Capital ROI

Revenue (in Millions)	Expenses (in Millions)	Labor Costs (in Millions)	Human Capital ROI
$800	$740	$600	1.10 ($800M − [$740M − $600M])/$600M

is **employee turnover,** which should be monitored and discussed on a regular basis. The turnover rate depends on the "number of separations" in an organization over a given time period. Calculating the overall turnover rate requires calculating the number of full-time equivalent employees. The formula is as follows:

Turnover rate = (Number of separations / FTE at midpoint)×100

The "number of separations" refers to the number of former employees who left the organization during a particular time frame. For example, if a company had 40 separations in a given year and had an FTE of 200 on July 1st of that year, then the company's turnover rate for that year would be 20 percent ([40/200] × 100). The turnover rate for a company can tell a lot about how employees are managed therein. Turnover is generally viewed in negative terms in the health care industry, particularly because there is a shortage of qualified applicants in so many health care positions. If the turnover rate is increasing, then the company is faced with numerous undesirable consequences.

There are numerous costs associated with turnover. If the turnover is the result of terminations or layoffs, then the company may be paying out severance packages or providing outplacement services to help the laid-off workers find employment elsewhere; the company may also be experiencing higher unemployment compensation costs because more former employees may be collecting unemployment, and there might also be the possibility of a wrongful termination lawsuit. If an employee quits for any reason, the company may be losing a highly productive worker. Continuity of care for patients may be interrupted as well. Furthermore, if a respected employee leaves the company, then other employees may wonder if they should consider looking elsewhere for employment. Regardless of the cause of the separation, companies will be faced with replacement costs, including lost productivity while the job remains vacant, recruiting expenses, and the costs associated with the selection process. The company will also be spending additional resources on training and orientation expenses.

Companies that are concerned with turnover often break it down into two categories: voluntary and involuntary. Voluntary turnover encompasses the separations that were initiated by employees rather than the employer. Voluntary separations are commonly associated with employees' quitting to work for another employer, but they can also include employees' leaving the company for health reasons, to retire, due to the relocation of a spouse, or to go back to school to pursue a career change. Because the vast majority of voluntary turnover occurs when employees leave to work for another employer, it is an indication of the desirability of the company. Employers that are experiencing an increase in voluntary turnover should conduct exit interviews with these former employees. Patterns may emerge in these exit interviews that identify certain negative attributes of the company (such as below-average pay or benefits) or problems in a given department or area (such as abusive management or few career advancement opportunities). The causes of voluntary turnover are often within the control of the company and thus worth monitoring to limit this undesired event.

Involuntary turnover is also a valuable metric to calculate and evaluate. Involuntary turnover represents the separations initiated by the employer rather than the employees. An involuntary separation is the result of either a termination decision or a reduction in the workforce. If an organization's involuntary turnover rate is increasing due to more terminations than in previous years, the organization should explore the causes of this undesirable trend. Involuntary turnover may be the result of a poor staffing system. For example, the company may not be taking hiring seriously enough, a situation that can manifest itself in numerous ways. The company may be rushing to fill vacancies and thus not taking the extra time to attract and identify the best applicants. In addition, the company may not be using the best practices in the hiring process, leading to poor hiring choices that do not work out. (For example, the company may be relying heavily on letters of reference and unstructured interviews, which are problematic for reasons discussed in Chapter Ten.) Moreover, the company may be allowing internal politics, such as nepotism, to influence selection decisions. Beyond staffing, the involuntary turnover could be caused by inadequate time to train and orient the new hires or approaches to these activities that are poorly thought out. Perhaps new hires are being put into the job without adequate preparation and are struggling significantly, which in turn may lead to more and more terminations. Finally, involuntary turnover could be the result of poor management. New hires may not be receiving adequate direction and leadership from employees in positions of authority. Or maybe the supportive environment the new hires need to become acclimated to the job and company is not present, and they are failing on the job. Overall, numerous causes of involuntary turnover are possible and potentially correctable. Organizations need to track both types of turnover over time. Turnover metrics can be as valuable as employee productivity metrics in assessing the effectiveness of human resources management.

A final component can be added to the process of evaluating the management of a company's workforce. Both employee productivity indices and turnover rates examine outcomes related to the workforce. A recommended additional metric that provides a different perspective on the company's workforce is an employee opinion survey. Numerous topics pertaining to employee relations have been addressed in this chapter: job satisfaction, organizational commitment, and the psychological contract. Employee attitudes have an impact on job performance and turnover. An organization that has strong employee productivity, low turnover rates, and positive employee attitudes is clearly one that manages its human resources effectively. As mentioned previously, employee productivity can be influenced by external factors (such as the economy and competition). The same is true for turnover. For example, both types of turnover can be affected by the labor market. Companies may be reluctant to let someone go whom they know will be difficult to replace (involuntary turnover), or an employee may be reluctant to quit when the job market is tight (voluntary turnover). Collecting and assessing employee attitudes provides insight into workers' motivation to be productive and their intention to remain with the company.

Before collecting data on employee opinions, the company should carefully decide what opinions are the most valuable. There are countless questions that can be asked. Companies publish numerous documents that indicate what type of company they want to be, such as the vision, mission, and values and ethics statements. Assuming these documents represent how these companies truly see themselves, these documents should be valuable in identifying the key opinions to assess among employees.

Once the key topics are defined, the company should decide how it wants to collect these data. Generally there are two options in collecting employee opinions: employee focus groups or employee opinion surveys. Focus groups are attractive because they allow employees to provide rich responses concerning these topics. The group dynamic may stimulate feedback as well. In addition, employees often find participating in a focus group to be more meaningful than filling out another survey. This option sends the message that their opinion really counts. Unfortunately, focus groups are much more labor intensive than opinion surveys and therefore more costly and time consuming. Further, some employees may be reluctant to share their true feelings without the anonymity of a survey. Finally, a focus group can devolve into an employee gripe session if the focus group's leader loses control.

Employee opinion surveys are valuable for many reasons. All employees can be given a survey and thus an opportunity to voice their opinions. In addition, surveys allow for quantification of opinions much more readily than do focus groups. Therefore, if the company wants to track employee attitudes over time, much as it would employee productivity and turnover, employee surveys are much better designed for this task. Surveys also have the advantages of costing less than focus groups, they enable faster data collection, and they allow the respondent to have either anonymity or at least confidentiality. Surveys can, however, have poor response rates if they are administered too often, require too much time to complete, or are not seen as taken seriously by management. If surveys are developed, administered, and assessed properly, they can be an excellent tool for gaining insight into the psyche of a company's workforce.

In conclusion, an employer should evaluate its workforce on a regular basis. Evaluating the productivity of the workforce has obvious benefits. Relying only on employee output, however, is shortsighted. A company should also include in its assessment both a critical measure of employee behavior, such as employee turnover, and employee opinions and attitudes. By including all three components in the evaluation, the organization has taken a comprehensive view of how well it manages its most valuable resource: its people. Because the health care industry is labor intensive, this perspective is paramount to managing human resources.

SUMMARY

This chapter has provided an overview of human resources management for health care organizations. The primary message is that for a health care company to be successful, it needs to acquire, develop, and retain a highly talented workforce. Achieving this goal is especially difficult due to the shortage of qualified employees in many health care specialties. In addition, organizations need to understand the rights of their employees (statutory, contractual, and implied) in managing their workforce. Proper management should lead to positive employee attitudes in the form of job satisfaction, organizational commitment, and a relational psychological contract. Poor management can lead to dissatisfaction, employee turnover, and possibly unionization. Finally, organizations should track such key measures of their labor force as workforce productivity, employee turnover, and critical employee attitudes.

KEY TERMS

collective bargaining

employee turnover

employment-at-will

job satisfaction

organizational commitment

psychological contract

unionization

whistleblowing

wrongful discharge

REVIEW QUESTIONS

1. In spite of difficult economic times, numerous health care jobs are considered to be in high demand. The compensation and mobility associated with a number of health care positions should encourage many people to pursue these career paths. Based on your knowledge of the health care industry, what do you expect over the next ten years or so in regard to the health care job market? Do you expect demand for health care professionals to increase, decrease, or remain stable in the years to come? Please explain.

2. The key message in this chapter is that any company should view its employees with respect and as a potential competitive advantage in the marketplace if managed properly. Human resources professionals should assist the organization in identifying highly qualified people for job openings, provide relevant training and orientation activities to assist new hires, design a compensation and benefits package that will motivate and retain quality workers, and so on. Due to time constraints, office politics, and budgetary limitations, is this a realistic expectation for most organizations? Please explain.

3. The topic of employee discipline comes up in relation to the subject of employer and employee rights. Most people do not look forward to disciplining others, and those responsible for administering discipline measures often try their best to be fair. Fairness is a perception that can vary from one affected party to another. Consistency in discipline is easier to attain if the company develops a comprehensive and objective policy that has clear penalties for specific violations (for example, "The second time you're late within a one-month period, you get a one-day suspension"). These policies, however, do not leave much room for other factors that may influence perceptions of fairness, such as seniority differences, tragedies in one's personal life, or one's past performance record. What do you see as the main employee discipline issues in health care organizations? Do you think most organizations handle these issues fairly and consistently? Do you have any recommendations to improve this process?

4. Employee retention and its counterpart, turnover, are critical issues in many health care organizations. What do you see as some of the critical costs associated with turnover in health care? What do you see as the key factors influencing retention in health care?

9

Staffing Health Care Organizations
Recruitment and Selection

Marc C. Marchese

LEARNING OBJECTIVES

- Be aware of the options organizations have in filling job openings
- Be able to evaluate the pros and cons of internal versus external recruiting
- Be knowledgeable of the various internal and external recruiting methods
- Be able to evaluate the relative success of various approaches to recruitment
- Be aware of the factors influencing the selection process
- Be familiar with major selection methods for health care organizations
- Be able to evaluate the relative success of selection procedures

The previous chapter presented one of the major challenges of human resources management, the growing demand for health services due to an aging population and the shortage of qualified professionals in many health care areas. This challenge makes the organizational process of recruiting and selecting employees extremely critical to providing quality care to patients. If health care organizations cannot hire highly talented employees, the overall quality of care will suffer, as will the reputation and success of the company. The purpose of this chapter is to highlight the critical issues involved in staffing a health care organization. The first part of this chapter will discuss the options organizations have in filling job openings. Then the role of the recruiting function in attracting the best and the brightest for any organization will be explored. The chapter will end by discussing in detail the selection process once a qualified pool of applicants has been established.

BEGINNING THE STAFFING PROCESS

Let's begin this chapter with the beginning of the staffing process. Someone in the company, whether he or she is a department head, division manager, or team leader, perceives the need to hire someone. This person requests permission to hire someone from the individual who is responsible for authorizing the start of the hiring process. The person who can give this authorization will vary from company to company. He or she may, for example, be the head of the affected division or location. In smaller organizations approval might require the consent of the vice president of business affairs or the chief financial officer. In other companies the head of human resources may play a role as well in granting a department permission to hire.

Alternatives to Hiring Full-Time Staff

Whoever has the authority to grant permission to hire should at least consider alternatives to hiring. When an organization seeks to hire a full-time employee it is making a commitment that may or may not work out. In most organizations full-time employees receive a variety of benefits from their employer, typically including health and other types of insurance (for example, vision, dental, disability, life); retirement benefits; and paid time off. These benefits can be quite costly to the employer. In addition to offering these benefits, an employer will have to match social security contributions based on the employee's pay. The employer will also be responsible for worker's compensation costs if the employee gets injured or ill in the course of employment. Furthermore, the employer may have to let the employee go at some point down the road, and consequently the former employee may collect unemployment compensation and severance pay. If the employee that does get hired ends up not working out and the employer fires this individual, the employer may have to defend itself against a wrongful termination charge. Considering all of these drawbacks to hiring a full-time employee, it is not surprising many employers at least entertain other options for fulfilling staffing needs before granting permission to hire.

One of the alternatives to hiring a full-time employee is outsourcing. Instead of filling a position with an employee, some companies may enter a contract with a third party to obtain various services. Outsourcing can have many advantages over a traditional staffing approach. For example, contracting with a vendor may afford access to better technology for certain forms of medical testing, provide high-level expertise in an area in which it may be expensive or difficult to hire, allow for greater workforce flexibility in areas in which staffing needs are variable, and yield overall savings for the organization. Health care organizations are likely to consider outsourcing such noncore service functions as purchasing, billing and collection, and maintaining tax compliance (Danvers & Nikolov, 2010). In terms of human resources management, there are several areas that may be outsourced: payroll, outplacement services, employee assistance programs, employee training and development, benefits administration, and candidate background checks (Fallon & McConnell, 2007). In terms of health care specifically, a recent study indicated that hospitals are likely to outsource business office services, food services, laundry services, and assessment of patient satisfaction (Danvers & Nikolov). Although many of the hospitals investigated in this study engaged in outsourcing, the results did not consistently reveal cost savings for them. However, other research has shown that outsourcing can lead to improvements in patient satisfaction in regard to the quality of the services provided (DerGuarahian, 2007). Outsourcing is not without risks and challenges. Companies engaging in outsourcing are relinquishing control over a function and entering a contract with a third party.

Finding the right vendor for the right price and for the right length of time is not easy. However, outsourcing is nevertheless worth considering when staffing demands are not being met.

An option related to outsourcing is employee leasing. Under an employee leasing agreement a vendor will supply personnel to provide services on-site for an organization. For example, a hospital could use employee leasing in food services. The vendor will supply workers to prepare, distribute, and collect food items at the hospital. The hospital can oversee these employees and even give performance feedback on them. However, these workers are not employees of the hospital and thus do not receive hospital benefits or get paid by the hospital. The vendor is also responsible for expenses related to worker's compensation, social security, and unemployment compensation. The downside of employee leasing for the hospital is that because these workers are not hospital employees, the hospital neither selects the "best and the brightest" nor has the same ability to influence these workers' productivity through performance management, which will be discussed in the next chapter.

Another option that is specific to the health care industry is the use of **locum tenens,** a Latin expression for "one holding a place." Locum tenens are temporary workers, and they are usually certain physicians or nurses. The use of locum tenens can help meet the needs of a health care organization that is experiencing a shortage of qualified personnel in these areas. Locum tenens typically get paid a daily rate. Some of these arrangements are made through a staffing service, whereas others are created through more informal means. The growing number of locum tenens among physicians was initially attributed in large part to the rising number of female physicians looking for employment that could be flexible to their personal needs (Croasdale, 2002). However, a research study of over 1,500 such physicians found that most were male (70 percent), in their fifties (with a mean age of fifty-three), and primarily motivated to be locum tenens to continue to practice on a part-time basis (62 percent). Moreover, many use this employment opportunity as a way to augment their retirement income (Simon & Alonzo, 2004).

A final alternative to hiring full-time employees is hiring part-time employees. Part-time employees usually are not eligible for benefits, and their schedules are easier to adjust as staffing demands fluctuate. Part-time employees can be used for any job in a health care organization. Many people incorrectly assume that most part-time employees want to be full-time workers. However, according to the Bureau of Labor Statistics (2011), there were approximately twenty-seven million part-time workers in May 2011. Almost 70 percent of these part-time workers were part-time by choice to accommodate family demands, to supplement their retirement income, or because of personal preference. Hiring part-time employees is thus another viable option for health care employers to consider before seeking full-time employees to fill vacancies.

Although several worthwhile alternatives to hiring full-time employees have just been presented, however, most of the time organizations will attempt to meet staffing needs with full-time employees. The advantages of this choice are aligned with the goals of human resources management. If the key to providing high-quality care is to have a high-quality workforce, then the health care organization needs to attract, motivate, and retain highly talented employees. To achieve this objective, offering attractive full-time positions with competitive salaries and benefits provides the greatest opportunity for companies both to identify talented applicants and to reward top performers with new and more challenging positions. In addition, there are several drawbacks of hiring part-time employees, locum tenens, temporary workers, and so on. The nature of these arrangements leads to a higher turnover rate among these workers than among full-time employees. Therefore, part-time health care workers are more often "learning on the job," which may compromise the continuity of care. Employee training, mentoring, and orientation are less likely to be systematically applied to these groups as well. Furthermore, the commitment to organizational success of a worker who sees an assignment as his or her *job* for right now may not be as strong as that of a full-time employee who hopes for a *career* with the organization. For all of these reasons, this chapter will emphasize creating a staffing process for full-time employees that benefits both the organization and the individual.

The Value of Job Analysis

When the company begins the staffing process it is tempting to start advertising the position and collecting employment applications. However, jumping too quickly into recruiting can be a big mistake. From a human resources perspective, the first step in the staffing process should be to clearly define the job opening and the type of person best suited for this position. Thus, the person or persons involved in the hiring process should take a close look at the job description before taking any recruiting steps. Is the current job description accurate? The company may want to solicit feedback from other employees who hold the same position as the one that requires filling in regard to the accuracy of the job description. Due to technological advances and new business processes or policies, the job may have changed significantly since the job description was last revised. In addition, the company may have different expectations for its incumbents in this position. The hiring person or committee needs to spend time clearly defining the tasks, duties, and responsibilities of the job opening.

When reviewing and revising the job description, employers must also be cognizant of the Americans with Disabilities Act (ADA) of 1990. This law prohibits discrimination against people with disabilities who can perform the essential functions of a job with or without reasonable accommodation. Therefore, when companies are reviewing the tasks, duties, and responsibilities of a given job, they must clearly identify which of these functions are essential and which are not. The ADA defines a function as essential if it is a primary reason why this job exists. Typically, essential functions require specialized education and training and are performed on a regular basis by job incumbents (DiLorenzo & London, 2006). Employers do not want to consider nonessential functions in evaluating applicants to fill job openings.

Once the job description is accurate and ADA compliant, the next step in the hiring process should be to align the job specifications with the revised job description. The job specifications are often attached to the job description, defining the knowledge, skills, abilities, and other characteristics (KSAOs) desired for this job. When reviewing the essential functions of the job opening, the employees responsible for filling it should identify which KSAOs are needed to perform these critical tasks, duties, and responsibilities. Employees that are very knowledgeable about the given job, often referred to as subject matter experts, should be consulted and asked to examine or create the list of KSAOs associated with this job.

Human resources professionals make distinctions between skills and abilities. Skills are directly observable capabilities, such as operating a piece of equipment (for example, an X-ray machine) or performing a manual task (for example, drawing blood from a patient). Abilities are cognitive capabilities that are inferred from behaviors (such as making a diagnosis or interpreting MRI results). Other characteristics that are included in the job specifications are such aspects as required licenses or certifications, desired or required education, and previous work experience. For many jobs these are difficult decisions to make. For example, job announcements usually indicate that previous work experience is desired, but how much is required is debatable. Often companies will advertise that a job requires five years of previous work experience. Is this requirement stated in the job specifications? How was this number decided on? Does something magically happen to employees when they go from four to five years of work experience? Obviously not, but these hurdles are commonly used in the staffing process to distinguish among applicants. Organizations should rely on subject matter experts to guide job requirements as indicated in the job specifications. It should be noted that requirements for licenses and certifications in health care are guided by state law or by professional standards.

As an alternative to a KSAO analysis pertaining to a specific job, a competency-based approach to job analysis has been adopted by some health care organizations. Competencies are broad characteristics that are relevant across many jobs. Common competencies include leadership, oral communication, problem solving, data management, and customer relations. As you can surmise, these competencies pertain to a wide variety of positions. To illustrate how this could be applied in a health care setting, an advanced practice nurse will be used as an example. Advanced practice nurses have both the basic nursing education (with licensure) and specialized experience and certification (Fried & Fottler, 2011). An advanced practice nurse might be a certified nurse midwife, a clinical nurse specialist, or a certified nurse anesthetist, among other occupations. Several competencies have been identified among advanced practice nurses: ethical decision making, consultation, clinical and professional leadership, and research skills (Hamric, 2005). Health care organizations can use these competencies to guide their selection process in evaluating their applicants. Employers need to determine if a traditional KSAO approach or a competency-based approach is best suited for their staffing and performance management process.

Many health care organizations are accredited, or seek accreditation, by The Joint Commission (TJC). Approximately nineteen thousand health care organizations and programs are currently accredited by TJC ("About The Joint Commission," 2011). Accreditation by TJC is considered a mark of distinction and quality throughout the United States. Health care organizations must comply with numerous standards to achieve and maintain this accreditation. One section of these standards applies to human resources. The first two standards in the human resources section pertain to the staffing process. TJC requires employers to make sure employees' qualifications are consistent with their job ("Health Care," 2010). The hiring process can be subject to review in an accreditation visit. Updated job descriptions and job specifications are expected documentation to satisfy this part of the review process.

Overall, job analysis is critical to guide numerous decisions that will be made in recruiting and selecting applicants for the job opening. The job description and specifications, if accurate, clearly define job requirements and indicate key qualifications for applicants. Further, the process of reviewing and revising these documents is important to complying with ADA regulations. Finally, this process and documentation are important for health care organizations seeking to attain or maintain TJC accreditation. Skipping this step would be unwise in many ways and is likely to lead to a poor hiring decision. Once the job analysis review is completed, the next step in the staffing process is recruitment.

RECRUITMENT

The primary goal of recruitment is to create a pool of qualified applicants for a given job opening. In general, companies prefer the applicant pool to be large, thereby providing them with more choice in the hiring process. However, too many applicants can create a daunting task for an organization to sort through. As mentioned earlier, in many health care positions there is a shortage of qualified applicants. Having too large of an applicant pool is not very likely for most health care positions at this time. The biggest challenge for health care organizations in recruiting is deciding the most effective way to create this pool. There are many options for organizations to consider. Before discussing these options, however, it bears mention that there are important recruiting decisions that need to be made before the position is advertised.

The first decision the organization has to make is how to present the job opening to potential applicants. Companies often have tried to make the job and the organization seem as attractive as possible to potential applicants. This approach can lead the applicants and ultimately the new hire to have overly optimistic views of the new position. When the new hire has been in the position for a little while and soon realizes that this job is not as perfect as he or she was expecting, that person may become disenchanted and start thinking about moving on to another organization. Human resources management research on this topic has led many companies to turn to the **realistic job preview (RJP)** in the recruiting process. An RJP indicates that applicants will be informed of both the positive and negative aspects of a job opening. For example, due to nursing shortages, many hospitals know that their nursing staff will be expected to work overtime on a regular basis. Informing applicants of the overtime demands of a job opening for nurses would weed out applicants who strongly dislike working overtime. In this way the applicant and the organization do not waste each other's time in the hiring process. Many jobs in health care are highly stressful, are subject to staffing shortages, have considerable travel demands, and experience budget constraints. Fully disclosing to applicants the pros and cons of the job opening is an effective way to reduce turnover and yield many other positive consequences for the company (Phillips, 1998). This has been found to be true in many industries, including health care (Crow, Hartman, & McLendon, 2009). In conclusion, an RJP is recommended for recruitment.

The next significant decision in recruiting applicants is where to look for them. There are two main options in recruiting: internal or external. An internal recruiting approach indicates that the company wants to use a current employee to fill the job opening, whereas an external recruiting approach indicates that the company wants a new hire to fill the job opening. There are advantages and disadvantages to both of these choices.

Internal recruiting has many positive aspects. This approach to recruiting sends the message to the workforce that the company wants to provide opportunities for its employees to take on new challenges and thereby grow and prosper in this organization. To make this happen, larger organizations often have career planning systems or career ladders for their workforce that allow employees to move up the corporate hierarchy. Internal recruiting is required to make any career ladder feasible. A related concept is succession planning, whereby specific employees are targeted for upper-level positions. In both career and succession planning, employees will need opportunities to move into new positions to develop the skills required for advancement. For example, in many hospital settings the chief medical officer began his or her career as a physician (Fried & Fottler, 2011). While employed as a physician, this individual probably embraced numerous administrative roles (such as that of the department head) and completed an advanced degree in business or health care administration. There are comparable career paths for other health care professionals as well, including nurses and therapists (Flynn, Mathis, & Jackson, 2007). Internal recruiting therefore has the advantage of developing the organization's human capital and at the same time being an effective retention device.

Another advantage of internal recruiting is that it is typically much more cost effective and timely than external recruiting. Moving a current employee into a new position can be much quicker than offering a job to a new hire who needs time to leave his or her current position and may expect additional time and reimbursement for relocation. In addition, internal recruiting provides greater information about the applicants than external recruiting. Because the internal applicant is already an employee, the company has knowledge of several critical aspects of this applicant. Is this person dependable? Does this person work well in a team environment? Can this person multitask effectively? How does this person deal with confrontation from patients or their families? A job interview or a background check may provide some insight into these questions in regard to external applicants, but internal applicants have a proven track record through their history of attendance, performance reviews, or other internal documentation systems. Finally, internal candidates have a much better idea of the department or division associated with the job opening, and they have a much more realistic job preview. Their expectations are likely to be more accurate than those of an external candidate, which in turn should help with retention.

There are also many advantages, however, of recruiting externally rather than internally. Recruiting externally is more likely to result in a larger pool of applicants, whereas internally there may only be a few employees who would even be eligible to apply for the job opening. In health care, provider jobs are often specialized and require a particular educational background, certification, or license—or a combination of these. Finding internal applicants may be unrealistic for staffing certain health care jobs, such as a surgical position. Even if there are potentially several internal applicants, external recruiting is more likely to lead to a larger pool of applicants, possibly including many highly talented candidates to select from. Moreover, external candidates are more likely to bring fresh perspectives into the organization, and external recruiting may also provide opportunities to increase diversity in an organization. What is more, external recruiting may simplify the recruiting process by avoiding the "domino effect" that could occur from an internal approach. The domino effect begins when an internal candidate fills a high-level job opening in the company. Now this person's job needs to be filled. Another internal person fills this job, which leads to another job opening, and so on. An external approach avoids this cascade of job openings. A final advantage of external recruiting is that it may lead to more objectivity in supervisory positions. For example, if a nursing manager's position becomes available, an internal approach may result in moving up a nurse into this job. This new nursing manager has established both positive and negative relationships with the other nurses. In his or her new role as a nursing manager, this person may have a tough time objectively leading employees whom he or she knows very well. An external person may be a better choice, especially if the department requires immediate and difficult personnel decisions.

In thinking about internal and external approaches to recruiting, companies do not have to commit to one choice over the other. Some organizations will always attempt to recruit internally first, and then if no desirable applicants come forward they will pursue an external approach. Other companies will adopt both approaches simultaneously and look for the best applicants regardless of whether a candidate is a current employee or not. Finally, some organizations will adopt an internal approach for certain jobs and an external approach for other jobs on a case-by-case basis. There is not one perfect answer to this issue. Organizations need to be aware of the advantages and disadvantages of both choices and think carefully about this decision before committing to a desired recruiting approach. The human resources department should work with the person or persons responsible for hiring and discuss the pros and cons of each option to help the company adopt the best recruiting strategy. Once the strategy has been decided on, the hiring manager or committee can move on to the next stage of the staffing process, which is to decide which recruiting methods will be used to create the pool of applicants—whether they are external or internal—for the job opening.

Internal Recruiting

Internal recruiting methods are not as diverse as external recruiting methods, but organizations do have some choices if they adopt an internal recruiting approach. A common internal recruiting method is an internal job posting. Companies can make their employees aware of a job opening by posting it in some manner that has wide accessibility for employees. For example, many companies have their own Web site with a link to the human resources department. On the department's Web page there can be another link for job openings. Similarly, organizations can rely on the company's e-mail system to advertise internal job openings. In addition to using these technology-based options, companies may simply put up flyers in popular areas of the business (for example, near the time clock, in the lunch or break room, on a bulletin board) or stick job announcements in paycheck envelopes.

Besides using job postings, companies may engage in internal recruiting based on their career or succession planning system. Requests for promotions and transfers can be examined in relation to the required qualifications of the job opening. Experience in certain jobs may prepare employees to move into the job opening. The human resources department should work closely with department managers to establish career paths for employees. When a position opens up, the department can communicate with the relevant department head to indicate which employees have the qualifications necessary to be considered for the job. Human resources professionals may also create a talent or skills inventory for the company's workforce to ascertain which employees across the organization meet the qualifications of the job. These employees can then be contacted directly to see if they want to be considered for the transfer or promotion. A well-designed career planning system can be mutually beneficial to the employer and the employees. For the employer, this system helps prepare employees for future job openings and thus develops talent in the workforce. A lack of succession planning can leave a company in a difficult spot, especially if a senior leader leaves unexpectedly. Such initiatives as mentoring, coaching, and leadership development can pay off in the long run. Employees may also be more likely to remain in the company if they know they will have opportunities in the future to move into new positions (Hauff, 2007).

The other common approach to internal recruiting is more informal. Internal networking (also known as the "grapevine" method) can be an effective way to find internal applicants. Many jobs are filled based on "whom you know." This approach can be highly subjective if it's based primarily on having "friends in high places," or it can be more systematic if the company allows employees to make internal referrals based on the job requirements. Some organizations will even reward employees for successful referrals of their coworkers if their referral is awarded the new position and he or she works out (Heneman & Judge, 2003). Whether or not this approach results in the promotion or transfer of a successful applicant is largely based on the extent to which qualifications influence the applicant pool over friendships or personal relationships. Overall, there are several choices in internal recruiting. Companies have to decide which methods are aligned with their values in regard to managing their people as well as the quality of their options in staffing the job opening.

External Recruiting

There are so many options when deciding on external recruiting methods that an entire chapter could be devoted to this topic. This chapter, however, will only touch on the major external recruiting methods. Before delving into the various choices for external recruiting, the first step an organization should undertake is to identify the relevant labor market for the job opening. The relevant labor market is determined by where the company expects applicants to come from for this position, and is generally based on geography (Mathis & Jackson, 2009). Organizations, with the help of their human resources department, will determine if applicants for this job opening are likely to come from the local area, from this region of the country, from somewhere else in the United States, or even from another country. With the shortage of health care professionals in many areas, the relevant labor market can be quite large, especially if an organization has job openings for surgical specialties. The choices of external recruiting methods will be influenced by the relevant labor market. For example, it would make little sense to advertise only in the local newspaper if the relevant labor market is international.

A review of the traditional external recruiting methods must include help-wanted ads in newspapers. This method has been around for a long time and is still popular today. Newspapers are an excellent choice to reach the local market, and the advantages of this recruiting source are numerous. Advertising in a local paper is usually very quick. The help-wanted ad may appear the next day in the classified section, which is a well-known place for job seekers to look. This method is also very flexible. Human resources professionals or others representing the company can tailor the ad however they see fit, which may or may not mean including the company's logo, salary information, the job description, company information, an equal opportunity employer notice, the deadline to apply, and so on. Furthermore, this method does not require the applicants to use any technology to access the ad, which may unnecessarily eliminate some desirable applicants who are not skilled at using the Internet for job searching. Moreover, newspapers ads typically have an online version as well. Employers can therefore advertise both in print and online using a single service.

One of the most successful traditional external recruiting methods is employee referrals. In terms of external recruiting, using employee referrals entails having your employees spread the word about job openings to their friends and family who do not currently work for the employer. This method has been found to be highly effective for finding qualified applicants. The turnover rate for employees who found out about the job opening through this method is lower than for those hired using other recruiting methods (Berry, 2003). Part of the success of this method is attributed to the fact that employees are not going to refer someone to work in their organization who will reflect poorly on them. Because the person they are referring is a friend or family member, employees screen out ahead of time the possible applicants who they expect would not be a good fit in their company. Moreover, employees also give their friends or family members a realistic job preview, so the potential applicant knows more about the work environment before applying for the job. As already mentioned, in many companies employees are given a reward for a successful referral, which usually means the person they referred is hired and is still employed for a certain amount of time, and this offers further incentive to make quality referrals.

There are two issues companies should consider before committing strongly to employee referrals, one of which is diversity. If the organization is concerned about a lack of ethnic or racial diversity, employee referrals may not be an effective mechanism to improve this situation. Employees typically have friends and family members from similar ethnic and racial groups. The other issue to consider is nepotism. If employees are referring friends and family members, the company has to decide to what extent it wants employees to work side by side with their relatives. Nepotism can lead to organizational conflict in companies if other employees perceive favoritism in the workplace among relatives (Bohlander & Snell, 2010). Many companies will impose antinepotism policies that prohibit family members from working in the same department or under the direct line of supervision of a relative. Despite these considerations, employee referrals can be an effective way to recruit applicants externally.

Another traditional external recruiting method that can be applicable for health care organizations is college recruiting. College recruiting has the advantage of a large pool of potential applicants who will be looking for employment in the near future. In addition, most college graduates have limited work experience and thus are expecting entry-level positions with entry-level pay for their chosen field. Furthermore, a quality higher education program should be producing graduates with the latest knowledge and skills pertinent to that profession. As hospitals or other types of health care employers looks for nurses, physician assistants, nuclear medical technologists, or physical therapists, highly respected college programs are a common external recruiting choice. The major drawback of college recruiting is that students are not available to work until graduation, which may be several months away, but the organization may need someone immediately. The other drawbacks of this method include the cost of sending the company's recruiters to various colleges as well as competition from other health care organizations that also desire these soon-to-be-graduates. Overall, however, college recruiting can be an excellent external recruiting choice.

Among other traditional external recruiting choices is advertising on television or on the radio. This option has the advantage that these two industries regularly monitor the demographics of their viewers or listeners. Organizations can use this information to target a particular applicant pool. Another traditional method is job fairs. Job fairs attract a large group of potential applicants, especially in difficult economic times. Unfortunately, employers are never sure whether the quality of the applicants at job fairs will match their job requirements. A free traditional external recruiting source for employers is the local unemployment office. Here again the quality of applicants may not meet the employers' needs. Another way to go about external recruiting that is free is for employers to retain unsolicited resumes and application forms. Oftentimes job seekers will target employers when looking for job openings, and organizations will keep these documents for six months or so in case positions open in the future. One more traditional external recruiting method deserves some attention here. Executive search firms or private employment agencies can be a valuable option, especially if the company needs someone in a high-ranking position. The assumption of executive search firms, sometimes crudely referred to as "headhunters," is that the best executives are employed. For a substantial fee (which can be as high as 33 percent of the person's base salary paid by the employer), these firms will persuade executives to leave their current job for the open position. Because top leaders of any organization can have a substantial impact on the financial well-being of the company, many employers find it worth paying these high fees to get the best and the brightest for these types of positions. In conclusion, there are several traditional external recruiting methods that are viable options for health care organizations to consider in attracting applicants.

More recently technology has opened up new avenues for employers to attract applicants in the form of **Internet recruiting.** There are hundreds of Web sites dedicated to recruiting. Most people have heard of Monster. com, but there are countless others. According to a recent study, approximately 4.2 million Internet help-wanted ads were available each month in 2011 ("Online Help-Wanted," 2011). Many recruiting Web sites focus exclusively on the health care industry. A quick Google search results in such Web sites as

www.healthcarejobs.org

www.healthcarejobsite.com

www.healthcare.careerbuilder.com

www.healthjobsusa.com

www.healthcareerweb.com

As mentioned previously, newspapers will often have a Web site corresponding to their print help-wanted ads. So job seekers can go to such places as www.jobmarket.nytimes.com, www.nationaljobs.washingtonpost.com, or www.latimes.com/classifieds/jobs. Moreover, health care employers will use their own company Web site to advertise job openings, such as www.mayoclinic.com/health/employment/AM00012, www.hopkinsmedicine.org/employment/index.html, or www.bcbs.com/careers/. Finally, health care professional associations will advertise employment opportunities online for their members. For example, one can find many job openings for physicians through the American Medical Association using a program called FRIEDA online. The American Nursing Association also has a link, www.nursing-world.org/careercenter/, that can help job seekers in this area. Similar Web sites can be found for physician assistants, such as that of the American Academy of Physician Assistants (www.aapa.org/find-a-job), as well as most other health care professions.

The advantages of using the Internet to recruit applicants are numerous. To begin with, Internet help-wanted ads can appear almost immediately after they are created. Also, online job postings can virtually reach the entire world and therefore may produce a large applicant pool. As indicated earlier, health care employers can target workers in certain health care professions using particular Web sites, thereby reaching specific types of applicants based on the job opening. Further, Internet sites may include links that allow interested applicants to submit a résumé or complete an online application. This can save the employer considerable time in processing applications. In addition, if the résumés or applications are submitted online, employers could adopt scanning software to eliminate unqualified applicants.

The disadvantages of Internet recruiting are also worth mentioning. Because the Internet can reach all corners of our globe, Internet recruiting has the potential to result in an overwhelming number of responses. Even with a résumé-scanning software program, the vast quantity of applications received may be extremely time consuming for an employer to process. In addition, the Equal Employment Opportunity Commission ("Recordkeeping," 2004) has defined an applicant as anyone who has followed the company's application procedure and expressed an interest in the job opening. Thus all online job applicants may need to be accounted for in case there are any equal employment opportunity (EEO) challenges to the company's hiring system. Another concern with Internet recruiting pertains to the assumption that applicants have computer access and expertise to use this technology. For some positions in health care organizations, most likely lower-level positions, this assumption may not be relevant to the job and may result in an adverse impact on people from lower socioeconomic groups. A final concern with Internet recruiting is that if the relevant labor market is local, the company may not want to consider applicants from other parts of the country or even from other countries. Internet recruiting is a valuable and popular external recruiting tool, but the drawbacks of this option should be considered before using this method.

Other nontraditional external recruiting tools also have to do with technology. The proliferation of social media outlets on the Web has opened up new recruiting options for employers. For example, Facebook, MySpace, LinkedIn, and Twitter can be used to communicate job openings. Research on these options is limited in regard to employers' success in finding quality applicants through these outlets. Recent studies have indicated that over 80 percent of employers do use social media for various purposes, with recruitment being the most popular use. LinkedIn was the most popular of the social media tools just listed for recruiting purposes ("Recruiting," 2010). As more and more people use social media tools, it is likely that the growth of external recruiting via these options will rise. The challenge for employers will be deciding if these choices are as effective at reaching the relevant labor market as traditional external methods or well-known Internet recruiting sites. Furthermore, employers will want to be certain that these Web sites reach a diverse enough audience to avoid claims of discrimination based on race, ethnicity, disability, or age. From an EEO perspective, at this point organizations would be wise not to rely heavily on social media outlets for recruiting. A few years from now, however, this statement may be completely inaccurate.

There also external recruiting methods that are specific to the health care industry. Due to the demands of many health care provider positions in regard to training and education, health care professionals may be required to participate in certain programs before they can begin regular employment. These programs provide opportunities for health care employers to "test out" potential applicants before they are ready to enter the workforce on a full-time basis. For example, pharmacists and nurse practitioners may complete a preceptorship or internship as part of their professional preparation. Physicians are required to perform clinical rotations to become certified. Fellowships are also available to health care professionals seeking development for managerial positions (Flynn et al., 2007). All of these programs give employers access to these individuals in a work setting, thus allowing companies to identify applicants with high potential. Of all of the external recruiting methods mentioned up to this point, these options specific to health care could be the most successful, especially if the demands of the program and the demands of the job are similar.

In conclusion, there are many internal and external recruiting methods for employers to consider in creating an applicant pool. Because many of these choices have strengths and weaknesses, it would not make sense for a health care organization to rely exclusively on only one or two of them. However, as organizations strive to control costs and improve quality, it does make sense for them to evaluate the success of the recruiting methods used. The final subsection on recruitment will address evaluating the recruiting function.

Evaluating the Recruiting Function

There are many ways to evaluate recruiting methods. These evaluation approaches are applied to external rather than internal recruiting methods because external methods often have significant costs associated with them (as with executive search firms) and may be quite time consuming (as with job fairs and college recruiting). Due to the time and costs associated with recruiting, two of the more common metrics to evaluate recruiting are "time to fill job openings" and "recruiting cost per hire." If speed in filling job openings is critical to the company, then "time to fill job openings" can be a valuable assessment of a recruiting method. Similarly, most employers are very cost conscious, and thus examining the "recruiting cost per hire" for each recruiting source can make sense as well. The drawback with both of these metrics is that quality is not factored in. Filling a position quickly is only desirable if the new hire is successful. If an employer hires someone who doesn't work out, then the employer is back to refilling the position. Moreover, the employer may take on certain costs associated with turnover, such as unemployment compensation, lawsuits for wrongful termination, severance pay, and lost productivity. Many employers would prefer to take more time and hire someone great than just get a "body" on board to fill a vacancy. It may therefore be better, for example, to wait a few months on a soon-to-be graduate of a respected nursing program than to hire an applicant with a long history of job hopping who responded to a help-wanted ad. Similarly, the recruiting cost for each hire is usually calculated by taking the direct cost of the recruiting method (for example, $500 for an ad on Monster.com) divided by the number of new hires who applied from that method. This metric often does not take into account other costs associated with the staffing process. For example, if a job posting on a Web site generated 200 applications but only 10 were quality applicants, the organization had to process 190 unqualified submissions. However, if another method generated only 30 applicants but 25 were impressive, the company's resources may have been better spent on the second method, even if the cost per hire was higher than with the first method.

One of the best approaches to assessing the effectiveness of recruiting methods is called a **yield ratio.** Simply put, a yield ratio is a percentage of success from a given recruiting source (Bohlander & Snell, 2010). The employer decides on some measure or measures of success in the recruiting function (for example, the number of applicants worth interviewing, the number of applicants offered a job, or the number of applicants who get hired and remain with the company for at least one year). For each recruiting method used, the measure or measures of success are determined and then divided by the number of applications generated by that method, and this number is then multiplied by 100:

$$\text{Yield ratio} = (\text{Number of successes} / \text{Number of applications}) \times 100$$

Table 9.1 provides some fictitious data for a hospital in regard to the recruitment of occupational therapists. The hospital considers a quality hire (a success) someone who is offered a job and stays at least six months.

Table 9.1   Recruitment Data

Recruiting Source	Number of Applications	Number Hired Who Lasted at Least Six Months	Yield Ratio
College campus	100	20	20 percent
www.otjoblink.org/*	30	15	50 percent

*This is the employment link from the American Occupational Therapy Association.

Based on the data in the table, the yield ratio for campus recruiting is only 20 percent, whereas the Web site from the American Occupational Therapy Association generated a yield ratio of 50 percent. In this fabricated example, therefore, the Web site is a more effective external recruiting source for this job. The value of yield ratios is contingent on a solid means of defining and measuring quality. Determining the quality of the applicant pool is the key to evaluating the success of a recruiting method, especially for health care organizations that depend on having a talented workforce.

SELECTION

The last part of the staffing process is selection. Selection is one approach to hiring, whereby the organization assesses applicants and "selects" the best applicant for the job. Hiring can be done in this manner, but unfortunately it can be done in other ways as well. Instead of determining the most qualified person for the position and offering the best candidate the job first, some organizations are influenced by internal politics in the hiring process. For example, nepotism may affect who gets offered the job regardless of qualifications. Personal biases against women, people of color, older applicants, or individuals with certain other characteristics may contribute to a person's not being given a job opportunity. In addition, some companies may be in such a rush to get someone as quickly as possible that they may not take the time to assess carefully the quality of the applicants. An authentic selection process requires a systematic evaluation of the job and the applicants. Objective scoring should play a role in identifying the attractiveness of the applicant in relation to the job. The KSAOs of the job should guide the selection methods used and the evaluation of the applicants. Consistency and fairness should be evident throughout the selection process. Such an approach is crucial for health care organizations that need to obtain highly talented providers to create and sustain high-quality patient care. Moreover, this approach will also lead to greater retention, which is crucial given that turnover costs in health care organizations are extremely high. As an example, research has estimated that the turnover cost per nurse ranges from $22,000 to $64,000 (Jones & Gates, 2007). Involuntary turnover is inversely related to strong hiring practices.

Before discussing the various selection methods companies may use to identify the best applicants, a review of some of the legal concerns with selection must be addressed. Numerous EEO laws have identified protected characteristics that cannot be used in the hiring process or in other employment decisions except in some rare circumstances. For example, one of the early pieces of EEO legislation that is still relevant today is the Age Discrimination in Employment Act (ADEA) of 1967. In terms of the hiring process, employers cannot discriminate against persons forty and older. If an applicant is forty or older, age cannot be a determining factor in the hiring decision. To comply with this law, employers should not ask for an applicant's age at any point in the hiring process. Employers can, however, ask if the applicant is at least eighteen years of age to comply with child labor laws. The ADEA applies to employers with at least twenty employees.

As mentioned in Chapter Eight, the landmark piece of EEO legislation is Title VII of the Civil Rights Act (CRA) of 1964. This law identified five protected characteristics that should not play a role in the hiring process: sex, race, color, religion, and national origin. The CRA applies to employers with fifteen or more employees. A common question with the CRA is, Why are both race and color listed in the law? At the time this law was passed, certain employers were hiring black applicants. However, a subset of these employers would make hiring decisions based on the darkness of the applicant's skin. Thus both race and color were included in the CRA (Moran, 2011).

Title VII of the CRA defined two main types of discrimination. The first type of discrimination is called disparate treatment, whereby an employer treats applicants differently based on a protected characteristic. For example, if a health care employer would not consider any woman for an executive position, this would be disparate treatment. In addition, if an employer made it harder for women to be considered for an executive position (for example, making only female applicants demonstrate their ability to read a balance sheet), this would also be disparate treatment. Disparate treatment would be permitted, however, if the employer could prove a particular characteristic to be a **bona fide occupational qualification (BFOQ).** A BFOQ is a necessary job qualification for the safe and efficient operation of a business. For example, if there is a nursing home for women and a nurses' aide is required to bathe patients, the nursing home may require all nurses' aides to be female. This would be a legitimate instance of a BFOQ. Please note that a BFOQ cannot be based on customer preference. Moreover, neither race nor color can be a BFOQ (Moran, 2011). Overall, most employers would be unable to prove a BFOQ for the vast majority of jobs.

The other type of discrimination is called disparate or adverse impact, whereby applicants are treated equally, but that treatment gives an unfair advantage or disadvantage based on a protected characteristic. The most well-known case illustrating disparate impact was *Griggs v. Duke Power Co.* in 1971. In this case the power company used a high school diploma and an intelligence test to select employees for higher-paying positions in the company. These requirements resulted in fewer black employees in the higher-paying positions compared to white employees. The company was unable to show that the high school diploma and the intelligence test were business necessities for these jobs, and thus the company lost this case (Berry, 2003). Employers are advised to conduct a bottom-line analysis to compare selection ratios (success rates) based on protected characteristics to see if certain groups have a more difficult time landing a job than others. If there are substantial differences in selection ratios based on protected characteristics (for example, sex and race), then an employer is vulnerable to disparate impact claims.

In addition to the ADEA of 1967 and the CRA of 1964, there are several other key pieces of EEO legislation related to selection. In 1978 the Pregnancy Discrimination Act made it illegal for employers to discriminate in any aspect of employment based on pregnancy (Steingold, 2007). Employers should not ask an applicant in the employment interview if he or she is pregnant, plans to have children, has child care responsibilities, and so on.

In 1986 the Immigration Reform and Control Act (IRCA) made it illegal to discriminate in hiring against individuals who are not U.S. citizens but are legally authorized to work in the United States. Employers cannot, however, hire undocumented workers. In the hiring process, employers must have all new hires complete an I-9 form to certify that they are legally authorized to work in the United States. Moreover, this law does permit employers to give preference to U.S. citizens over equally qualified legal aliens (Berry, 2003).

Four years after the IRCA was passed, the Americans with Disabilities Act influenced hiring across our country. As mentioned earlier, the ADA prohibits discrimination in employment against people with disabilities who can perform the essential functions of the job with or without reasonable accommodation. Organizations need to know that disabilities can be either physical or mental. Companies must review job descriptions to make certain the essential functions of the job are identified before recruitment begins. What constitutes reasonable accommodation is contingent on the nature of the disability and the financial strain of that accommodation on the organization. Employers do not have to provide accommodation if they can show that it would cause undue hardship (Berry, 2003). Most forms of accommodation, such as redesigning office space to make it more wheelchair friendly or offering magnified screens for computer monitors to help the visually impaired, do not meet the threshold for undue hardship. Employers should not ask applicants about whether or not they have a disability. Employers can have applicants demonstrate their ability to perform essential functions and offer reasonable accommodation if applicants request it.

A recent piece of legislation, the Genetic Information Nondiscrimination Act (GINA), passed in 2008, prohibits discrimination in employment for private employers on the basis of genetic information. Executive Order 13145 was passed shortly thereafter and extended this protection to federal employees (Fried & Fottler, 2011). Employers should not use medical exams in the selection process to avoid violating GINA or the ADA.

As a result of these EEO laws, organizations may be tempted to avoid the appearance of discrimination at all costs by making sure their hiring process creates equality across the protected characteristics. To achieve equality, some employers will give applicants points for being members of a protected group, thus increasing the likelihood of those group members' being selected for a job opening. This practice is referred to as race norming. In 1991 another Civil Rights Act was passed, and this practice was made illegal (Moran, 2011). To assist companies in complying with EEO legislation, the Equal Employment Opportunity Commission (EEOC) does publish guidelines for employers. The most well-known publication by the EEOC is the 1978 *Uniform Guidelines on Employee Selection Procedures.* This document is available online at www.access.gpo.gov/nara/cfr/waisidx_10/ 29cfr1607_10.html.

In summary, there are numerous EEO issues associated with the hiring process. Health care organizations need to scrutinize their employment practices to make sure no protected characteristics are affecting the selection process in terms of disparate treatment or disparate impact. Further, keep in mind that the aforementioned laws constitute federal legislation. States often have their own EEO laws, which can be more restrictive, not less restrictive, on employers in granting rights to applicants concerning freedom from discrimination. For example, some states (such as Hawaii, New Jersey, Maryland, and Vermont) have identified sexual orientation as a protected characteristic (Steingold, 2007). So although there is no federal protection for sexual orientation, employers in these states must comply with these regulations. Moreover, some cities and towns have local ordinances that may also have an impact on employment. Health care organizations should consult an employment attorney to make sure they are aware of all relevant EEO legislation for all of their locations.

Commonly Used Selection Methods

There are many selection methods to choose from. As indicated earlier, the goal of the selection process is to determine which applicant is best for the job opening. To make this determination, organizations need to assess the applicants' qualifications in relation to the job specifications. The challenge is of course determining how best to assess the KSAOs pertinent to the job. Each selection method is geared toward assessing certain KSAOs and thus should influence which selection methods are adopted for a given job. In addition, some methods take longer to implement than others, and some are more costly than others as well. Companies need to balance the numerous selection options with their relevance to a particular job, time constraints, and budgetary limitations. Hiring systems that are greatly influenced by time and cost considerations, however, can in the long run result in a greater percentage of poor hires and end up being the most costly due to such factors as low productivity, poor customer satisfaction, high turnover, and liability issues.

The selection process usually begins with having applicants complete an application form or submit a résumé and cover letter, increasingly in online rather than paper formats. Online application forms and résumés as opposed to traditional paper versions give employers an advantage because the online forms can be processed electronically. Companies can use scanning systems to weed through submissions to eliminate applicants who do not meet minimum qualifications (for example, those without a college degree). A concern with requiring online applications or résumés is the assumption that applicants have the necessary technology skills to apply. Does the job he or she is applying for require applicants to possess such skills? Another concern relates to how the company will evaluate the information provided on application forms and résumés. For example, for the vast majority of jobs previous work experience is a desirable attribute in an applicant. How much experience is required versus how much is preferred is often a judgment call. After a certain amount of experience, does more experience really matter? Employers need to consider how they will evaluate information provided on application forms or résumés prior to collecting these documents.

The most significant challenge with application forms and résumés for employers is fraud. Some applicants will exaggerate their qualifications, whereas others may blatantly lie on these forms (Berry, 2003). An employer that hires someone who lacks the proper qualifications is vulnerable to litigation. If that employee harms someone (a patient, for example), the organization can be sued under the legal concept known as **negligent hiring.** A well-known example of negligent hiring occurred in 1991 when Jesse Rogers was hired as a home health care aide. He claimed to have a clean criminal record as well as a degree in nursing and relevant experience with the state. All three of these claims were false, but his employer never verified any of this information and hired him anyway. In the course of his employment Rogers viciously murdered a patient and the patient's grandmother. The patient's family was awarded $26.5 million in damages paid for by the employer (Lewis & Gardner, 2000). Thus another critical selection practice is conducting background checks. Conducting a background check may involve verifying the applicant's education, work experience, certifications, licenses, and so forth. Some organizations will also run a criminal background check to make sure the applicant does not have a history of violence. This practice would be especially relevant in health care. Credit checks may also be considered in jobs that give employees access to organizational funds. If credit checks will be included in the selection process, companies must comply with the Fair Credit Reporting Act (Steingold, 2007). This law requires employers to get permission from the applicants to conduct a credit check, ensure the confidentiality of the findings, and permit the applicant to see the results of the credit check if the applicant is rejected on the basis of this action.

Letters of reference constitute another well-known selection device. Often employers will ask for three letters of recommendation from applicants. One of the most consistent findings in the human resources literature is that letters of reference are poor at predicting job success (Berry, 2003). Rather than advocating wasting valuable company time reading countless glowing letters, many human resources professionals recommend contacting previous employers as part of the background check to gather more useful information on the applicants. Although this is a recommended practice, many previous employers are reluctant to provide negative information about a former employee. They are concerned that if this former employee finds out about the negative reference, he or she will sue for defamation of character. In spite of this limitation, companies should attempt to solicit feedback directly from former employers about the applicants as an alternative to collecting recommendation letters.

Testing is another selection tool for companies to consider in hiring. One of the many types of tests for use in the selection process is performance tests. Employers can make applicants demonstrate their ability to perform job-relevant tasks as part of the selection process. A performance test may involve an applicant's using a piece of technology (such as a CT scanner); simulating a critical job incident (such as role-playing breaking bad news to a patient's family); or making important decisions (such as providing a diagnosis based on simulated patient data). Before implementing performance tests in the selection system, the company should make sure that any performance task being tested is critical to the given job and is something applicants need to be able to perform prior to being hired rather than something that they can easily be trained after being hired. Moreover, a scoring rubric for the performance tests should be established before implementation to reduce potential biases.

Cognitive ability tests are also used in selection systems. Research on intelligence tests has consistently found that mental ability is a strong predictor of job success across a wide array of jobs (Bohlander & Snell, 2010). One of the most popular intelligence tests used for employment is the Wonderlic. This twelve-minute, fifty-question multiple-choice test is a very convenient instrument, and it has been successful at identifying applicants with high potential (Berry, 2003).

Personality tests are another option. The personality of a health care provider can be very important in dealing with patients and their families, especially during stressful times. Personality research has identified five personality dimensions, commonly referred to as the "big 5," that have been consistently associated with job success (Bohlander & Snell, 2010). These five are

1. *Openness to experience.* The individual is willing to try new things, and is creative and curious.

2. *Conscientiousness.* The individual is dependable, perseveres, and does things completely and correctly.

3. *Extraversion.* The individual is outgoing, sociable, and talkative.

4. *Agreeableness.* The individual gets along with others, and is friendly and approachable.

5. *Neuroticism (the opposite of emotional stability).* The individual is overly sensitive and emotional.

The NEO-R is the most well-known instrument for assessing the big 5 personality dimensions (Berry, 2003).

The final selection method that will be discussed here is the **employment interview.** The interview is often the key selection method that determines who is the best applicant. Many of the previous selection methods are used to eliminate candidates for the job, whereas the interview is seen as an opportunity for one of the finalists to stand out from the rest. The interview is a very popular selection device. For most health care jobs interpersonal skills are an important part of one's job performance, and the interview provides insight into the applicant's interpersonal skills. The interview can also reveal an applicant's work motivation, job-relevant knowledge, and character (for example, whether he or she is dependable, takes calculated risks, is honest, and is willing to go above and beyond the job description). Seeking out all of these characteristics is critical in identifying the best person for the job.

The employment interview, however, has two major challenges. In most employment interviews the applicant wants to be offered the job, and is therefore motivated to present the best possible image of himself or herself to the employer. So when an applicant performs well in the interview (appearing to be highly motivated, enthusiastic, reliable, and so on), how does an organization really know if this is a true reflection of that individual or a manufactured positive impression that can be conjured when needed but will not appear on the job?. The other challenge with the employment interview is that an interviewer can be influenced by personal biases and stereotypes. The interviewer's opinion of the applicant can be swayed by factors irrelevant to the job opening and thus may lead to poor assessments and ultimately the wrong choices.

Research on the employment interview has led to some key recommended practices. One of the most valuable improvements that can be made to an employment interview is to structure it (Bohlander & Snell, 2010). In a structured employment interview the company predetermines the questions that will be asked, decides on the order of those questions, and establishes a scoring guide for the interview. Structured interviews are likely to have only job-relevant questions (the questions are predetermined), will treat all applicants consistently (the order of the questions has already been decided), and will promote fairness in evaluating applicants (the predetermined scoring key minimizes potential biases). Another recommended interview practice is to ask applicants behaviorally based and situationally based questions (Gatewood, Feild, & Barrick, 2008). With behaviorally based questions applicants are asked to recall events in their work history that are relevant to the job opening (for example, "Describe to me a time when you had to break bad news to a patient. How did you do this? Would you do anything different next time?"). These types of questions are useful for employers in predicting how applicants will behave on the job based on how they acted in the past. Similarly, situationally based interview questions ask the applicants to imagine themselves in a critical incident on the job, and to indicate what they would do in that situation (for example, "You are walking down the corridor to your office, and as you turn the corner you see someone passed out on the floor. What would you do?"). The situationally based questions present hypothetical scenarios, whereas the behaviorally based questions rely on the applicant's past. Both of these options provide insight into the applicant's decision-making abilities and probable behaviors if hired. Using these questions properly requires designing them based on essential functions of the job opening and predetermining a scoring system so responses can be assessed consistently and accurately. Overall, the employment interview can be a quality selection method if these recommended practices are used.

Overall, health care organizations have several selection methods that may be used to hire new employees. Whichever methods are implemented, the employer needs to consider the job requirements, the legal context, and the quality of the selection method. To determine the quality of the selection methods used, organizations need to carefully evaluate the success of their selection process. The last subsection of this chapter examines this issue.

Selection Evaluation

After the selection system has been in place for a while, an organization should take time evaluating the success of this system. The best way to assess the quality of a selection process is to evaluate its **validity.** Validity refers to the accuracy of the selection process, as measured by how closely it relates to the position being filled. Collecting validity evidence is somewhat complicated. The EEOC's *Uniform Guidelines on Employee Selection Procedures* mentioned earlier in this chapter does devote a large section to obtaining validity evidence. The two types of validity evidence most commonly obtained are called content validity evidence and criterion-related validity evidence.

Content validity evidence refers to the degree of overlap between the content of the job and the content of the selection process (Gatewood et al., 2008). This evidence requires the employer to identify subject matter experts (SMEs) who by definition know the job demands extremely well. These SMEs render opinions based on the connection they perceive between what the applicant is required to do to get the job (for example, taking a performance test of an essential function) and what the critical demands of the job are. The stronger the perceived connection between the selection process demands and the job demands, the higher the content validity.

Criterion-related validity evidence represents a much more quantitative approach to validity. In gathering such evidence, statistical connections are made between scores achieved during the selection process (such as ratings of a résumé or test scores) and some measure of job success (such as performance appraisal scores, revenue generated, or the number of patients served). A correlation coefficient between these two indices is a common statistic used to determine criterion-related validity. In a quality selection system, a strong positive correlation would provide evidence that applicants who are impressive in the hiring process have a strong tendency to be impressive on the job. This would indicate that the company is basing its selection system on job-relevant factors that are resulting in predictive accuracy. If the data do not reveal strong relationships, then the company should reevaluate the selection methods used and make changes as needed (Gatewood et al., 2008).

Regardless of which approach to obtaining validity evidence is implemented, health care organizations need to make sure that what they are doing to hire people is accurate and relevant to the job. It helps protect them legally, but, even more important, it helps them cultivate a talented workforce.

SUMMARY

The overall objective of this chapter is to present the process by which health care organizations can staff themselves. In certain situations health care employers may rely on alternatives to seeking full-time employees. These alternatives may include hiring part-time employees or locum tenens, employee leasing, or outsourcing. If an organization does not want to use these alternatives, then the staffing process should begin with a careful examination and revision, if need be, of the job description and specifications for the given job opening. From there the employer has to decide if the recruiting should be done internally, externally, or both to create a pool of qualified applicants. There are many internal and external recruiting options, each with advantages and disadvantages. The recruiting function should be evaluated as well, with a particular emphasis on yield ratios. After the recruiting process has been completed, the organization needs to create a selection system to identify the best applicant. In designing this system, the organization should revisit numerous EEO laws to reduce the possibility of a discrimination lawsuit. The selection process should be crafted in such a way as to determine which applicant is most qualified for the job and will be a good fit in the company. Numerous selection methods to meet this objective were presented in this chapter. Finally, the selection process should also be evaluated to make sure it is valid, resulting in high-quality hires. Health care is a labor-intensive industry. The effectiveness of the staffing process will have a considerable impact on the quality of services provided and thus the overall success of the organization.

KEY TERMS

bona fide occupational qualification (BFOQ)

employment interview

Internet recruiting

locum tenens

negligent hiring

realistic job preview (RJP)

validity

yield ratio

REVIEW QUESTIONS

1. Job analysis is often considered the foundation of human resources management. If an organization has an updated and accurate job description, this document can guide the hiring process, performance review, training, compensation, and so on. Ironically, job analysis is often ignored in many organizations. The job description can be inaccurate in terms of the tasks, duties, and responsibilities required for employees. What has your experience been with job analysis? What do you see as the contributing factors affecting the accuracy of job descriptions?

2. This chapter presented alternatives to hiring full-time employees (hiring locum tenens and temporary workers, hiring independent contractors, outsourcing, and so on). Have you seen these alternatives work well, or not so well, in health care? To what do you attribute the success or lack thereof of these alternatives?

3. Legal aspects of the staffing process were presented earlier. Which of these legal issues do you believe are the most challenging for health care employers? Why? What should an employer do to manage this challenge?

4. The selection section of this chapter made the clear distinction that although selection is one approach to hiring, not all hiring approaches involve selection. Hiring can be influenced by whom one knows, time pressures to get someone on board as soon as possible, or people who prefer to rely on their "gut" to make this kind of decision. A selection process should be a planned effort to evaluate applicants' qualifications and fit for a job systematically and objectively. For most health care organizations, do you think a true selection process is present? Realistic? What are the implications for these organizations if your answer is no?

10

Employee Performance Improvement
The Pursuit of Quality Care

Marc C. Marchese

LEARNING OBJECTIVES

- Understand the value of employee orientation and mentoring
- Recognize the importance of training and development to maintaining a high-performing workforce
- Be able to recall the components of the ADDIE model for training
- Appreciate the numerous critical decisions required in creating and evaluating employee training programs
- Distinguish among the various uses of performance appraisal in managing a workforce
- Acknowledge the various sources of performance feedback for employees
- Differentiate among the various performance rating options

The value of quality care has been emphasized throughout this book. This chapter focuses on developing and sustaining quality job performance in a health care organization after the staffing process has finished. The previous chapter discussed the process by which health care organizations recruit and select talented employees. In this chapter the primary objective is to explore how organizations can orient, train, and manage the performance of their workforce to meet and exceed job performance expectations. The chapter will begin by reviewing key elements of employee orientation and socialization. Then, employee training will receive considerable attention as a way to help prepare new hires for their job demands as well as to assist employees with organizational changes. Development programs will also be included in this discussion to address future employee needs in the company. The second half of the chapter will turn to performance management issues, including uses of performance appraisal data and major issues in conducting formal performance appraisals.

EMPLOYEE ORIENTATION AND MENTORING

Most large health care organizations have some kind of formal employee orientation program. Although the goals of such programs will vary, most formal orientation programs are intended to introduce new hires to key company policies and procedures, educate them on significant company features to provide them with an overview of the organization, and assist them in adjusting to a new job. Some of the topics covered in formal orientations are

- The company's history
- The organizational chart
- Community partnerships
- Major employee policies: sexual harassment, smoking, Internet use, and employee discipline
- Major employee benefits: health insurance, retirement, paid time off, and sick leave
- Compensation information: paycheck distribution, frequency of pay raises, and overtime

- Facilities (possibly including a tour of key offices and buildings)
- Company leaders
- Contents of the employee handbook

One of the biggest criticisms of formal orientation programs by new hires is that these programs are often long and boring. Unfortunately, for the sake of expediency and convenience, formal orientation programs are usually crammed into one or two days. The new hires sit through numerous presentations that cover many of the aforementioned topics. After a while their attention span is weakened, and they are not learning the key information. Formal orientation programs ideally should be spread out over several days in small increments, and they should incorporate some activity for the new hires that will engage them in this learning process.

In addition to attending a formal orientation, which is usually coordinated by the human resources department, new hires also receive an informal orientation from their coworkers and immediate supervisor once they start working. This informal orientation is influential in terms of establishing a new hire's performance expectations, as he or she quickly learns the department's norms concerning key aspects of employee behavior (for example, the speed at which one works, the acceptance or rejection of taking risks, the level of cooperation among coworkers, and expectations about working past one's shift). Too often undesired behaviors are conveyed to a new hire as being "normal." The senior employees who take a new hire under their wing either can help capitalize on a great hire, resulting in high-quality performance, or can hurt the motivation of a new hire, resulting in a marginal worker. Health care organizations should therefore examine the cultural differences by department to ensure new hires are properly socialized, or else the value of an effective staffing process is marginalized.

Some health care organizations are using **mentoring** in addition to orientation to help new employees succeed in their position and become comfortable with their surroundings. Mentoring generally involves a relationship between a junior employee (sometimes referred to as a protégé or mentee) and a seasoned employee, who often is in a higher-level position in the company (the mentor). Mentoring can occur informally in an organization, such as when a new hire establishes a bond with a higher-level employee, leading to the evolution of a protégé-mentor relationship over time. Many organizations, however, have created formal mentoring programs in which protégés are intentionally paired with mentors. In this case a mentor is required to meet with his or her protégé a certain number of times over the length of the program. Further, the protégé establishes goals with his or her mentor for the mentoring program, which often include career development plans. It's beyond the scope of this chapter to go into the specifics of matching protégés with mentors, but it's worth mentioning that experienced employees should never be forced to be mentors (Fallon & McConnell, 2007). If an employee does not want to take on this responsibility, then he or she should be excluded from this process. In mentoring relationships, mentors provide protégés with numerous benefits. Protégés will learn technical information concerning job responsibilities, but, just as important, they will learn about interpersonal and organizational skills that will help them be successful in developing effective working relationships. Moreover, research on mentoring has shown that the mentors also benefit from participating in these programs. Mentors often find these relationships satisfying and report enjoying the opportunity to share their wisdom with employees who have less experience (Flynn, Mathis, & Jackson, 2007).

A relatively recent study highlighted a mentoring program targeting nurses working in four California hospitals (Mills & Mullins, 2008). This study indicated that the vacancy rate for nurses in the western United States was 15 percent. The cost of replacing a medical-surgical nurse was estimated to be $42,000 per vacancy, and the cost was $64,000 per vacancy for nurses in other specialties. A formal mentoring program was developed that required a three-year commitment from both the mentors and the protégés. Furthermore, the nursing mentors were required to complete a sixteen-hour certification program. The results of this mentoring program were quite impressive. Only 8 percent of the nurses who participated in the mentoring program as protégés left their hospital, compared to 23 percent of nonparticipating nurses. In addition, both mentors and protégés reported high levels of job satisfaction and professional confidence. Overall, the mentoring program was estimated to have saved the hospitals between $1.4 million and $5.8 million.

Another study described a creative mentoring program targeting physicians (Cohn, Bethancourt, & Simington, 2009). In this study a medical group established an on-boarding program, which is a form of comentoring. Newly hired physicians were assigned several mentors rather than participating in the traditional one-on-one mentoring relationship. For example, one veteran physician would help the new hire socialize with other physicians, whereas another mentor would coach the protégé on the hospital's management and culture. The on-boarding program lasted one year for new hires. Although the hospital regularly experienced a 10 percent turnover rate for physicians per year, none of the physicians who participated in the on-boarding program had left the hospital at the time the study was published.

EMPLOYEE TRAINING

To perform at a high level, employees need to be motivated and able to meet their job requirements. In the staffing process, top talent should have been identified and secured for the organization. Regardless of the quality of the new hire, however, most recently hired employees need at least some training to learn the specifics of the company's processes and technology. In addition, organizations are regularly changing equipment, technology, procedures, policies, and work arrangements. Employees will need training to adapt to the constant changes in the workplace if they are to maintain high performance. Thus employee training deserves considerable attention in any discussion of employee job performance.

Before delving into the training components, a review of key concepts relevant to this section is necessary. Employee training is a systematic process to enhance an employee's capabilities, with the goal of improving his or her job performance. A series of blood-borne pathogen workshops for licensed practical nurses (LPNs) to address this job component would be an example of a training program. A related concept is employee development, which refers to a systematic process to enhance an employee's capabilities for future jobs or new responsibilities. Employee development focuses on moving the employee in new directions within and beyond their current job. A managerial skills development program for physicians would be one example. Organizational development refers to an initiative to improve organizational performance that may involve large-scale learning by employees. For example, if a hospital implements an information system using electronic medical records that requires most hospital employees to go to a seminar, this would be considered organizational development. Employee education is another concept that often falls under the training umbrella. An employee education program is usually designed to increase the overall competence of an employee. The education received may not be job specific, but it helps broaden the employee's knowledge and skills that may be applicable in a wide variety of jobs. Many health care organizations will provide tuition reimbursement for their employees who are pursuing a master's degree in health care or business. Overall, these four related concepts (employee training, employee development, organizational development, and employee education) pertain to different perspectives on programs that are intended to improve employee learning and ultimately influence employee performance. In some organizations training professionals are viewed as performance consultants or coaches (Flynn et al., 2007). The main objective of the trainer is to design programs to help employees overcome difficulties in their current job as well as to provide them with opportunities (seminars, conferences, and education programs) to help them achieve career goals.

As mentioned in Chapter Nine, many health care organizations seek accreditation from The Joint Commission (TJC). A key standard in achieving and maintaining this accreditation is ensuring staff competence (Flynn et al., 2007). The training and development programs of a health care organization are central to meeting this standard. A health care organization needs to show TJC its training and development plans aimed at enhancing its employees' job capabilities.

For any form of training to be effective, the program requires a well-thought-out plan to achieve its objectives. The best-known approach to creating training and development programs is called the **ADDIE model**

(Fried & Fottler, 2011). ADDIE stands for assessment (or analysis), design, development, implementation, and evaluation. A brief review of each of the components follows.

The first part of the ADDIE model is analysis, which is also referred to as **needs assessment.** The objective of this part of the model is to determine what type of training is needed in the company. Before examining the possible training needs in an organization, however, needs assessment begins with an examination of the level of support for training in this company. If training is not supported, then there is no point in trying to identify training needs. For example, if a number of employees are struggling to perform their jobs to company standards, the company has two options. One option would be to design a training program to enhance their job skills. Another option would be to relieve these employees of their job and replace them with new hires. Thus needs assessment begins with identifying the level of support for training: Do executives provide the necessary resources for training and development programs? A training budget will typically equal around 2 percent of payroll (Noe, 2010). Companies that are highly committed to training often have a training budget closer to 4 percent of payroll. Training programs can have considerable costs associated with them. For example, training employees to use a new piece of technology will often demand funds set aside to purchase extra equipment on which trainees can practice. In addition, other expenses may include the cost of renting out space to conduct the training; the cost of materials (such as handouts, photocopies, and folders) and refreshments for the trainees; the cost of training equipment (such as computers, projectors, and screens); and the opportunity costs inherent in paying employees to go to training rather than paying them to work). In addition, there are costs associated with hiring training consultants to carry out certain training programs. Some training programs will also cover the cost of travel, including reimbursements for airline tickets, hotel fees, and meals, if the company is geographically dispersed. As you can see, without financial support for training, the value of assessing training needs is marginal. Support for training also extends to perceptions by managers and employees. Even with a sufficient training budget, if managers and employees do not hold training in high regard, then training's ability to yield true performance improvement will be hampered by poor attendance or low motivation by trainees. Overall, needs assessment should include both a financial analysis of training resources and an assessment of the level of support for training from executives, managers, and employees. If both of these analyses are positive, then identifying specific training needs should begin as part of this component of the ADDIE model.

It can be somewhat challenging to identify specific training needs, which may be classified as being at either the micro or macro level. Micro-level training needs are those pertaining to one employee or a small number of employees. For example, hiring a new physician assistant who needs training in hospital safety procedures would represent a micro-level training need. Macro-level training needs pertain to the entire organization or a large segment of employees (such as employees in an entire division or location). For example, a hospital's implementation of a new system of electronic medical records would represent a macro-level training need because a large number of employees would have to go through a training program.

The sources of micro-level training needs are either employees in new positions (recent hires or those just promoted or transferred) or performance problems (poor job performance ratings, a workplace accident, or a customer complaint). Managers often look to training to solve performance problems. The challenge is to identify the cause of the performance problem and then to determine if training is the appropriate response based on this analysis. As an example, an LPN might improperly assist a patient into a hospital bed, resulting in an injury to that patient. If this occurred more than once, her manager might want to send her to a refresher training course on this job responsibility. However, if the cause of this poor performance was that the LPN does not care about her job, then the performance problem was the result of low motivation. Sending her to training will not resolve the situation. Furthermore, the performance problem could have been the result of alcohol or drug abuse. It could also have been caused by faulty equipment or machinery (a broken lift assist device). Overall, performance problems can be caused by numerous factors (such as low motivation, personal issues, and equipment failures). Training would only be the correct response if the performance problem were the result of an employee or employees' lacking the needed knowledge, skills, abilities, and other characteristics (KSAOs) demanded to undertake the job responsibility.

Macro-level training needs arise from organizational problems or organizational development initiatives. Some examples of company problems that might lead to training solutions are a decrease in revenue, an increase in patient complaints, a lawsuit being filed against the company, an increased rate of hospital-acquired infections, or a decrease in patient survival rates. All of these problems are significant for any health care employer. As with micro-level performance issues, the challenge for the organization will be to determine the causes of the problem. If it turns out that employees lack the proper KSAOs to deliver quality patient care, then a large-scale training program would an appropriate response. If, however, this problem is the result of an organizational culture that does not reward high performance, conscientiousness, and professionalism, training would not be effective. Organizational development initiatives that might result in training needs are the implementation of a new company-wide computer system; the acquisition of or a merger with a competitor; the expansion of health services (for example, in a new pediatric wing of a hospital); or the opening up of new company locations. For any of these initiatives to enhance organizational performance, a large number of employees would require some type of training.

Overall, needs assessment is the critical first step in training. If done properly, the company has determined whether or not it has the necessary resources and support for employee training. If the company does have the required support, it has identified any micro- and macro-level training needs that require employees to improve their KSAOs. Both of these components—ascertaining the level of support and identifying needs—are necessary before the next steps of training. Without undertaking needs assessment, the company is risking spending time and money on training programs that employees may not attend, that may have no impact on performance, and that may not resolve an organizational problem or assist the organization in meeting one of its objectives.

In the design component of training, the employer makes numerous critical decisions. One or more training needs have already been identified for this organization, and in the design component these training needs are translated into training objectives. The training needs indicate some aspect or aspects of job performance that require improvement. Training objectives take these needs and specify the performance expectations for them. A quality training objective will indicate what the trainee will be able to do at the completion of the training program. For example, if opticians are struggling with fabricating lenses, a quality training objective could be, "At the end of training, trainees will be able to create lenses according to prescription specifications within one hour." A training objective that just says "Trainees will be better at making lenses" does not provide the necessary information to lead to performance improvement. Indicating a performance standard in the training objective has numerous advantages. For one thing, this training objective will assist training professionals in other aspects of training design (for example, selecting training methods). It will also help show the value of the training program to potential trainees and their managers. Moreover, specific training objectives help guide the evaluation phase of training to determine the training's overall effectiveness. Therefore, a key part of training design is specifying training objectives based on training needs (Noe, 2010).

Once the training objectives are established, the next part of training design involves identifying key aspects of learning to achieve these objectives. Training and development programs are aimed toward enhancing employee learning to improve job performance. So understanding how employees learn is essential to accomplishing the training goals. It's beyond the scope of this chapter to provide a comprehensive review of the learning literature, but a few major components will be discussed. One aspect to consider in designing a training program is that people have different learning styles, or ways in which they learn the best. The VAK model is the most well-known breakdown of learning styles. The "V" stands for visual learners—people who learn best by watching (visual spatial) or by reading (visual linguistic). The "A" stands for auditory learners—people who prefer to learn by listening and talking. The "K" stands for kinesthetic learners—people who prefer to learn by doing. Kinesthetic learners want to be active in the learning process, which may entail completing practice exercises, participating in group activities, or even taking notes and quizzes. A training design question is, then, To what extent does the training program appeal to all types of learning styles? In addition, research in **andragogy,** the study of adult learning, has shown that adults prefer learning events that have clear practical value to their job or their lives, allow them to share their experiences as they learn, and provide them with opportunities to be active in the learning process (Noe, 2010). All of these findings have direct application to training design. Finally, social learning theory has shown that people learn skills and abilities by observing others (Blanchard & Thacker, 2004). This theory clearly advocates for the inclusion of demonstrations, videos, or even role playing in training programs that are intended to improve observable employee behaviors (for example, dealing with potentially violent patients). Overall, research on learning yields several practical suggestions for training design:

- Make the training program meaningful to trainees (via clear training objectives).

- Allow for active learning rather than making training purely passive.

- Incorporate a variety of training methods to accommodate various learning styles.

- Use modeling (or demos) to help trainees see desired behaviors.

- Provide opportunities for trainees to practice new skills or abilities in advance of actual on-the-job experiences.

The last major component of training design is selecting the training methods that will be used for this program. The training methods should be chosen primarily based on the training objectives defined previously. Training objectives that specify skills and abilities needed for performance improvement really should correspond to training methods in which the trainees will have opportunities to practice these new skills or abilities. Training objectives that refer to increasing an employee's knowledge can be accomplished by passive training methods (for example, via reading materials) or active training methods (for example, through question-and-answer sessions). Another factor that will influence the choice of training methods is the company's willingness to incorporate recommendations from the learning literature as previously mentioned. Further, the training budget and time constraints might also have an impact on training methods because some methods are more expensive or more time consuming to develop and implement than other methods. Ideally, time and money should be the least important factors in selecting training methods. If the company truly wants to improve employee performance, training design should be influenced primarily by an ethos of doing things right the first time rather than trying to cut corners and hoping things work out.

Training methods can be classified into two main categories: on-site or off-site. On-site training methods, which can also be referred to as on-the-job training methods, occur at the same place where the job is performed. Off-site training can occur on the company's premises, but the trainees do not experience the training at their work site. On-site training methods have advantages over off-site training methods. Because the training happens on the job, the transfer of learning from training to the workplace is not a concern. On-site training methods are clearly applicable to the job, and thus the trainees see the immediate value of the training. Further, on-site training methods do not require the additional equipment, materials, and space that are often associated with off-site training methods, thereby saving resources. Off-site training methods have their advantages as well. Some, such as those involving e-learning, allow trainees to learn at their own pace and can accommodate trainees' schedules and preferences for learning. Other off-site training methods allow for training to be administered to groups (for example, in a classroom setting), which can convey a common message and experience to all trainees. Moreover, off-site training methods can allow skills and abilities to be practiced in a safe and controlled environment (for example, in a place where trainees have access to simulators or cadavers). Because both on- and off-site training methods have their advantages, in many training programs organizations may begin with off-site training methods and then move to on-site training methods near the program's completion.

On-site training methods in health care can be quite diverse if one includes medical education in this discussion. Health care professionals are typically required to engage in various forms of the on-the-job learning in the course of completing their education and certification. This may include such experiences as internships, preceptorships, clinical rotations, and fellowships. Once the health care professional is an employee and the company wants to improve his or her job performance through training, an on-site training method could be a shadowing program in which the trainee watches a highly accomplished coworker perform the duties to be learned. Coaching is another on-site training method that refers to a reversal of roles in relation to shadowing. The trainee is being watched while he or she performs job tasks and is given advice by an experienced coworker who assists the trainee in improving his or her performance. Mentoring could also be considered an on-site development method if the mentor gives the protégé opportunities to expand his or her skills.

Off-site training methods have a great deal of variety. Off-site training traditionally occurs in a classroom. Lecturing, question-and-answer sessions, manuals and books, and visual aides (including PowerPoint presentations, handouts, or even overhead projectors) are still heavily used to train employees in virtually all industries. Classroom training can be enriched by the use of other off-site training activities, such as role-plays, group exercises, business games, team-building exercises, and demonstrations. In addition, many training programs use videos (in DVD format or online) to distribute training across a geographically dispersed organization. In health care, computer simulations are growing in popularity to help health care professionals understand and practice medical procedures in a safe and controlled environment. As an example, the University of Calgary has a $1.5 million virtual reality room in which a program called CAVEman allows a physician to walk inside a 3-D image of a human body. This program simulates our anatomy and physiology (Binns, 2009). Finally, various forms of **e-learning** are being used in health care training programs. E-learning refers to using Internet-based resources for training or education, which may include Web sites that allow trainees to read materials, videoconference with other trainees or trainers, engage in chat room or bulletin board discussions, take tests or quizzes, and watch video clips. Online training programs can also track the activities and performance of trainees and can determine when the trainee has successfully completed the training. As an example of e-learning, there is an online program that provides nurses with information on cytotoxic drugs, which can be used in chemotherapy ("Developing," 2011). The program is broken down into five modules, each of which ends with a required examination. A nurse's score must be 100 percent to move on to the next module. So far the program has been viewed as highly successful.

In conclusion, training design requires the employer to identify specific training objectives that are related to performance improvement. Training design should factor in best practices in regard to learning. Finally, training methods should then be selected based on these training objectives and learning principles. The methods may be on-site, off-site, or a combination of both.

The next phase of training is development. In development the organization first decides if the training will be internal or external. Internal training indicates that the training program will be created in-house. Members of the training staff, human resources professionals, or other employees will develop the training program. External training indicates that the employer will contract out the development of the training to a consultant or training firm, or will purchase an existing program. This decision will be affected by the types of training methods desired for this program (on-site training methods are conducted in-house, whereas off-site methods may be developed internally or externally); the expertise (for example, in e-learning or computer simulations) and size of the in-house staff; time pressures to get the training program implemented; and the level of control the company desires to have with this program.

If the company decides to develop the program in-house, the next step will be to develop a lesson plan for the training. Lesson plans are most closely tied to classroom training programs but can also be used for other types of training. In a lesson plan the training is laid out visually in a table format. The lesson plan indicates what will be done; when it will be done (first, second, third, and so on); why it will be done (how it is connected to training objectives); the trainer's role for each event (for example, giving a lecture or facilitating a group discussion); the trainee's role (for example, watching a video or partnering with other trainees to complete an exercise); and the time allotted for each event. The lesson plan is important because it provides an overview of the training program to ensure all of the training objectives are being addressed. It also helps the trainers be prepared and organized so that the training will be professional and efficient. Further, it gives the company an idea of the time demands of the program. After the lesson plan is completed, the next part of development is the actual creation of the program. The training staff will then prepare the methods for this program, which may include developing lectures, creating PowerPoint presentations, building team exercises, and other tasks. Then the company is ready to implement the training.

The implementation phase of the ADDIE model involves a series of decisions for the employer. Based on the time demands identified in the lesson plan, the trainer will decide if the training will be implemented using a massed approach or a distributed approach. In a massed approach the training will occur in the fewest number of days possible, whereas in a distributed approach the training will be spread out over a longer time frame. For example, a six-hour program on safe patient handling procedures could be conducted in one day, from 9:00 a.m. to 4:00 p.m., with a one-hour lunch break (massed approach), or it could be spread out in ninety-minute increments over four days (distributed approach). Research has consistently shown that a distributed approach is better for learning (Bohlander & Snell, 2010); however, a massed approach is more convenient for scheduling and thus, unfortunately, is more popular (Blanchard & Thacker, 2004).

Implementation also involves selecting a training location for training programs that are off-site and are not in an e-learning format. An attractive training room would be one that can accommodate the size of the training group, has the necessary equipment, is free of distractions, and is conveniently located. Implementation will also involve advertising the training program to potential trainees. Although there are many options in advertising (such as sending an e-mail to all employees), the most effective way to generate interest in a training program is to contact managers directly. If they are enthusiastic about the training program, they are more likely to encourage their subordinates to attend it. Other aspects of implementation involve preparing the room (arranging the seats, testing out the equipment, ordering refreshments, and so on) and registering trainees to make sure they get credit for attendance.

The last phase of training is evaluation. The most well-known approach to training evaluation is the Kirkpatrick model, which has four levels of evaluation (Noe, 2010). In a level I evaluation, training effectiveness is assessed by administering a survey to trainees at the end of the program. Trainees are asked questions about their satisfaction with the training, how useful they perceived the program to be, and the quality of the trainers. This level does indicate employees' satisfaction with training and may provide valuable ideas to improve the program for future trainees. This level does not, however, offer evidence that the trainees actually learned what the program was designed to teach. A level II evaluation involves testing the trainees before and after the training to ascertain the extent to which they learned what was intended. This level is important because if the trainees did not learn the desired material, then the program was not effective at all. The purpose of training, however, is to make a significant performance improvement in the trainees. A level II evaluation may show learning, but it does not guarantee that this learning will be applied in the workplace. Transfer of training requires that the trainees not only learn the new KSAOs but also can retain this information and can apply it to their job. Thus, a level III evaluation requires the employer to assess the performance of trainees before and after the training in regard to the behavioral aspects of the training objectives. A substantial improvement in performance as a result of the training would be compelling evidence that the training was successful. The challenge at this level is determining when to assess performance after the training, and how often. The performance improvement ideally would be both considerable and long-term. A level IV evaluation would attempt to show the value of a training program in monetary terms. To what extent was the training program cost effective? The costs associated with a training program are relatively easy to determine (for example, the cost of materials, equipment, space, and food; consultant fees; and travel expenses). The harder challenge in a level IV evaluation is to assess the financial benefits of a training program. For example, if a training program for nurses was intended to build teamwork, and if this program was a result of exit interviews revealing that the lack of teamwork was a main reason why many nurses leave the hospital, then improvements in retention could represent the financial benefits of the training. Thus, if a team-building training program cost the hospital $75,000 but the hospital's turnover rate dropped, resulting in a savings of $150,000 per year, this would provide support that the program was worth it. Level IV evaluations are more debatable than level III evaluations because any financial indicator may be influenced by many factors (for example, the economy or competitors) in addition to the training program. In conclusion, the goal of training is to improve the performance of an employer's workforce. A thorough training evaluation is necessary to determine to what extent this goal was accomplished.

In summary, employee training programs are intended to improve employee performance. To accomplish this goal, a lot of planning and careful decision making must occur to assess training needs, design an appropriate training program, develop this program, implement it, and then ultimately evaluate its effectiveness (Figure 10.1 provides a summary of the ADDIE

Figure 10.1   ADDIE Model

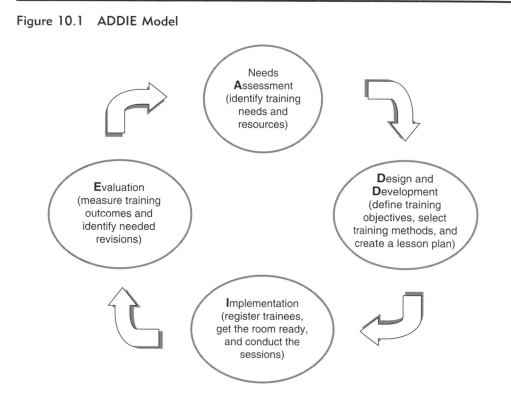

model). Successful organizations recognize the value of this key human resources management function.

PERFORMANCE APPRAISAL

The focus of this chapter is on performance improvement. Providing quality training and development programs can be an effective way to improve employee performance. To be successful in any approach to performance improvement, however, job performance must first be defined and assessed. Performance appraisal is a systematic approach to accomplish this objective. Employers take many approaches in assessing the performance of their workforce, making numerous critical decisions that will have an impact on the company's productivity and ultimately its financial well-being.

Conducting a performance appraisal of one's staff can help establish a baseline for use in benchmarking initiatives that are intended to improve job performance. There are many other advantages to conducting performance appraisals as well. Assuming the performance appraisal system is well designed and implemented properly, the information gained can be used to identify a company's best employees. These employees can then be rewarded with financial incentives, growth opportunities, or both. Similarly, the weakest employees will also be identified, making training needs apparent. Examples of other personnel decisions that can be guided by this assessment are layoffs, terminations, or demotions. It is imperative, however, that companies think very carefully about the message the performance appraisal system is sending to their employees. In a classic management article, "On the Folly of Rewarding A, While Hoping for B" (Kerr, 1975), the author points out that too often a company's performance appraisal and reward system sends the wrong message to its workforce. An example in this article refers to medicine. The "best" physicians for a health care organization should be those who accurately and efficiently diagnose their patients. However, performance appraisal and reward systems may encourage physicians to prescribe unnecessary tests and medication to avoid malpractice claims. Overall, identifying the true dimensions of the "best" employee takes time and careful consideration.

In addition to their use in guiding personnel decisions, performance appraisal data can be helpful to employees in increasing their awareness of how their performance is viewed by their employer. This feedback communicates to employees what their employer perceives to be their strengths and weaknesses. Just by receiving this information employees may be motivated to improve on their weaknesses and capitalize on their strengths.

Performance appraisal systems have benefits that go beyond the individual employee. Performance appraisal results can be used to assess organizational programs. As mentioned earlier, a level III training evaluation requires a performance appraisal before and after the training to see if there has been significant performance improvement. As another example, if an employer wants to evaluate the quality of its selection system, performance appraisal data are used to determine the predictive success of the hiring methods. In addition, performance appraisal can be used as documentation for litigation purposes. If a former employee sues his or her previous employer for discrimination, performance appraisal data may be helpful in defending the organization's termination decision as being job relevant rather than motivated by illegal factors, such as the person's race, sex, age, and so on. Overall, there are numerous reasons why many employers conduct regular performance appraisals of their employees. The value of using this process for performance improvement will be the emphasis in this chapter.

In designing a quality performance appraisal system, one of the first decisions that has to be made is what the content of the appraisal should be. The job description should be reviewed in making this decision. An accurate job description should define the major behavioral responsibilities of the given job. These responsibilities are likely to be included in the performance appraisal and thus are the main areas in which performance may be improved. In addition, some employers also may want to include desired traits for certain jobs. For example, health care providers need interpersonal skills when dealing with patients and their families. Such personality traits as friendliness, approachability, and being a good listener are all justifiable components to include in the appraisal. Ratings of quality patient care are affected by the personality of the individual who delivered that care. The challenge with including personality characteristics in a performance appraisal is that they are subjective. The true difference between a rating of 4 or 5 in friendliness can be difficult to ascertain.

Finally, some employers may be tempted to use financial outcomes in the performance appraisal process as well. For example, a hospital may want to consider adding revenue generated in its performance review of a physician. In addition, the hospital may want to factor in the number of tests the physician prescribes for his or her patients. Health care, like other industries, has been pressured to become more efficient. A physician's bringing in more revenue or being more cost-conscious than other physicians may constitute the type of performance the health care organization wants to reward. This decision needs to be made very carefully. A physician's job may include many activities that do not generate revenue (such as administrative duties, public outreach, and research). Does the employer not want to recognize the value of such components? If these are not included in the performance review, then the message to the physicians is that such activities are not that important. Moreover, how much control does the employee have over the financial outcomes? A health care provider's shift schedule (morning versus evening); facility location (and the population of the local community); and the number of competitors can greatly influence the number of patients served as well as the procedures performed. Finally, patient safety should never be sacrificed to cut costs. Health care organizations should proceed very carefully in including and weighing these outcomes in the performance appraisal process.

Another important decision in implementing a performance appraisal system is how often performance appraisals should be conducted. In general, performance appraisals are conducted annually. There are two main options in annual evaluations. In some organizations all employees in the company, division, or department are assessed at the same time of the year. In other organizations, employees' job performance is evaluated near their anniversary date of hire, which results in employees' being evaluated throughout the year. Evaluating all employees at the same time of the year has the advantage of promoting consistency for a manager who may have to complete numerous assessments of his or her staff. In addition, this option may also be beneficial in terms of budgeting if the performance reviews have an impact on pay raises that will be implemented in the upcoming fiscal year. However, this option may place a tremendous amount of work on a department head who has numerous staff members to evaluate, possibly resulting in the manager's not taking his or her time to carefully complete the performance appraisals and the subsequent performance review meetings that follow. The anniversary date option spreads the time demands of the appraisal process out for the department head and may result in a higher-quality review. On the downside, this option may not be as consistently applied throughout the year, and it may not correspond to budgetary implications (Fallon & McConnell, 2007).

In addition to the annual review, in many organizations new employees are given "probationary status" when they begin work. The probationary period typically lasts around three months. At the end of the three months the new hire's performance is appraised. Based on this review, the new hire may be let go or moved to regular employee status. A similar three-month performance appraisal may be applied to employees who have been promoted or transferred to a new position. Finally, performance appraisals may be conducted more than once a year if an employee's performance was viewed as unsatisfactory based on his or her last review. The company may give the employee three to six months to show performance improvements in certain areas or risk termination. So the frequency of performance appraisals may vary depending on the situation.

This discussion of the frequency of performance reviews has implied that the employee's manager is the sole person responsible for completing the appraisal. This is the traditional approach to performance reviews (Aguinis, 2009). The manager is the person in charge of assigning the employee work to do and is in a position to oversee how that employee completes his or her assignments. Relying on the opinions of only one person for an employee's performance review does, however, make the appraisal potentially vulnerable to inaccuracies. An employee's manager's animosity or friendship may distort his or her review of that employee. In addition, a manager may be influenced by ulterior motives in rating his or her subordinates. For example, a nursing manager may not want to risk losing a highly valued employee under his or her supervision to a promotion to another section of the hospital, and thus may be tempted to rate an excellent nurse as "satisfactory." The manager may also feel stress from headquarters to keep pay raises under control, and may consequently keep performance ratings artificially low to minimize salary increases.

Moreover, there are numerous **rating errors** that can be made in performance evaluations. A manager who has limited contact with his or her subordinates may want to "play it safe" and give ratings in the middle of the scale to avoid trying to justify high or low ratings, which is called the central tendency error. Other managers might want to appear rigorous to their superiors and subsequently give their subordinates lower ratings than deserved, which is referred to as the severity error. In contrast, the leniency error occurs when managers want to be overly nice to their people and give higher ratings than warranted. The recency error occurs when a rater bases his or her ratings only on recent performance (for example, from the last couple of months) rather than performance over the entire review period (for example, the whole year). The primacy error is the opposite of the recency error. The ratings are based primarily on the beginning of the review period rather than the entire time frame. Finally, the halo error occurs when a rater is influenced substantially by one impressive aspect of an employee's performance and allows that aspect to incorrectly inflate ratings in other areas. For example, if a particular physician assistant was excellent in terms of attendance (never late, no sick days, always willing to work overtime when needed), that person deserves a high rating in dependability. However, if that person's manager was so impressed with this aspect of performance that it resulted in this person's getting high scores in other areas that were not very impressive (for example, in answering patients' questions or in organizational skills), then this would be an example of the halo error. Overall, there are numerous possible rating errors that may limit the value of performance appraisals (Aguinis, 2009).

Due to concerns over potential biases, ulterior motives, and rating errors, many organizations are expanding the performance review process to include feedback from others. The use of more than one person in the review process is commonly referred to as **multisource feedback** (Spurgeon, 2008). One possible additional source of feedback is the employee himself or herself. In some companies employees will rate themselves and then meet with their managers and compare ratings. Allowing employees to self-rate sends the message that the company wants to get their perspective on how well they believe they are doing. This option makes employees reflect on their strengths and weaknesses, and it can be a valuable jumping-off point in a performance review meeting in which an employee's self-ratings vary dramatically from the manager's ratings. Research has revealed an increase in the use of self-ratings in performance reviews (Fox, 2009).

The use of peer or team ratings is another alternative in performance reviews. Research has shown that peer appraisals are often the most accurate (Bohlander & Snell, 2010). For many employees, their peers have more contact with them than does their manager. Some employees will "act busy" when the boss is around and then revert back to weak performance once he or she leaves the area. Peer ratings can therefore provide more insight into employee performance than can the manager's perspective. If employees are assigned to a team, the advantages are similar. Teams, by their very nature, require close and regular interaction, which means that team ratings may be very accurate. The challenge with peer and team ratings is that peers or teammates can also develop friendships, which could impair objectivity in the ratings. Also, team ratings have the danger of eroding teamwork if a teammate is criticized by his or her teammates.

Another option is customer or patient ratings. Patient satisfaction is critical in our highly competitive society. Many health care organizations will survey the satisfaction of their patients or their families. Feedback from patients can be quite informative in regard to what an employee does well (for example, he or she has a good bedside manner) or needs to improve (for example, the employee has trouble explaining the health effects of certain medications). Oftentimes these surveys will address many aspects of the patient's experience at the health care organization (the time spent in the waiting room, the courteousness of the staff, the physical comfort of the setting, and so on). The measurement of patient satisfaction is also important to attaining and maintaining accreditation by TJC (Yellen, Davis, & Ricard, 2002). These approaches to patient satisfaction are not usually directed toward a specific individual and thus may be difficult to use in an employee's performance review. Health care employers would need to include specific questions in patient satisfaction surveys that identify individual employees if they intend to use them as part of the appraisal process. Another alternative, albeit questionable, is to use Web sites that claim to have patient satisfaction information on health care providers. These Web sites, such as RateMDs.com (www.ratemds.com/) or HealthGrades (www.healthgrades. com/), allow one to enter and view patient opinions of physicians, dentists, or health care organizations. Unfortunately, these Web sites do not verify whether or not the person entering the information was actually a patient, and people can enter information pertaining to a given practitioner or facility numerous times. Because of the limited controls on these Web sites, organizations would be better off creating their own system to solicit patient feedback.

For performance appraisals of managers and department heads there is another option as well. Some health care organizations will have subordinates provide feedback on their immediate supervisor, commonly referred to as **upward feedback.** This information can be helpful for an organization in identifying managers with excellent leadership skills. This approach could also motivate managers to improve relationships with their staff, because they know that their staff will be evaluating them in the future. Finally, this information could help managers learn which areas of their performance they need to work on to be more effective. The primary concern with this option is a possible negative reaction by the manager to being criticized by his or her staff. The manager might attempt to retaliate against those he or she believes were not highly supportive of him or her.

Health care organizations should carefully weigh the pros and cons of including multiple sources in the review process. If the primary objective of the performance appraisal is to conduct a thorough analysis of an employee's performance with the intent of improving job performance in the future, multiple sources should be included in the process. At the extreme, all five sources just mentioned (manager, self, peer, patient, and subordinate) could be used simultaneously for certain employees (usually managers or department heads). This process is called a 360-degree review. Although it is time consuming, a 360-degree review can be a highly effective employee development tool (Aguinis, 2009).

A final major decision employers must make in the performance review process is how the employee's performance will be assessed—and what types of data will be collected in the performance review. A narrative method is one approach to addressing this issue, whereby the employee's manager records throughout the review period critical incidents of performance by the employee. These critical incidents are events in which the employee performed exceptionally well or poorly in completing an important aspect of his or her job. For example, if a physical therapist stayed beyond her shift and spent several hours helping a patient rehabilitate an injury, then this might be noted in her file by her manager. At the end of the review period, all critical incidents are reviewed with the employee, and his or her overall performance is based on the totality of these events. This nonquantitative approach is vulnerable to the recordkeeping and writing skills of the evaluator. However, this can be an effective manner of documenting favorable or unfavorable significant performance (Mathis & Jackson, 2012).

With a comparative method, by contrast, employees are compared to one another, usually in terms of overall performance. In its simplest form, the comparative method involves a ranking of employees in a given department. The head of the department creates a rank order of his or her employees from best to worst on overall job performance. Additional rankings could be based on major job components, such as patient relations and clinical skills, to provide more feedback. The **forced distribution** method is another alternative. Jack Welch, during his time as the CEO of GE, popularized the concept of the forced distribution system in his attempt to turn GE around from financial crisis (Aguinis, 2009). In a forced distribution system the evaluator assigns his or her staff to a limited number of categories based on set percentages. For example, the department head identifies the top 20 percent of his or her staff and the bottom 10 percent, and by default the remaining 70 percent are considered to be in the middle. So using these percentages, a department of twenty employees will have four employees "exceeding expectations," fourteen employees "meeting expectations," and two employees "falling below expectations." Comparative methods can make certain personnel decisions, such as who gets the largest pay raise, who gets promoted, and who get laid off or terminated, much clearer for the employer. This option does not, however, provide much guidance for performance improvement. Employees know where they stand in comparison to others, but what they need to do to improve their ranking is often uncertain. This option can also create a highly competitive work environment and thus limit teamwork and communication.

The most common approach to scoring in a performance appraisal system is a rating method. The simplest rating scales are referred to as graphic rating scales (GRS). In a GRS approach, listed in the left-hand column of the appraisal form are the performance indicators, which are usually key tasks, duties, traits, and responsibilities. In the right-hand column is a scale with a handful of data points, usually ranging from 3 to 9. Figure 10.2 contains some examples of GRS.

The attraction of the GRS approach is that these rating scales are easy and quick to create and complete. From a performance improvement perspective, though, GRS do not provide much detail into the behavioral components of the ratings. An employee may be told that he or she is "satisfactory," but what does that employee need to do to be "good"? Also, some raters may have different standards that correspond to the various terms.

Figure 10.2   Examples of Graphic Rating Scales

Strongly disagree	Disagree	Neutral	Agree	Strongly agree
1	2	3	4	5

Needs improvement	Satisfactory	Good	Excellent
1	2	3	4

Very poor		Acceptable		Average		Strong		Top performer
1	2	3	4	5	6	7	8	9

Does not meet expectations	Meets expectations	Exceeds expectations
1	2	3

An alternative to the GRS approach is to use a behavioral observation scale (BOS). A BOS describes ideal performance on a given job dimension. Then the rater will indicate based on the BOS how often the employee meets the desired level of performance. For example, the BOS may look like this:

Employee correctly completes requisitions for additional supplies

5 = All of the time

4 = Most of the time

3 = About half of the time

2 = Seldom

1 = Never

Sometime the BOS ratings correspond to percentages:

5 = 100 percent of the time

4 = 75 to 99 percent of the time

3 = 50 to 74 percent of the time

2 = 25 to 49 percent of the time

1 = Less than 25 percent of the time

The BOS categories are less subject to interpretation than the GRS performance indicators, and the BOS does provide feedback to the employee concerning why he or she scored at a given level. It does not, however, provide behavioral feedback on how to perform the given task more effectively. This approach also assumes that the raters are keeping track in some numerical way of every employee they rate on every rating dimension for the entire review period. This may be unrealistic.

A final rating approach is to use a behaviorally anchored rating scale (BARS). In a BARS approach, each critical task is described in behavioral terms for low, average, and high performance. The top of the scale describes ideal performance for this job dimension, the midpoint of the scale describes acceptable performance, and the bottom of the scale describes poor performance. See Table 10.1 for an example.

The BARS approach provides the most detail for employees in terms of behavioral feedback, which is helpful for performance improvement. This

Table 10.1   Behaviorally Anchored Rating Scale Example—Job Dimension: Responding to Patient Questions About Medical Exams

5	Consistently asks patients if they have any questions. Responds to questions accurately and pleasantly. Reassures patients before leaving the room.
4	
3	From time to time will inquire if patients have any questions. Usually responds completely and correctly to patient questions. Generally has friendly exchanges with patients. Will occasionally leave patients' room abruptly.
2	
1	Does not solicit questions from patients. Often provides incomplete or inaccurate information to patients. Comes across as rushed when responding to questions.

system also reduces subjectivity in the performance ratings across raters. The main drawback of the BARS approach is that it takes the greatest amount of time to create at the outset. Research has indicated that the BARS approach yields the most accurate ratings among the rating options (Bohlander & Snell, 2010).

Overall, health care employers have three major options in choosing the process by which they evaluate the performance of their employees: using a narrative method, a comparative method, or a rating method. Table 10.2 outlines the major advantages and disadvantages of these three options. Keep in mind that all three of these options require judgments by one or more evaluators. Combinations of these three options can be used as well. In addition, the employer can reduce the influence of performance judgments by relying heavily or exclusively on results or outcomes. As mentioned previously, however, performance evaluations based on outcomes often do not cover an employee's job completely. Further, results can be influenced dramatically by forces outside an employee's control (for example, changes in health insurance can affect reimbursement rates). Finally, rewarding employees based primarily on outcomes may lead to unethical or undesirable consequences. If a hospital evaluates physicians based on their reduction of the number of tests performed on patients, then the possibility of a physician's

Table 10.2   **Performance Review Approaches**

	Key Advantages	Key Disadvantages
Narrative method	Significant job performance (positive and negative) events are emphasized over the course of the review period.	Data are not easy quantifiable, and thus comparisons across employees can be debatable.
Comparative method	The best and weakest employees are identified, which could make personnel decisions clearer.	Performance improvement feedback is lacking; this method may also artificially inflate performance differences.
Rating method	By providing feedback on key aspects of performance, this method promotes employee development.	Reviewers' reluctance to give high praise or low marks, as well as rating errors, may damage employee morale.

missing a key piece of medical information becomes greater and patient care may suffer. A more specific example occurred in 2009. A large health insurer, Wellpoint, evaluated the performance of its employees based on the number of policies held by very sick patients they were able to cancel. The practice is referred to as rescission. The more rescissions the employee was able to make, the more positive his or her performance review. The rescissions often were based on minor errors in the patient's initial application for health insurance. Many of these technical errors were issues of which the patient was unaware. As a result of canceling the policies, the insurance company saved millions of dollars, and sick patients suffered financially and physically ("Largest U.S. Health Insurer," 2009). Health care employers need to consider carefully the basis of employee performance reviews. If the main objective of a performance appraisal system is to help improve employee performance, then the review should be a thorough assessment of the employee's job that includes input from all relevant parties and is aligned with organizational goals.

After all of the relevant data have been collected from all of the parties involved in the review, an appraisal review meeting is scheduled with the employee. This meeting is often very anxiety provoking because most employees do not like to be evaluated and most managers do not like confronting and criticizing their staff, even if the criticisms are easily justified. For this meeting to be successful, the manager or department head running the meeting needs to be well prepared. The manager should be ready to tell the employee what he or she has done well and what needs improvement, and should have specific behavioral examples in mind to back up both positive and negative comments. The manager should also ask the employee for his or her perspective on performance areas that need improvement. The implications of the employee's failure to improve his or her performance deficiencies should be articulated in this meeting as well (Aguinis, 2009). From there, the manager and employee should agree on an action plan in which performance goals, along with a clear timetable for accomplishing these them, should be established. Resources (including training and development opportunities) should be identified to help the employee achieve the performance goals. The manager and employee should also set several target dates prior to the next formal appraisal to check on the progress of the employee in meeting these performance goals. This approach to the performance review meeting is commonly referred to as management by objectives (MBO). According to Bohlander and Snell (2011), MBO has been around since the 1950s, when it was introduced by well-known management consultant Peter Drucker in his book *The Practice of Management* (1954). It is worth noting that many advocates of total quality management have significant reservations about MBO. Quality guru W. Edwards Deming considered performance reviews one of the "deadly diseases" (p. 97) of management (Deming, 1982). MBO could lead to a short-term orientation for employees (next review in six months) rather than a long-term continuous improvement perspective, which in turn may result in employees' sacrificing quality to meet performance goals (Dean & Evans, 1994; Soltani, Van der Meer, Williams, & Pei-chun, 2006). Health care organizations therefore need to train their managers to make sure the performance management system is properly implemented and is aligned with the company's long- and short-term goals.

SUMMARY

The intent of this chapter has been to present ideas related to improving employee performance in health care. A high-performing workforce is essential to providing quality patient care. To achieve this objective, health care organizations need to have in place well-thought-out programs to enhance employee productivity, perhaps beginning with a new hire orientation program to get employees on the right track when they begin their employment. A solid mentoring program can also provide employees with valuable insight and opportunities from well-intentioned and highly competent mentors. Training programs can be crafted to prepare employees for new positions as well as to correct performance deficiencies. Moreover, employee development programs can be instrumental at cultivating the workforce for future positions and higher-level responsibilities. A systematic and carefully thought-out performance appraisal system has numerous performance benefits for the company. First and foremost it provides a snapshot of how well employees are currently doing their job. It also represents an opportunity to identify areas for improvement and establish action plans to reach performance goals. Overall, these practices are vital to attaining and retaining a vibrant and competent health care workforce and ultimately a productive organization.

KEY TERMS

ADDIE model

andragogy

e-learning

forced distribution

mentoring

multisource feedback

needs assessment

rating errors

upward feedback

REVIEW QUESTIONS

1. There are considerable advances in medicine and medical technology that call for employee training. Research has shown that health care organizations spend less on employee training than do other organizations (Flynn et al., 2007). Do you believe this finding? If yes, why do you think this is happening?

2. The use of e-learning is becoming more common in both undergraduate and graduate education. To what extent should our education system embrace e-learning for future health care professionals? Does your answer change if the purpose is for employee training in a health care environment?

3. There is considerable pressure on health care organizations to control costs. The drive to improve efficiency has resulted in some health care professionals' having their job performance evaluated in terms of dollars and cents. What is your view of including monetary criteria in the performance review process for health care professionals? Does your answer vary based on the person's job level? What are the implications for employees if money is a key factor in their performance reviews?

4. There are, as you know, three approaches to evaluating an employee's performance: a narrative method; a comparative method (for example, forced distribution); and a rating method. Which of these approaches do you believe is best for promoting high-quality health care? Why?

PART 5

Special Areas of Health Care Management

The last section of this new health care management book is devoted to special areas of health care management. The four chapters found in this section of the text address the topics of health care marketing, financial management, ethics, and the future of the health care delivery in our country. These are areas that are quite often neglected in traditional books about health care management.

The first chapter in Part Four deals with marketing concepts taken from business and their application to the health care setting (Chapter Eleven). It begins with a discussion of marketing theory, requisite marketing skills, and the entire process of marketing found in business organizations—but now applied to health care organizations. Then there is an overview of marketing concepts in general and their application to both health care organizations and the health care consumer. There's also a great discussion about marketing strategy and the use of marketing research in the development of a marketing plan for a single health care facility or an enterprise encompassing multiple entities. This chapter ends with a discussion of emerging marketing trends and specific issues that apply to the health care industry. The chapter includes an actual ad that is currently being used by a health care organization.

The second chapter in Part Four deals with several areas of importance for a health care manager in regard to financial management in health care organizations (Chapter Twelve). The health care manager must have a very good understanding of how health services are financed, and Chapter Twelve offers an in-depth look at the history of government intervention in health care as well as health insurance. A great deal of time is spent discussing the role of government financing in regard to both Medicare and Medicaid, including the attendant management issues for the health care facility. The chapter concludes with a thorough discussion of the unique characteristics of health care finance, and addresses the topic of cost-effectiveness and reform of the financing mechanism used to pay for health services.

The third chapter in this section of the book moves to an in-depth discussion of the various ethical issues surrounding health care management (Chapter Thirteen). Ethical concerns have become a very important part of our current health care environment, and they will continue to require our attention in the years to come. This chapter begins with an introduction to ethics and ethical decision making in the world of health care. Such topics as autonomy, nonmaleficence and beneficence, justice, and morality are discussed at length in this chapter. The development of a code of ethics and the formation of ethics committees are also brought into play. The chapter concludes with an evaluation of discrimination issues in health care and the subject of technology and ethics in health care settings.

The final chapter of Part Four—and of the entire text—explores future challenges for health care facilities and, of course, the health care manager (Chapter Fourteen). This chapter begins with the various economic issues that should be important for any health care manager to consider. The idea of cost escalation in health care delivery was first covered in Chapter One, and Chapter Fourteen extends that discussion into the topic of improved efficiency and the reduction of health care costs through the adoption of reengineering principles in health care delivery. The chapter then addresses the role of leadership and culture development in any reengineering effort. This final chapter ends with the topic of innovation in health care delivery, followed by a discussion of the importance of trust, brand, and reputation.

11

Health Care Marketing
Speaking the Language

Amy L. Parsons

LEARNING OBJECTIVES

- Understand basic concepts of marketing and the marketing process and how they apply to health care organizations
- Acknowledge what makes health care marketing unique
- Be familiar with the different types of marketing strategies used in health care organizations
- Understand the importance of ethics in health care marketing
- Know the steps involved in the marketing research process
- Recognize the important role the health care consumer plays in health care marketing
- Be aware of emerging trends related to marketing in the health care industry

Understanding **marketing** is important for any health care manager. According to the American Marketing Association's official definition approved in October 2007, "Marketing is the activity, set of institutions, and processes for creating, communicating, delivering, and exchanging offerings that have value for customers, clients, partners, and society at large" (Keefe, 2008, p. 29). **Health care marketing** involves applying marketing practices to the health care field (Rooney, 2009), which can be challenging because there are many aspects of the field that make it unique. Marketing may be officially performed by the marketing department, but all members of the organization contribute to the success or failure of the organization's marketing strategy.

Marketing is an important function within the health care organization. Health care organizations need to develop trusting relationships with their patients because health care is an intangible product that is also private and sensitive (Renfrow, 2009). Health care marketing needs to become more personal and more narrowly targeted, and it should involve more two-way communication and dialogue (Renfrow). In general, a marketing department can accomplish three things: (1) creating public awareness by developing a brand (or brands) and communicating through advertising and public relations, (2) generating leads and encouraging consumer action, and (3) providing support to allow salespeople to close the sale (Krauss, 2010) Although budgets are more constrained, the need still exists for marketing, and health care managers must monitor what their employees are doing and manage their budgets more efficiently while also exploring ways to generate new revenue (Paton, 2010).

THE MARKETING PROCESS

Identifying the **target market** or target audience is crucial to the success of any marketing strategy. The target market refers to who might consume the product or service. A target market can be broad in nature, such as eighteen- to forty-nine-year-olds, residents of Philadelphia, or mothers, or it can be more specifically defined, such as eighteen- to twenty-two-year olds; residents of Lombard Street in Philadelphia; or mothers ages thirty-three to forty who live in Newark, New Jersey. Challenges with identifying the target market include finding a market that is large enough to be profitable and defining the target market specifically enough to be able to market relevant products and services efficiently. For a hospital, a target market might be defined by geography or perhaps by the types of patients to whom services are offered. For example, children's hospitals specialize in catering to the needs of children. The target market would be families who need medical services for their children. For an individual private practice in health care, a target market might focus on geography but could also focus on the types of patients according to gender, age, or the nature of the care required. A family doctor would most likely have a broader target audience in terms of age and gender than would a cardiologist who offers more specialized services.

Related to the identification of the target market is the concept of **market segmentation.** Market segmentation involves looking at a large market and identifying smaller groups or segments of that market that may have similar needs. Once the segments are identified, the organization can decide whether to develop different offerings to reach each segment or to focus on the larger market. Segments can be identified based on demographic factors, such as age, gender, ethnicity, geography, lifestyle, social class, frequency of use, or brand loyalty (Berkowitz, 2004). In the health care marketplace there are likely to be some segments that value friendly, personal care, and other segments that look for a convenient location (Steblea, Steblea, & Poklea, 2009). Today there is a need to clearly identify and understand consumer segments to effectively develop product offerings in health care because consumers are becoming increasingly involved in the health care delivery process (Simons, 2009). For managed care organizations, segments could include hospitals, retailers, and wholesalers as well as employers and unions (Dancer, Fisher, & Wilcox, 2011). Another approach to segmentation that is gaining popularity in the health care industry is generational targeting. Generational targeting identifies four main groups of adult health care consumers: the Greatest/Silent Generation (born in 1942 or earlier), baby boomers (born between 1943 and 1960), Generation X (born between 1961 and 1981), and Generation Y (born since 1982), with each group having different needs, different criteria for selecting health care providers and evaluating health care experiences, and different media consumption habits. For example, Virginia Commonwealth Medical Center used

Table 11.1 Potential Segments for a Health Plan

Segment Category	Potential Segments
Types of customers	Large businesses (1,000 employees or more)
	Medium-size businesses (300–1,000 employees)
	Small businesses (fewer than 300 employees)
	Individuals
	Families
Types of needs	Wellness
	Senior care
	Routine or preventative care
	Inpatient services
	Outpatient services
Geographic reach	City
	County
	Region

generational marketing in its "Every Day, A New Discovery Red Letter Day" campaign by incorporating patient stories that were relevant to each of the four generational segments (Igaray & MacCracken, 2011). Table 11.1 presents potential segments for a health plan.

When making decisions about segmentation, managers need to be sure that the segments are identifiable, accessible, inclined to buy the product or service, profitable, desirable, consistent with other segments, and available and able to buy the product or service (Berkowitz, 2004). Effectively reaching each segment may require developing different product strategies and creating different communication approaches (Paton, 2010). The challenge in today's marketing environment is finding creative and less expensive ways to reach each segment (Paton). A segment must have characteristics that distinguish it from the larger target market—characteristics that are different enough to warrant creating new marketing strategies specifically targeted at that segment.

KEY MARKETING CONCEPTS

One of the key concepts in marketing is the marketing mix. This refers to four different aspects about which organizational managers need to make decisions. These aspects are often referred to as the "four P's"—product, price, promotion, and place. Another "P" that may be especially relevant for health care refers to people, which should also be included in the marketing mix. Table 11.2 provides possible considerations related to each of the four P's, plus people, for a hospital. It is crucial that managers understand each

Table 11.2   Marketing Mix for a Hospital

Marketing Mix Element	Possible Considerations
Product	Surgery
	Nursing care
	Prescription drugs
	Extended stays
	Intensive care treatment
	Medical testing
Price	Co-pay for a prescription drug
	Cost of overnight rooms
	Insurance reimbursements
Promotion	Brochures
	Newsletters
	E-mail
	Blog
	Facebook page
Place	Main location at 100 Main St.
	Emergency room location at 125 Main St.
	Regional or local coverage
	Accessibility of service
People	Physicians
	Nurses
	Orderlies
	Administrative staff

aspect of the marketing mix and consider how the elements relate to each other when seeking to gain a competitive advantage in the marketplace. For example, when making decisions about which products or services to offer, it is important also to consider how pricing, place, promotion, and people play a role in determining the viability of those products or services.

Product

The term *product* refers to the goods, services, and ideas offered by an organization. Goods refer to the tangible offerings of an organization. Services refer to the intangible offerings of an organization. Ideas refer to concepts related to goods and services.

Many types of goods and services are offered by health care organizations, such as medical services delivered by nurses and physicians, pharmaceutical products provided for patients, hospital stays, medical testing, and health plans for individuals and employers, along with such ideas as wellness, disease prevention, and health awareness. Unlike a consumer products company that offers shampoo, toothpaste, potato chips, lawn furniture, shirts, socks, or household cleaners, or an industrial products company that offers steel, roof shingles, ball bearings, or automotive parts, health care organizations primarily offer services, whereby the consumer does not bring home a tangible product. For example, a hospital may perform surgical procedures, offer extensive medical testing, provide nursing care to patients, offer emergency room care, sell food in its cafeteria, and so on. A health insurer will offer different plans to employers and individuals. A pharmaceutical company works with doctors to recommend products for patients. Each of these product offerings may involve a different type of marketing approach.

Products can be categorized in many different ways—as goods versus services, durable versus nondurable, and consumer versus industrial, and in terms of the breadth and depth of the product or service lines offered. Durable products, such as housing, furniture, appliances, or automobiles, will last over the long term, whereas nondurable products, such as food, clothing, entertainment, or toiletries, are consumed in the short term. Breadth refers to the variety of different products or services offered (for example, Walmart sells clothing, paint, food, household items, garden supplies, toiletries, and other items); depth refers to the variety of offerings within a specific product category (Walmart might offer ten brands of toothpaste to its customers). In the health care industry, products can also be conceptualized based on the following dimensions: the level of care, the level of urgency, inpatient versus outpatient services, medical versus surgical services, diagnosis versus treatment, clinical versus nonclinical services, and elective versus nonelective services (Thomas, 2005).

Another product-related consideration is the brand. "A brand is a conceptual identity that focuses the organization of marketing activities—usually with the purpose of building equities for that brand in the marketplace" (Bendinger et al., 2009, p. 10). Brands can be expressed through a name, a logo, a symbol, a color, an idea, or some combination of these. Some brands periodically may need reevaluation to reflect changes in the marketplace, changes due to mergers and acquisitions, the introduction of new products, or a need to change strategic direction. The University of Texas MD Anderson Cancer Center is an example of a health care organization that pursued a rebranding strategy, which led the organization to reevaluate how it was presenting itself and resulted in an updated logo that lists the name of the organization, draws a red line through the word "cancer," and includes the tagline "Making cancer history." The new logo and the MD Anderson Cancer Center have become synonymous, and the logo has helped the organization provide a more consistent message (Flory, 2011).

Price

Pricing decisions involve developing a price for each product or service that an organization offers. An important determinant of a product or service's success is whether or not it is appropriately priced in the marketplace. Pricing decisions must take into account the cost of producing or delivering the product or service and what the consumer is willing to pay. The nature of health services makes pricing a challenging issue, as consumers, employers, insurance companies, and health care providers all play a role in determining the price of health care. The challenge for hospitals and physicians is to determine the right formula to offer high-quality care that is also cost effective (Wilson, 2010). For the consumer and the consumer's employer there are issues related to the cost of insurance coverage, whereas for the insurance company and health care provider there are issues related to covering the cost of health care delivery and production. Health care providers must strive to balance the costs associated with health care delivery (including human costs, such as the salaries of doctors, nurses, and other staff members; expenditures for malpractice insurance, medical equipment, and overhead; and investments in information systems) with insurance reimbursements, the demand for services, and the willingness of consumers to pay for services.

Insurance companies also play a role in determining the price of health care, as they negotiate rates with health care providers (Wilson, 2010). Insurance companies have traditionally used quality, access, and cost variables when determining rates and prices for health insurance policies. However, quality is now mandated through government licensing, and access to health care has been hard to limit due to health plan member and employer demands, making cost the primary consideration when determining price (Davila, 2010). As an example of an insurance company that addressed this issue, Blue Cross and Blue Shield of North Carolina was looking for a way to control medical care costs to improve health care delivery for its customers. It launched a campaign called "Let's Talk Cost" that encourages all participants in and consumers of health care delivery to stop looking for scapegoats and to work together to share the responsibility for keeping medical care costs more reasonable (Kochman & Calabria, 2011).

For the individual consumer, the price of health care might include the cost of the health plan, co-pays, deductibles, and other out-of-pocket expenses. Consumers may pay different prices for individual health services depending on the scope of their insurance policy (Davila, 2010). Consumers may also delay seeking out health care because of the cost (Galloro, 2011). For an employer looking to purchase health care for its employees, the price would be the cost of the premium and required reimbursements.

Promotion

Promotion focuses on delivering a message about a company's product. As with pricing, it is essential to consider how the product or service will be promoted, because even if a product or service is exactly right for what the target market demands and is priced competitively, sales will be low if the target audience is not aware that the product or service exists. Communication is an essential component of promotion, and it is important to develop an appropriate message as well as the right strategy to deliver that message. Four key tools of promotion (also known as the promotional mix) are advertising, public relations, personal selling, and sales promotion, which can all be used strategically as part of an integrated marketing communication plan. Integrated marketing communication involves setting goals and strategies as well as developing and executing the communication tactics needed to achieve these goals by coordinating, prioritizing, and optimizing available options (Bendinger et al., 2009).

Advertising

Advertising is a paid form of nonpersonal communication delivered by an identifiable source. Advertising decisions focus on creating messages to reach the target audience and designing media strategies to reach that audience most effectively and efficiently. The objective of advertising is to "use persuasion to sell, inform, educate, remind and/or entertain the target about a product or service" (Blakeman, 2009, p. 14). For health care organizations, advertising can be used to generate awareness, recognize donors, encourage growth, announce new buildings and locations, enhance an organization's reputation, and promote advocacy (Feinberg, 2011).

Health care organizations must decide whether to develop their own advertising in-house or hire an advertising agency. The advantages of in-house advertising are that it can cost less, information can be kept confidential, and employees are already familiar with the business and industry. But in-house advertising may not always be objective, it may not always be able to deliver fresh ideas, and employees may lack expertise in advertising (Bendinger et al., 2009). Advertising agencies give clients objective opinions, provide a wide variety of services, and are experts in the field, but hiring them can be expensive, and conflicts do arise between agencies and their clients. When selecting an advertising agency, there is the option of choosing either a full-service agency that services a wide variety of clients or a specialized agency that focuses on the needs of health care clients; focuses on a particular function, such as media or creative; or covers a specific geographic area or a specific type of marketing, such as Internet marketing. Full-service agencies fulfill four basic functions: account management, creative, media planning and placement, and research (Bendinger et al., 2009). Regardless of who develops the advertising strategy, choosing the right message to reach the right target audience is crucial. As an example of a successful campaign run by an advertising agency, New York Presbyterian Hospitals along with the agency Munn Rabôt created a campaign called "Amazing Stories" that focused on telling the stories of real patients in their own words. This campaign resulted in increased awareness, more Web site visits, and positive feedback inside the organization (Feinberg, 2011).

Just as important as the creation of the actual message is media management, which involves choosing the type of medium—traditional (such as television, radio, newspapers, magazines, or out-of-home advertising); non-traditional (such as social media, mobile marketing, Internet marketing, search engine marketing, guerilla marketing, word-of-mouth marketing, or direct marketing); or some combination of these. Other relevant issues with media management once a medium has been chosen include strategically choosing which vehicle within the medium to use, when the message will run, and for how long it will run. All media decisions need to consider the most effective way to reach the audience, how frequently to place a message, and how to do so in the most cost-efficient way.

Each type of media vehicle has different advantages and disadvantages. *Television* is good for reaching mass audiences, can tell a story effectively through visuals and sounds, can be targeted to reach specific audiences, and offers the advertiser both network and cable programming to choose from. Television also can be expensive to produce, ads need to be creative enough to stand out from the clutter, and television commercials only last for a short period of time. *Radio* can be adapted for both national and local audiences, can be used frequently to get a message across, is effective at targeting, and can be relatively inexpensive. Radio is not, however, as popular as it once was in terms of audience size, it can only provide audio and not video, and it can be seen as background noise. *Newspapers* can provide a good deal of information, work well for local audiences, offer a variety of ad sizes, have loyal readers, are relatively inexpensive, allow the advertiser to advertise frequently, and visually display information. They are also declining in readership, especially among the younger generation; the print quality may not always be high; ads may not get noticed by readers; and ads have a short shelf life. *Magazines* give the advertiser the ability to target specific audiences. Magazine ads also last longer than other forms of media; they are relatively high-quality; and they can use color more effectively than do newspapers because of improved paper quality, making them useful for image advertising, which focuses on using visuals to create awareness and build a brand's image. *Out-of-home advertising* can include mobile and stationary billboards, advertising in transit shelters, bus advertising, advertising on benches, advertising in airport and train terminals, and taxi advertising. In other words, it gives the advertiser a wide variety of options. Out-of-home ads are there twenty-four hours a day, they can have a strong visual impact, and they enable the advertiser to reach a large audience—including the target market—through the choice of the right location. However, out-of-home advertising delivers a relatively short and fleeting message, may not be noticed, and requires a strategic choice of location—and it is difficult to measure the impact of the message.

There are also many advantages and disadvantages to using a nontraditional medium. *Social media* is a growing way to reach audiences, with more and more people starting to use at least one social network on a regular basis. However, advertising using social media is still in its early phases, and especially for health care organizations there are privacy issues and the legal obligation to warn consumers that any information they share about themselves or their conditions becomes public once it appears in social media (Burke & Goldstein, 2010).

Mobile advertising is also gaining in popularity as more people purchase smartphones and tablet devices, such as iPads. There are different options available with mobile advertising, such as banners, mobile Web, mobile search, mobile video, text messaging, downloadable applications (apps), and games. Baptist Hospital East in Louisville, Kentucky, developed a mobile Web site that provides physician and visitor information for consumers, allows access to directories, and gives consumers a place to check and monitor symptoms (Solomon, 2011). Mobile advertising is seen as a way to interact instantly with consumers, and when consumers choose to receive content by "opting in," messages can be sent to a receptive audience. However, as with social media, mobile advertising is still in its early developmental stages, there are size limitations on the ads themselves, and consumers may see it as annoying.

Internet marketing has many forms and can be transmitted through banner ads, e-mail, Web sites, webisodes, and pop-up ads. Internet marketing can be effective for targeting individuals with customized messages, is relatively inexpensive, offers flexibility, allows for interactivity, and can engage the consumer. However, some types of Internet marketing can get lost in the clutter, consumers may find it annoying, not all consumers have access to the same level and quality of Internet access, and Internet marketing efforts are still difficult to measure in a meaningful way.

Search engine marketing is a subcategory of Internet marketing. The goal of search engine marketing is search engine optimization, which is "a long-term, holistic . . . approach that uses skilled web site edits and other third-party relationships and commentary to influence the ranking of your web site in organic or natural search results" (Gronlund, 2010, p. 20). Search engine marketing can effectively target audiences, and can be a low-cost way to generate leads and awareness. Search engine marketing requires strategic planning to reach the right target audience in a cost-effective manner. There are two types of searches. One is nonpaid or organic, and results of this type of search appear naturally when a consumer is searching for information on a search engine. Nonpaid searches do not require the advertiser to pay for page placement. The other is paid, and requires the company to bid on keywords to ensure that its listing rises to the top of the consumer's search results. These types of searches may appear as "sponsored results" at the top of the page. Search engine results can also be tracked by using a tool such as Google Analytics, which helps answer questions related to the effectiveness of organic, nonpaid search versus paid search; what keywords visitors use that lead them to the Web site; where visits come from; who is visiting; and what visitors look at (Solomon, 2010).

Guerilla marketing is "the use of nontraditional promotional methods to attract attention, increase memorability, and make sales" (Blakeman, 2009, p. 278). Guerilla marketing by definition requires creativity. It can be effective at generating interest and targeting specific audiences, is very interactive, and does not get lost in the clutter. However, guerilla marketing can be seen as intrusive, can be expensive, and may not reach the intended target audience.

Word-of-mouth marketing, or viral marketing, occurs when people share positive or negative information about a product or service with others (Gombeski, Britt, et al., 2011). Effectively using word-of-mouth marketing requires both delivering a quality product or service and continuous monitoring. In the health care industry physician recommendations for care and prescriptions and as well as referrals from family and friends are forms of word-of-mouth marketing (Fredricks, 2011; Weiss, 2011). *Direct marketing* uses databases to identify and then reach customers through direct mail, e-mail, or telephone, and is an interactive way to target specific audiences. It can be personalized, results can be measured easily, and specific customer needs can be addressed through the use of databases. Also, if done right, direct marketing can generate a fair amount of attention. Conversely, direct marketing can be expensive given the costs and time associated with production and postage, and consumers may view it as clutter and dispose of it without reading it.

There are, of course, many specific issues related to using these types of media vehicles for health care organizations. All choices will involve some financial constraints, which may ultimately influence which vehicle the organization chooses. The choice of vehicle will ultimately depend on the target market because of variations in media consumption across demographic groups (Paton, 2010). A few of the key issues for both traditional and nontraditional media will be discussed here.

When selecting traditional media there are a number of decisions to make. For example, pursuing television advertising necessitates making a decision about what programming is appropriate and what type of message is appropriate, as advertising for health care needs to be more informative and less entertaining than advertising for other types of products. Advertising on the radio involves deciding what stations to use and determining whether to focus on building name recognition or promoting specific services offered by a health care organization. Advertising in the newspaper is similar to advertising on the radio in terms of deciding which paper and what services to focus on. Another issue with newspaper advertising is determining the size of the ad, what types of illustrations or photos to include in the ad, how much copy (text) to include, how the visuals should relate to the copy, in which section of the paper the ad should be placed, and whether to use color or black and white. When opting to advertise in magazines, a few strategic issues include which magazines the ads should be placed in, how much copy to include, how the visuals should relate to the copy, whether or not to use color, how many pages to run, where to place the ad within the publication, how much to spend, and how to deal with production time constraints and deadlines. (See Figure 11.1 for an example of an ad that could appear in a newspaper or a magazine.) For out-of-home advertising, decisions need to be made about what format to use, the location,

Figure 11.1   Blue Mountain Health System Print Advertisement

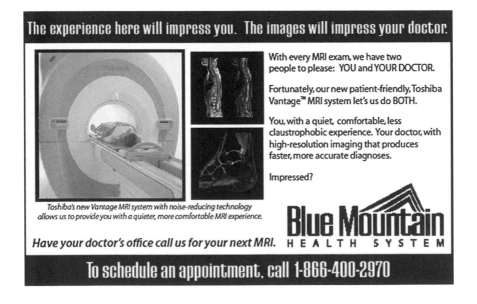

the size of the message, the nature of the message, and how long the message will run.

When selecting nontraditional media, advertising using *social media* may involve maintaining a page or profile on a particular social network, and this may be a function of either the marketing or advertising department or the public relations department. Banner ads or sponsored ads may be placed on pages within social networks, which will involve making decisions concerning to whom the ads should be targeted and where the ads should appear. Social network sites, such as Facebook, allow advertisers to specify which users will see their ads based on demographic information and member interests.

Pursuing mobile advertising entails deciding on what type of device to target, as smartphones have much better messaging capabilities than do traditional cell phones. Whether to use just text or to add video or other visuals to the message is an additional consideration. Another decision has to do with what type of mobile advertising to use, there being different options available for the placement of advertisements, including mobile search, apps, display ads, and text messages.

There are many different facets of Internet marketing. Most companies have Web sites whose design and content are strategically important. Companies may also decide to develop smaller, focused microsites to address specific concerns. They can also place advertising on other Web sites through banner ads and links that must be strategically placed and designed to attract the attention of the desired audience. Search engine marketing also requires the strategic placement of ads to reach the right audience, a process that includes identifying and managing the selection of keywords to purchase and bid on from the hosting search engine (Google, Yahoo, Bing, and so on) to influence where their business appears in search results; finding the right place on a Web page to place an ad; and finding the search engine that is the best strategic fit for the organization (Gronlund, 2010).

Guerilla marketing involves determining where the marketing will happen, how consumers will interact with the brand, and the cost of implementation. For word-of-mouth marketing the challenge is monitoring it, because communication is generated by consumers and not by the organization. Family and friend referrals are perceived by many consumers to be more valuable than physician referrals (Fredricks, 2011). UK HealthCare strategically monitors word-of-mouth marketing by asking outpatients who influenced them in their health care choices in semiannual surveys (Gombeski, Britt, et al., 2011). Word-of-mouth marketing can also be monitored using interviews and social media analytic tools. For direct marketing there is a need to determine what format to use, such as a catalog, a brochure, an e-mail, or a postcard; what to spend on mailing, production, and distribution; what to promote; whom to distribute the message to; and where to access names and addresses.

Not all advertising targets a mass audience. To complement mass marketing strategies, many health care providers are turning to "gentle collisions" or personal interactions designed to get consumers to think positively about their brand in an effort to reach a narrower target audience (Stahl, 2010). The goal of gentle collisions is to encourage consumer action and foster a more meaningful interaction between the consumer and the brand. Creating appropriate opportunities for gentle collisions relies on understanding the target audience and being aware of how members of the target audience spend their time, understanding how they feel about health care and their situation, understanding how the brand can interact with consumers during their leisure time, identifying the consumer's support network and targeting messages toward that support network as well as the consumer, identifying where to deliver the message, and deciding who will be trusted to deliver the message (Stahl). The overall focus of all advertising is also changing from image advertising directed to a general audience to more targeted advertising promoting specific services to a more narrowly defined audience (Paton, 2010). Advertisers are increasingly turning toward nontraditional or media vehicles that deliver a message to consumers where they don't expect it—a message that can be effective if it is relevant, simple, and creative (Reyburn, 2010).

Public Relations

Public relations is a form of communication with both internal and external audiences that is designed to build relationships and strives to reinforce, define, or rebuild the image of a corporation, product, or service (Blakeman, 2009). Like advertising it delivers a message to a target audience, but it differs from advertising in that it is generally not paid for directly by the organization sending the message. Public relations is seen as a relatively low-cost and credible way to interact with the community. The effects of public relations efforts are difficult to measure, however. Public relations tools include press conferences, media kits, press releases, video news conferences, public service announcements, and sponsored events. One function of a public relations department may be to maintain the organization's Web site and perhaps to manage its interaction with social media outlets. Kaiser Permanente, for example, has a News Center to which stakeholders can go to find information (Lofgren & Cantu, 2010). Public relations helps the health care organization develop and maintain relationships with the community, including the media. As another example, City of Hope in the Los Angeles area works with the music industry to produce public service announcements using celebrities that create national and regional awareness for its cancer research and cancer care. City of Hope also works with the sports industry, partnering with local sports teams to promote cancer education and research funding (Maceo, 2011). Rancho Los Amigos Hospital in Los Angeles hosts annual conferences for the medical community and several events for the community at large in an effort to raise awareness for its programs and services and to enhance its reputation as a top U.S. rehabilitation facility (Orozco, Aisen, Limbaga, Waskul, & Waskul, 2011). Organizations can sponsor their own events or purchase sponsorships at other community events. Sponsorships provide opportunities for health care organizations to meet with potential customers and build relationships, and they can improve an organization's visibility in the community, create employee pride, foster goodwill, and promote health in the community (Gombeski, Wray, & Blair, 2011). Although sponsoring events does involve direct costs for the organization, the hope is that the event will receive media coverage that the organization does not directly pay for. Unfortunately, due to financial concerns in recent years, sponsorship budgets have been eliminated or reduced, and decisions related to which community events to sponsor have come under closer scrutiny by boards of directors and senior management.

There is also a risk of "ambush marketing," which is an attempt by unofficial sponsors to gain benefits without paying the event owner (Gombeski, Wray, & Blair, 2011; Paton, 2010). For example, an organization might pay for the rights to be an official sponsor of an event, and a competitor might set up a booth across the street from the event or distribute marketing materials to event attendees as they enter the event. Public relations can complement other efforts as part of an integrated marketing communication plan.

Personal Selling

Personal selling relies on personal communication between individuals rather than on communication between a marketer and a mass audience. Personal selling gives the salesperson the opportunity to get direct feedback from the customer, allowing the salesperson and the customer to work together to identify and solve problems. Health care employees may work closely with salespeople from organizations that provide pharmaceutical products and supplies, medical equipment, uniforms, cafeteria items, furniture, and so on. Healthcare organizations, such as health insurers and hospitals, also need to promote themselves and may rely on salespeople to generate new business and maintain relationships with current customers. For example, health insurers use salespeople to identify and recruit local businesses that purchase plans for their employees as well as individuals who might participate in these plans. Sales representatives create forced repetition by continually reminding customers about their products or services, and they have the ability to connect to and form relationships with their customers as well as to challenge the way physicians evaluate treatment options by asking the right questions (Moldenhauer, 2010). The effective salesperson must be knowledgeable about what he or she is selling and about the health care environment, and must be able to identify and address the needs and wants of potential customers. Problem-solving skills are also extremely critical in helping establish relationships with customers (Dancer et al., 2011).

The sales environment in recent years, especially in the pharmaceutical industry, has been changing. Companies have reduced the size of their respective sales forces, and the nature of the selling task and the skills needed to succeed are also changing. The target for pharmaceutical marketing messages is expanding beyond physicians to include patients who want information and payers who want evidence of product value (Evangelista & Poulin, 2009). Traditionally sales representatives were rewarded based on the number of calls made (reach), how often calls were made (frequency), prescription volume, market share, and revenue attainment, but the use of qualitative measures, such as selling skills and call quality, territory management, and teamwork, is growing (Fisher, Wallace, & Wilcox, 2010). Sales representatives have less face time with and access to physicians, so the nature of their communication with physicians is also changing, as effective sales representatives need to be able to deliver their selling messages in just a few minutes (Moldenhauer, 2011). Given the constantly evolving health care industry, pharmaceutical sales representatives will need to have skills in regard to business, marketing, negotiation, and finance. Further, they will have to develop core competencies pertaining to account management and business development rather than interpersonal skills (Evangelista & Poulin, 2009; Fisher et al., 2010). Managed care sales representatives need to keep current with changes related to health care reform, understand the implications of this reform for both payers and providers, and provide relevant health care economic data and analysis to help their customers navigate through the changing health care landscape. Managers need to ensure that their salespeople have the resources available to help their customers solve problems and should strive to create customer-focused environments that encourage learning by establishing listening programs, performing regular client reviews to encourage feedback, and recording progress (Dancer et al., 2011).

Sales Promotion

Sales promotion is generally considered a short-term strategy designed to temporarily boost sales by rewarding the buyer for making a purchase. Sales promotion can be targeted either at the direct consumer or at intermediaries in the distribution channel. Popular short-term, consumer-oriented sales promotional tools include coupons, rebates, free gifts or premiums, events, and contests or sweepstakes. Traditionally sales promotion has not been used extensively in the health care industry because it may lead to unnecessary consumption of health services (Berkowitz, 2004). However, sales promotional tools can be useful for encouraging medical screening and have been used extensively in the pharmaceutical industry in the form of samples and gifts. A reward program that promotes customer loyalty on a long-term basis would also be considered sales promotion. For example, the Henry Ford Health System in Michigan created Lifetime Connections, a patient reminder and loyalty program designed to encourage patients to make their routine health care appointments (Glenn, 2010).

Place

The emphasis of the fourth component of the marketing mix, place, is on distribution of the product or service. Distribution decisions can involve where to locate a retail outlet, where to sell a product or service, and how to deliver that product or service, among other considerations. Place incorporates all aspects of a transaction that determine how easily consumers can obtain a product or service. As with pricing and promotion, place-related decisions need to consider the impact of other aspects of the marketing mix. Such decisions for a health care organization may have to do with the facility's physical location, the layout of the facility, and where various services will be delivered within the facility; whether the organization wants to establish a regional or local presence; the hours the facility will operate; parking accessibility; waiting times; the availability of staff; and how many locations to have. For example, Vanderbilt University Medical Center in Nashville, Tennessee, needed a way to expand its services but was limited by the amount of urban space available, so it established an off-campus facility in a nearby shopping mall that offered convenience, an improved patient experience, and reduced traffic congestion (Austin & Wilson, 2011). Consumer perceptions of such place-related issues as online access to medical records, the availability of flexible or twenty-four-hour service or help lines, or flexibility in using out-of-system providers in emergencies may influence their evaluation of the services provided (Thomas, 2005).

When making decisions related to place, it is important to understand the four primary functions or categories of utility involved. *Place utility* has to do with decisions that add value to the product or service by making it more accessible for the consumer, such as the decision to add weekend hours at a clinic or to create satellite locations to target specific consumer segments. *Time utility* refers to how or when services will be made available and the costs associated with having services available. For example, operating an on-site pharmacy or staffing a twenty-four-hour help line will be more expensive for the organization but adds value for the consumer. *Possession utility* refers to how consumers acquire and finance their purchase. Some health plans require patients to pay up front at the time of their office visit, whereas other health plans prefer to bill the patient after services have been rendered. *Form utility* refers to what the organization does to change the product or service for the consumer (Berkowitz, 2004). In health care this may involve customizing services to address customer needs, such as by offering online or mobile access to medical records, changing the hours of service availability, or creating customized wellness and rehabilitation programs.

People

Services rely on people to deliver them. The quality of a service offered is often directly correlated with the performance of the person or people who deliver that service. For example, when a patient comes to a doctor's office, this may involve interacting with a receptionist, a nurse, a medical technician, a physician, and a physician assistant. A patient's evaluation of the service performed may be based on interactions with all of these different people involved in delivering the service. Even with the move toward using more technology in health care delivery, the human touch is still an important component in health care marketing: patients need to feel that those who provide health care products and services know and care about them and understand their challenges (Stahl, 2010). Employee engagement also contributes to improved customer service, and companies should strive to create a culture of engagement. For example, St. Luke's Health System in Idaho promotes engagement through regular visits by management to the various locations, an intranet site that encourages conversations between employees and executives, and an overall commitment by the organization to fostering employee engagement (Squazzo, 2011). The price of the service will need to take into account the cost of the people who deliver that service and where the service is offered (place).

The single most important factor for a consumer in selecting a hospital is not the location or the competition—it is the hospital's physicians. People clearly matter in health care delivery (Steblea et al., 2009). Physicians also play an important role in determining market share and profitability because they have a say in what types of services are performed, where the services are delivered, and for how long the services are administered (Weiss, 2011). It is also important from a managerial perspective to develop an organizational culture that exemplifies the organization's values across different departments and even different locations. For example, Carolinas Health-Care System wanted to "better link employees, physicians and volunteers to create one unified enterprise with common values relating to the delivery of patient care" (Brower, 2011, p. 17). To address this challenge the organization launched an internal branding campaign called "Care Without Compromise" that sought to communicate four key values—caring, commitment, integrity, and teamwork. Since the campaign was launched customer satisfaction rates have increased by 5 percent (Brower).

Although it is essential to understand the elements of the marketing mix and the various issues related to each one, the health care marketing manager must also strive to identify how decisions related to one aspect of the marketing mix influence or relate to decisions pertaining to the other aspects. A successful product launch depends not only on the product itself but also on how competitively it is priced, how effectively it is promoted, and how strategically it is distributed—and on the people who deliver the product to the customer. A wonderful advertising campaign for a product may generate customer interest and awareness, but if the product is of poor quality, inappropriately priced, and difficult to access, and if the people who deliver the product are rude and lazy, the product will ultimately fail.

THE HEALTH CARE CONSUMER

Today's health care consumers are often actively involved in researching and learning about the services they consume, and they want increasing control over their health care needs (Renfrow, 2009). They want to gather and share health information, and they demand tools to help them make decisions about their own health care—they want to be in charge of deciding what services they and their family members need or do not need (Beach Thielst, 2011). Patient experiences are the primary driver in shaping consumer perceptions of health care providers (Segbers, 2010).

Today's health care consumers are likely to be talking about their experiences with friends, family, coworkers, and anyone who will listen, so it is essential for health care providers to pay attention to word-of-mouth marketing (Fredricks, 2011). Consumers share their experiences by speaking to others; sending e-mails; posting videos on YouTube; or expressing their opinions on blogs, microblogs, and social media sites. Suburban Hospital in Bethesda, Maryland, learned this the hard way when a patient shared his negative experience with minor knee surgery via a blog and Twitter, causing a public relations headache for the hospital (Segbers, 2010).

How companies address and promote customer loyalty can be conceptualized in terms of the Customer Loyalty Pyramid (Lowenstein, 1997). This model suggests that companies operate at satisfaction-based, performance-based, and commitment-based levels. At each level companies approach customers in a different manner. Companies at the *satisfaction-based* level treat customers in a passive and reactive manner, have traditional bureaucratic management, and have ineffective customer processes. Companies at the *performance-based* level are more sensitive to and aware of customer needs, and they are more proactive. There are processes in place to address customer complaints, and customer satisfaction is often measured and used as a performance indicator for compensation purposes. Companies at the *commitment-based* level treat their customers as partners; they are customer driven. Employees are rewarded for the delivery of high-quality services and for customer retention. In terms of patient loyalty, the overall quality of care, the likelihood that the patient will recommend his or her hospital to others, and how well the hospital exceeded expectations all have an important influence on consumer loyalty. This loyalty influences return visits and recommendations, which are key to an organization's maintaining its fiscal health (Binder & Reeves, 2010).

Consumers are less responsive to advertising messages from health care organizations that push one-size-fits-all solutions, and they want ownership of their health care. Marketing should therefore make consumers feel that they have some control and that health insurers and the medical establishment are no longer dictating the course of their health care (Simons, 2009). These changes in consumer behavior have led to the development of the term *consumer-driven health care marketing*, which focuses on customer wants, needs, and expectations and recognizes the consumer's role in health care delivery as well as in the promotion of health education and wellness (Rooney, 2009).

Given the emergence of consumer-driven health care marketing, marketing communication should focus on the needs of consumers in terms of what they are thinking and feeling; it should show how the organization strives to deliver quality services and why the consumer is important to the organization (Paton, 2010). Consumers want to see messages that are about them, not just about the organization (Reyburn, 2010). In other words, they want to know how the organization's products and services will address their concerns and what benefits the organization can offer them (Rooney, 2009). A successful example is Kaiser Permanente's "Thrive" campaign," which uses integrated marketing communication that includes advertising through social media, Internet marketing, internal marketing, and direct marketing as well as public relations efforts to promote the concept of total health. This campaign reflects the organization's mission and its commitment to offering its members and patients high standards of care, focusing on benefits rather than features (Lofgren & Cantu, 2010).

MARKETING STRATEGY

Marketing strategy refers to the "approach taken in meeting the challenges of the marketplace" (Thomas, 2005, p. 247). An organization must decide how it will compete in the marketplace, and identifying the marketing strategy is a critical step in the strategic planning process. Marketing strategies can serve several purposes for the organization, such as providing direction; differentiating the organization; helping to tailor key aspects of the marketing mix and to organize and target resources; or affording the organization a competitive advantage (Thomas, 2005). An organization's marketing strategy may depend on the nature of the local market and whether the organization wants to compete on a local or national level. For example, in areas with multiple hospitals, those hospitals will need to consider different factors when developing their marketing strategy than would a hospital that is the only one in its area. It is important in competitive markets for the organization to determine how it wants to be positioned among its competitors. Adventist Midwest Health in Chicago, for example, launched a campaign in 2009 that positioned the entire organization as a trusted regional health care expert because it wanted to be seen as a regional health care provider, whereas in the past it had focused on promoting its four individual Chicago-area hospitals (Levy, 2011). Hospital for Special Care in New Britain, Connecticut, made a strategic decision to gain national recognition as a long-term acute care hospital by developing an integrative campaign that focused on five specialty practices (Ricci, 2011).

When planning marketing strategy it is important to ensure that that the offering matches a customer need; that the tactics chosen (using Facebook, mobile advertising, television, and so on) match the strategic goals; that proper incentives are offered to the sales force; and that the marketing department works together with other areas of the organization and outside partners if applicable (Topin, 2011).

There are also ethical questions related to health care marketing that must be taken into consideration when developing marketing strategy. Due to the nature of health care, some argue that it is inappropriate to market health care in the same way that other consumer products are marketed. However, if marketing functions as a way for the health care organization to communicate about the various services it offers, it can be ethical and appropriate (Nelson & Campfield, 2008). Health care marketers must consider the ethical standards of the American Marketing Association (AMA), the American College of Healthcare Executives (ACHE), and the American College of Physicians (ACP). According to the AMA ("About AMA," 2008):

As Marketers, we must:

1. *Do no harm.* This means consciously avoiding harmful actions or omissions by embodying high ethical standards and adhering to all applicable laws and regulations in the choices we make.

2. *Foster trust in the marketing system.* This means striving for good faith and fair dealing so as to contribute toward the efficacy of the exchange process as well as avoiding deception in product design, pricing, communication, and delivery of distribution.

3. *Embrace ethical values.* This means building relationships and enhancing consumer confidence in the integrity of marketing by affirming these core values: honesty, responsibility, fairness, respect, transparency and citizenship.

The ACHE *Code of Ethics* states that health care executives must "be truthful in all forms of professional and organizational communication, and avoid disseminating information that is false, misleading or deceptive" (*American College*, 2011). The ACP *Ethics Manual* states that "advertising by physicians or health care institutions is unethical when it contains statements that are unsubstantiated, false, deceptive, or misleading, including statements that mislead by omitting necessary information" (Snyder, 2012, p. 89). Nelson and Campfield (2008) suggest that marketers consider the following questions when designing a marketing campaign to ensure that the campaign meets ethical guidelines (pp. 44–45):

- Why is the marketing campaign being developed and potentially implemented?
- How does the service or activity being promoted address a community health need?
- Is the campaign fully truthful?
- Is it misleading?
- Is the marketing activity fiscally responsible?
- Does the tone of the marketing campaign fit the health care organization's image and standing in the community?

- If consumers know of the hospital only what they learn from the marketing campaign, are you OK with that?

Marketing strategy can be general, or it can be focused on specific aspects of the marketing mix. There are a number of different strategies available to marketers that vary in focus. One set of strategies involves identifying the market and the product (in the form of goods, services, or ideas). A *market penetration* strategy focuses on how to generate new business in an existing market for an existing product. An example of a market penetration strategy would be to encourage more women to get annual mammograms. A *market development* strategy focuses on developing a new market for an existing product. An example of a market development strategy would be to establish senior programs to recruit more seniors to join an existing health plan. A *product development* strategy focuses on developing new offerings for existing markets. An example of a new product development strategy would be to add wellness programs for current health plan members. A *diversification* strategy involves identifying a new market for a new product. For example, Hospital for Special Care plans to open a medical unit specially designed to meet the needs of the increasing number of patients with cardiac conditions (Ricci, 2011).

Looking beyond the strategies that focus on market *and* product, there are additional strategies available to marketers that focus primarily on the product. These strategies focus on the features and benefits of the product the organization offers. Options available include preemptive strategy, having a unique selling proposition, and positioning strategy. A preemptive strategy involves making statements about a product that a competitor is not likely to repeat to avoid being seen as an imitator. Such a strategy is appropriate if there are minimal differences between products. Having a unique selling proposition requires identifying product benefits that are distinctly different from those offered by the competition. Finally, an organization pursuing a positioning strategy strives to create a positive position for the company's offerings in the consumer's mind. Effectively applying a positioning strategy requires an understanding of the organization's competitors and the marketplace and of how the organization is perceived in that marketplace relative to the competition. For example, Blue Cross and Blue Shield of Florida launched an integrated advertising campaign during Super Bowl XLV with the tagline "In the pursuit of health" to focus on health solutions and reposition the organization after discovering that consumers primarily perceived it as a health insurance provider, which was not how the organization wanted to be positioned (Chordas, 2011).

Another important consideration relative to strategy is developing a corporate identity or brand. Brand names represent the companies that produce the products or services, and they help the consumer differentiate between similar product offerings. Establishing a brand identity is critical for all businesses, including health care organizations. For example, a strategic consideration for Blue Cross Blue Shield of Michigan during its 2008 campaign to motivate people to pursue positive lifestyles was to ensure that the Blue Cross Blue Shield brand was an important part of all marketing communication. The organization thus included a mock Blue Cross Blue Shield membership card in all of its advertisements (Riedman, 2008). City of Hope developed a successful brand campaign using the tagline "Canswer," which was based on the idea that people facing cancer diagnoses want answers. This campaign, designed to help City of Hope strengthen its national brand in cancer treatment and become a leader in cancer care in Southern California, resulted in higher volumes of patients over five years (Maceo, 2011).

USING MARKETING RESEARCH IN HEALTH CARE DELIVERY

Conducting **marketing research** involves the "planning, collection and analysis of data relevant to marketing decision making and the communication of the results of this analysis to management" (McDaniel & Gates, 2004, p. 14). Marketing research can be used in a variety of ways to help managers make important decisions related to health care delivery. Data can be obtained from patients, employees, shareholders, donors, patients' family members, or other stakeholders in the organization (Ricci, 2011). Today's health care industry is increasingly market driven, and the market for health services is more diverse. Health care providers should therefore use marketing research both to identify segments or niches of potential customers and to help deliver services to meet the needs of those identified niches (Thomas, 2005). Marketing research can be used to evaluate the effectiveness of a marketing campaign during the campaign development process and after a campaign has been launched, as Virginia Commonwealth University Medical Center did using consumer surveys during its "Every Day, A New Discovery Red Letter Day" campaign (Igaray & MacCracken, 2011). Marketing research can also gauge customer satisfaction and monitor customer feedback by measuring the relationship between customer satisfaction and physician skill. Physician skill can be measured by asking questions related to patient expectations about what a physician should do. These could include survey items pertaining to patient-physician interactions; clinical competency; and the management of system factors, such as teamwork, and the care management process (Gombeski, Rudy, Springate, & DePriest, 2010).

Marketing research in a health care context could be used to help evaluate the quality of services, to analyze competitive offerings, to determine locations for services delivery, to determine market demand and characteristics, to identify the types of services to offer, or to evaluate patient satisfaction (Thomas, 2005).

Step One: Problem Recognition

Problem recognition is the crucial first step in the marketing research process. Problems must be clearly defined to generate meaningful data when the research process is complete. Marketing research may be conducted to explore opportunities or identify existing problems. Problems can be related to the launching of new products or services or to issues arising from current products and services.

Step Two: Identification of Research Objectives

Once the problem is defined or the issues are identified, the researcher must determine what the objectives of the study should be. These objectives should be based on what the researcher wants to learn about the problem. They help determine the design of the research.

Once the objectives are identified, a decision needs to be made about what type of study to conduct. There are four main types of research, which have different goals and will provide the researcher with different outcomes. *Exploratory research* is conducted to further understand the nature of a problem or to help define a problem more narrowly. *Descriptive research* offers a snapshot of the situation to be studied and provides details without attempting to explain why the situation is occurring. *Causal research* does attempt to explain why a situation is happening and strives to identify important variables that are having an impact on a situation. *Predictive research* attempts to forecast what might happen in the future. The decision about what type of research to conduct will depend on the nature of the research problem as well as time and cost considerations.

Step Three: Research Design

Once the problems and objectives have been identified, the next step is to develop a plan that outlines what data will be collected, where and how the data will be collected, how the data will be analyzed and interpreted, and how the results will be presented. Important considerations in determining the research design will be access to data, the time involved in collecting the data, the availability of resources to analyze the data, and staff time and availability.

There are two main types of data used in marketing research. *Primary data* are collected for and designed by the researcher. These data are specifically tailored to help investigate the defined research problem, and the confidentiality of these data can be preserved. However, there are some limitations associated with primary data, as these can be timely and costly to collect and analyze. *Secondary data* constitute information, usually collected by someone other than the researcher, that has been gathered to address another research problem. These data can include publicly available information, such as government reports; internally produced information; U.S. Census data; and commercially available research. On the positive side, secondary data can be relatively inexpensive to obtain and involve significantly less time to collect than primary data, and secondary data can be more objective, especially if a third party produced them. On the negative side, the data available may not exactly provide what is necessary to solve the research problem, may be out of date, and may not be reliable. Overall, though, secondary data can be helpful in the early stages of a research project to help further define the research problem.

Step Four: Data Collection

There are a variety of methods available to researchers who want to collect primary data: observational research, experimental research, and survey research. *Observational research* provides information about individuals by employing other individuals or mechanical devices, such as cameras or monitoring devices, to observe behavior. *Experimental research* requires the researcher to manipulate key factors to determine a causal relationship between those factors. This type of research allows the researcher to evaluate the effects of one variable on another variable of interest. Although true experiments are difficult to conduct in nonacademic settings, quasi-experimental designs can be used in marketing contexts. A quasi-experimental design might include, for example, using different information (such as phone numbers, codes, and Web addresses) in different versions of advertisements and measuring response rates to the different versions used. *Survey research* is one of the most common methods for obtaining primary data. Surveys can be administered as telephone interviews, personal interviews, online or in-person focus groups, mail questionnaires, or online questionnaires. Designing the survey instrument is a crucial step in collecting data that are helpful and relevant for solving the identified problem. Researchers must give thought to the survey instructions, the types of questions asked, the wording of the questions, the order of the questions on the instrument, and the length of the instrument. Surveys have often been used in health care to determine what factors consumers believe to be important when evaluating health care options and to gauge patient satisfaction (Steblea et al., 2009). A concern when designing surveys is obtaining meaningful data, and one approach is to ask patients for verbatim comments about their experiences on satisfaction surveys so researchers can better understand the each patient's situation (Segbers, 2010). Another useful approach may be to use conjoint analysis to determine consumer preferences (Steblea et al.). The goal of conjoint analysis is to assess the sacrifices and trade-offs that consumers make in reaching a decision. It involves creating a list of paired attributes that you want to test against each other. For a hospital, important attributes might include location (located in your town or located in your region), physicians (exceptional or average), technology (state of the art or average), personal care (exceptional or average), or hospital reputation (exceptional or average). Respondents are asked to complete a series of questions that require them to make choices between the paired attributes until they ultimately select one option, which helps the organization assess which attributes seem to be the most relevant for selecting a hospital.

Step Five: Analysis and Reporting of Results

Once the data are collected, they need to be analyzed and interpreted. Data require coding, a process that may necessitate the training of staff members. Once the data are coded, and if quantitative data have been collected, the next step may involve using statistical techniques to interpret the data in a meaningful way. Qualitative data also need to be analyzed for trends and insights. Once the data are analyzed, a report needs to be created that summarizes the problem, the research objectives, the research design, and how data were collected. This report should also show the results of data collection. Reports may be prepared in a written format, be presented to key stakeholders in the organization, or both.

Once the report is complete, it is important to use research findings to learn about and connect with the target audience. For example, Kaiser Permanente does this to learn about what matters to patients:

> [Kaiser Permanente's] research indicated that, while people had negative impressions of health care as being an impersonal bureaucracy, they had positive associations with their own doctors and being healthy. This led to some new brand positioning: "We stand for Total Health. Kaiser Permanente's integrated health care delivery system and commitment to preventive care empower our members to maximize their Total Health—mind, body and spirit." (Lofgren & Cantu, 2010, p. 10)

It is also important to follow up on negative experiences and share results with patient ambassadors, patient advocates, and media and community relations departments to deal effectively with any negative findings and also to take advantage of potential opportunities (Segbers, 2010). For example, Centra State Health Care in New Jersey found through research that consumers rated the organization as not meeting expectations in terms of technology. In response, Centra State Health Care identified and proceeded with marketing a new robotics technology ahead of its six direct competitors, helping this organization establish a competitive advantage in technology (Mackesy & Zupa, 2011).

See Table 11.3 for an example of how the marketing research process can be applied to help identify potential segments.

Table 11.3   Application of the Marketing Research Process

Step of the Process	Tasks to Be Performed
Step One: Problem recognition	Ask, "Are there potential segments of our customer base that we could be reaching more effectively?"
Step Two: Identification of research objectives	Identify and evaluate our customer base in terms of key factors (demographic information, services used, frequency of visits, and so on). Assess the wants and needs of our customer base in regard to health services. Assess customer perceptions of current health care offerings.
Step Three: Research design	Develop a survey for existing customers to assess their needs and perceptions of current health care offerings. Analyze existing customer data for trends. Determine the time frame for the implementation of the study. Identify resources needed to complete the study (in terms of people, technology, time, and costs).
Step Four: Data collection	Distribute the survey via e-mail, during patient visits, and by mail. Extract key information from existing customer records.
Step Five: Analysis and reporting of results	Tabulate survey responses. Prepare a report of key trends identified from existing customer records.

EMERGING TRENDS IN HEALTH CARE MARKETING

In today's era of evolving health care reform, gaining and building patient loyalty are high on marketing priority lists. It is therefore essential for marketers to focus on three key objectives: (1) retaining existing patients by focusing on the overall patient experience, (2) attracting new insured patients by trying to establish a competitive advantage, and (3) drawing patients away from other providers by emphasizing the patient experience and developing expertise (Weiss, 2010; Yakubik, 2011). Marketing budgets, especially in the pharmaceutical industry, have been under tremendous scrutiny in recent years, and the challenge remains of how to reach the thirty-two million previously uninsured consumers whose coverage is now mandated by health care reform. Health care organizations want to know where to spend their marketing dollars and how to maximize their return on investment. There is also a need to continuously monitor patient feedback and measure patient satisfaction; a need to think more strategically, focus more narrowly, and target marketing communication; as well as a need to find imaginative ways to extend the corporate brand (Weiss, 2010). One option, especially for pharmaceutical companies but also for any company for which there are differences in market share across different areas of the country, is to consider regional rather than national marketing to address the differences in population, physicians, providers (managed care organizations, hospitals, and clinics), competitors, and payers (government payers, employers, or individuals) (Spanbauer, 2010).

Technology is changing how health care is delivered, how consumers learn about health care, and how health care is marketed. Being a leader in using marketing technology is a competitive advantage that allows a health care organization to differentiate itself from its competitors. Marketing dollars are increasingly being shifted away from traditional approaches and toward digital approaches (Weiss, 2010). According to Mickelberg (2010), with "the rise of 'ambient healthcare' . . . the organized implementation of the myriad digital, mobile and social tools available to us . . . we now have the real prospect of taking control and engineering an environment that actually fosters health" (p. 31). Successful ambient campaigns will have messages that "fit not just the consumer, but also the context in which the consumer encounters the message" (Reyburn, 2010, p. 10).

Technology-related opportunities in health care marketing include developing mobile health content and apps; using social network sites and other new media, such as YouTube; communicating over the Internet through e-mail, online forums, online videos, podcasts, and blogs; developing healthy gaming software that can promote healthy lifestyles, such as Wii Fit; or creating Web sites that allow for patient feedback (Fell, 2009; Renfrow, 2009; Rooney, 2009).

Mobile marketing is providing a new way for health care providers and patients to communicate, facilitating conversations and enabling the sharing of information between providers and patients and also between patients and their peers (Mickelberg, 2010). People are using their mobile devices to access instant information and to make decisions about health care (Anderson & Albritton, 2011). For example, Blue Cross and Blue Shield of North Carolina has developed an app for the iPhone called HealthNAV that provides information to consumers. This includes a DrugFinder, which offers discounts on prescription drugs, and an Urgent Care Finder. It also allows users to record notes related to their health care (Anderson & Albritton, 2011).

Health care organizations are becoming increasingly social media savvy and are trying to establish a social media presence and monitor social media activity for consumer feedback (Roberts, 2010). There is a growing need to communicate with customers where they are and to engage them in conversation through social media (Weiss, 2010). Each of the many options available has distinct features. Blogs provide an opportunity to reach out to the general community or to specific populations; microblogs, such as Twitter, can be helpful in emergency situations; social network sites, such as Facebook, can be effective for interacting with consumers with specific conditions or diseases; and podcasts or videocasts can help educate consumers and provide information (Beach Thielst, 2011). Using social media is a way for health care providers to be more transparent and to actively engage their patients and the community (Beach Thielst). For example, the Henry Ford

Health System ran a campaign to boost mammograms by encouraging Facebook users to remind their friends online to schedule a mammogram; the organization also created a blog about medical issues. Aetna established a national social networking platform for employers that allows their employees to access online information, schedule exercise sessions, and participate in competitions. The Humana Innovation Center in Louisville, Kentucky, created a fitness program called Twit2Fit, which uses Twitter "to provide support and encouragement to Twit2Fit members in need of physical and emotional support" (Chordas, 2010, p. 96; Glenn, 2010). Finally, Vanderbilt University Health Center used Twitter to promote awareness about its new location and to inform potential customers about the new location's improved security (Austin & Wilson, 2011).

As increasing numbers of consumers have access to the Internet, establishing a strong online presence is critical for health care organizations. For example, Adventist Midwest Health partnered with the Chicago Tribune to create a Web portal called Keeping Chicago Well (www.keepingchicagowell. com), which includes content that is written by physicians and driven by consumer input, in an effort by these organizations to position themselves as local health care authorities. Similarly, Harvard Pilgrim Healthcare in Maine, Massachusetts, and New Hampshire launched a Web site that allows consumers to share information about healthy living (Chordas, 2010; Levy, 2011).

SUMMARY

This chapter provided an introduction to key concepts and ideas related to marketing. Creating a marketing strategy requires an understanding of what the product or service is, how it will be promoted, where it will be delivered or offered, how it will be priced, and to whom it will be targeted. A health care organization may need to conduct marketing research before offering a new service, or to understand the nature of a current problem. Marketing research can help managers design strategies to address identified concerns. Understanding the different aspects of marketing research can help managers more effectively handle any issues and concerns the organization may face. Health care managers must continue to monitor the environment to adapt to changes in regulations, technology, and consumer behavior.

KEY TERMS

health care marketing

market segmentation

marketing

marketing research

marketing strategy

target market

REVIEW QUESTIONS

1. Apply the concepts of the marketing mix to the following types of health care organizations: hospitals, private practices, and HMOs. What are the key similarities and differences in the marketing mix for these organizations?

2. Find a recent example of a health care advertisement. Analyze its effectiveness in terms of the copy, the use of visuals, its ability to reach the target market, and the appropriateness of its media placement.

3. What ethical issues can you identify related to health care marketing, and how could you overcome each issue when designing your marketing strategy?

4. Suppose you wanted to evaluate the quality of services offered by your health care facility. Outline how you would study the problem using the steps of the marketing research process.

5. Which emerging trend related to health care marketing do you think is the most critical for health care managers to understand? Why?

6. What role do you think technology will play in the future for health care marketers, and why is technology increasingly becoming a critical component of health care marketing? What role do you think social media should play in the health care industry?

12

Financial Management
Show Me the Money

Mark H. DeStefano

LEARNING OBJECTIVES

- Acknowledge that a health care organization must leverage sound business principles to remain a going concern

- Understand government policies and initiatives that were designed to stimulate and later control health care system growth after World War II

- Know the history of public and private sector health insurance and their impact on the growth of the health care industry

- Become aware of health insurance cost containment and reform measures designed to reduce the growth in premium increases and improve access

- Be able to explain specific financial management and funding challenges affecting health care facilities

- Understand proposed measures designed to create efficiencies and enhanced quality in the health care system

Most Americans would probably assert that the primary goals of our health care system are to provide access, affordable and quality care, and the best possible outcomes for patients. However, health care is a business and, quite frankly, a big business. For a business to remain a going concern in the long run, it must do more than simply sustain current operations. The business and its leaders must establish a clear vision and mission; objectively measure progress and benchmark on a continuous basis; and leverage competitive advantages through reinvestments in its infrastructure, the latest technology, and, perhaps most important, its people. Only then may the business position itself for more than just survival in a competitive environment; and it really positions itself for future growth by effectively deploying sound business principles while delivering products or services that consistently meet or exceed consumer expectations.

In health care, the "profit motive" often creates a conflict when an organization and its administration are faced with balancing money and mission. Change appears to be the one constant, and gone are the days of maintaining the status quo and operating in a stoic, inflexible, and overly structured fashion. Fierce competition, scarce resources, tightened debt markets, and pressures from government and third-party payers to contain costs through less generous reimbursements and managed medical consumption coexist in an environment rife with rapid technological advancements and higher patient expectations. This market dynamic has influenced health care organizations to become more efficient and nimble, and to adopt a practical approach to disciplined fiscal management. In addition, competitive pressures and a requirement to eliminate unnecessary expenses and inefficiencies have prompted organizations to undergo continuous evolution to avoid extinction.

We have moved beyond the Baby Boomer Industrial Age into the Information Age, and health care organizations must embrace a culture that regularly challenges the entire health care team, embraces consumer activism, and strives for continuous reinvention. Technology is incorporated not only as a differentiator and a growth engine but also as an important basic element of everyday business operations. In health care, open leadership skills that leverage strong communication and relationship building among stakeholders will be a driving force for coordinating quality care and better positioning an organization for future growth and sustainability. Stakeholders ranging from physicians to nonclinical support staff to patients must be engaged to help shift the dynamics of the provider structure toward accountable care. **Consumerism** encourages individuals to be more active in and accountable for their health care management. Passing accountability and the associated economic impact from health care providers and third-party payers to consumers has the potential to promote the efficient use of the health care system and reduce total health care costs.

OUR HEALTH CARE SYSTEM: WHAT WE FUND

Health care organizations are either public or private entities. Public health care organizations are concerned with the well-being of communities and populations, and private health care organizations are concerned with individual consumers of goods and services. The U.S. health care system and its health care organizations are complex and involve a number of competing interests that drive demand, access, costs, quality, and outcomes.

Health care enterprises, which encompass providers including primary care and specialized physician offices, outpatient and urgent care facilities, and hospitals, are organized either horizontally or vertically. As the names suggest, horizontally structured health care enterprises combine entities with like characteristics, such as hospitals or physician offices, and vertically integrated health care enterprises combine entities with different functionalities, such as hospitals, physician groups, and nursing homes. In the case of vertical integration, the output of one entity is often the input of another based on patient flow and derived demand created by the treating physician or physicians. Health care enterprises may be formed via ownership, affiliation, joint ventures, on a contractual basis, on a leased basis, or through a combination of various structural options.

Financing and third-party and government payers have influenced the expansion of the U.S. health care system by providing access to the system and paying for the costs associated with movement through the system. Individuals with access to care are grouped into various segments, which include middle-class, poor, entitled, and military and VA groups. Members of the middle class are generally employed and either receive insurance through employers or purchase individual policies. The poor may or may not have access to care depending on their state's poverty-level benchmark. The poor who meet their state poverty-level benchmark may have access to **Medicaid** or public welfare insurance, whereas the working poor who do not meet state criteria may not have access to Medicaid or be able to afford to purchase individual health insurance. Medicaid does not provide a system of coordinated, comprehensive care, but is typically used by its participants who are responding to acute illness rather than focusing on prevention. Despite its shortfall in stimulating preventative and integrated care, Medicaid does offer a safety net and access to providers for the working poor. Members of the entitled class, which mainly comprises retired individuals age sixty-five and older, have access to **Medicare.** The military system tends to be proactive in nature, with medical testing and evaluation upon entry, promotion, and exit. Finally, the VA system provides access to distinct members of the population who have served in the military, and these facilities primarily focus on chronic illnesses, drug and alcohol dependency, and other mental health issues. Charity care may be provided to those individuals among the forty-five million uninsured who have no access to health insurance. It is important to note that these sources of health care, which have expanded due to increased financing over the years, often compete for a finite pool of federal and state health care dollars.

With these various entities in the U.S. health care system come benefits and challenges. As a benefit, access to health care is broadly available to middle-class, poor, and elderly individuals as well as to those who have served in the military. In many cases this access is provided at a nominal cost to the insured, particularly in the managed care models, which do not entail high-deductible plans. Accordingly, health services may be consumed without the barrier of prohibitive cost. Furthermore, patients who are engaged in the management of their health may receive coordinated and comprehensive diagnostic testing or other innovative procedures to detect a specific disease from physicians who are thorough in the delivery of care.

Paradoxically, however, these benefits also lead to challenges. Many consumers of health services have no incentive to concern themselves with the cost and quantity of the services they consume, which leads to the absorption of scarce economic and health care human resources. In addition, the health care consumer is often not the direct purchaser of the insurance and may only be contributing to a small percentage of the overall cost of the coverage. Providers also create demand and to a degree practice defensive medicine in our litigious society. These represent fundamental root challenges to an already fragmented health care system.

The health care system in the United States, which is complex and often disjointed, is influenced by strong lobbying groups and financed by both the public and private sectors. In general, we finance movements through the system of health care delivery. These movements comprise inputs, or those actually providing the health services; throughputs, or elements relating to the management of the health care system; and outputs, which should encompass good health and positive outcomes relative to illness. In a perfect economy, the role of policy should be to influence the latter goal: to improve the quality of life and enhance health outcomes; however, conflicts among concentrated interests often generate inefficiencies and stymie change in regard to the financing of our health care system.

As our government's tolerance for leaving forty-five million Americans uninsured has waned—and in light of public outcry due to the robust increases in the cost of medical insurance and health care delivery, a Medicare trust fund driven to the brink of bankruptcy by medical inflation— significant increases in the cost of health care—compounded by an aging baby boomer population, and an economic recession that has decreased tax revenues while causing Medicaid rosters to swell—health care reform has taken priority on the Obama administration's agenda. As the government evaluates and moves toward universal care, the up-front financing challenges and the anticipated resource shortages inherent in expanded health care coverage and any related proactive programs and services continue to take center stage in the reform debate.

THE COST OF HEALTH CARE, AND HISTORICAL AND PROJECTED NATIONAL SPENDING

In any competitive marketplace, consumers demand instant access to information and responsive service. That access is generally available within most industries, except in the health care arena. Despite immediate short-term patient goals of access and cure, primary longer-term goals in health care, which might sound simplistic, must include influencing healthy behaviors, reducing high-risk behaviors, and facilitating improved outcomes at a reasonable cost. However, the health care sector has failed to achieve these goals, in part due to inefficiencies created by government regulation and intervention, special interests, and often conflicting third-party-payer interests. There is arguably a price to progress and technological advancements, which have been significant cost drivers. This price to progress, along with enhanced patient expectations in a resource-starved health care system, may often conflict with the goals of providing valuable and affordable, quality services.

Quantitative data provide insight into chronic diseases, which continue to escalate at epidemic proportions and which represent a key driver of the expanding volume of procedures and serious problems facing health care delivery in the United States. Statistical information demonstrates that mortality rates improved materially over the course of the twentieth century, with a crude mortality rate at the beginning of the twentieth century of approximately 1,700 deaths per 100,000 people, with a life expectancy of forty-seven, versus 854 deaths per 100,000 people by the year 2000, with a life expectancy of seventy-seven (Turnock, 2009). This mortality reduction on both a crude and adjusted rate basis has been the result of such enhancements as improved environmental factors, advancements in medicine and medical technology, and access to quality health care. Public health initiatives have also contributed to improved health levels by facilitating activities ranging from the promotion of immunization against contagious diseases to education efforts and early prevention and screening programs. Clearly the improvement in health care, technology, and nutrition as well as other measures have increased longevity. As the data suggest, people in the United

States are living longer than they did a century ago, and this increase in life span continues to have an impact as complications from chronic illnesses compound costs and strain our health care system.

In 2009 $2.5 trillion was spent on health care. More than 50 percent of those dollars went to hospital and physician care; 10 percent went to prescription drugs; and only 3 percent went to government public health initiatives, which include education and prevention programs. Figure 12.1, which reveals data tabulated by the Centers for Medicare & Medicaid Services, provides a look at health care spending by various sectors.

The cost of our health care system and the amount spent each year on health care are difficult for the typical American to fathom. The attempts to decrease or even control costs over the years have ultimately failed. Furthermore, the financiers of these expenditures, mainly government and third-party payers, have historically reimbursed and incentivized health care

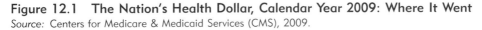

Figure 12.1   The Nation's Health Dollar, Calendar Year 2009: Where It Went
Source: Centers for Medicare & Medicaid Services (CMS), 2009.

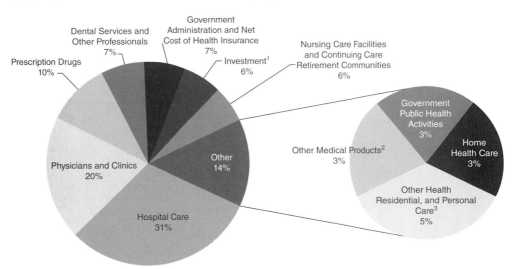

[1]Includes research (2%) and structures and equipment (4%).
[2]Includes durable (1%) and nondurable (2%) goods.
[3]Includes expenditures for residential care facilities; ambulance providers; medical care delivered in nontraditional settings (such as community centers, senior citizens centers, schools, and military field stations); and expenditures for Home and Community-Based Waiver programs under Medicaid.
Note: Sum of pieces may not equal 100% due to rounding.

organizations based on the volume and types of curative procedures rather than on proactive and preventative measures and outcomes. The explosive growth in health expenditures in this country has been driven by these same government and third-party payers. As the cost of health care continues to rise, along with the cost of accessing quality health insurance, it is clear that there needs to be a new focus on alternative ways to engage individuals in managing their own health, to promote appropriate and efficient use of medical services, and to encourage healthy behaviors. As medical inflation; inefficient use of the health care system; and sophisticated, state-of-the-art technological advancements continue to drive up the costs associated with health services, opportunities have arisen to reinforce the importance of healthy behaviors and to seek new ways to manage the health care system. As described earlier, only 3 percent of the $2.5 trillion in 2009 health care spending has been directed toward public health activities—at a time when we must invest in education and prevention to reduce high-risk behaviors and help "bend the cost trend" in our health care system.

Total health care spending represents a substantial expenditure category in the federal budget, second only to defense. Figure 12.2 provides a look at annual federal spending budget categories, with health expenditures totaling 23 percent of the federal budget in 2011.

Figure 12.2   U.S. Federal Expenditure, 2011: $3,819 Billion
Source: Chantrill, 2011a.

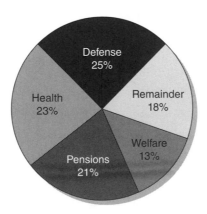

Health expenditures have increased dramatically over the past fifty years. The general trend of increased total health expenditures is projected to continue into the foreseeable future (Chantrill, 2011b).

Health care spending in 2006 totaled 16 percent of GDP (Marmor, Oberlander, & White, 2009). However, in 2009, for the first time in fifty years, the rate of spending slowed to an annual increase of 4 percent, versus 4.7 percent in 2008. The impact of a severe and lengthy recession and high unemployment contributed to a reduction in this year-over-year increase. Still, health care spending as a percentage of GDP rose to 17.6 percent in 2009, a full percentage point increase from 2008 and the largest one-year increase on record. The United States, including government and nongovernment spenders, had dedicated one-sixth of its available financial resources to health care by the end of 2009 ("Growth of Spending," 2011). More alarming is the projection by the Congressional Budget Office that by 2035, national health expenditures will total 26 percent of GDP ("CBO Projects," 2010).

Marmor et al. (2009) argue that seeking to control health care costs in this country has been an unattainable goal for the government and the health care industry. Clearly, a variety of controlling interests would vigorously lobby against any reduction in health expenses that would amount to a reduction in health care industry income for one or more system inputs. Marmor et al. note that although cost containment is a goal of reform, under any of the possible reform measures the federal government will increase costs in the short term with an expansion of the State Children's Health Insurance program, broad economic stimulus packages that fund insurance for the increased number of individuals who are unemployed, and possible investments in health information technology. Figure 12.3 displays the increased trend in national health expenditures as a percentage of GDP from approximately 5 percent in 1960 to nearly 18 percent in 2009.

Health care is funded by individuals, employers, and federal and state governments. Private spending generally represents out-of-pocket co-pays and private sector insurance. The ratio of private sector versus public sector insurance spending decreased after 1965, largely due to an expansion of federal government spending associated with Medicare and Medicaid pro-

Figure 12.3   Increased Trend in National Health Expenditures (NHE) as a Percentage of GDP
Source: Baker, 2011.

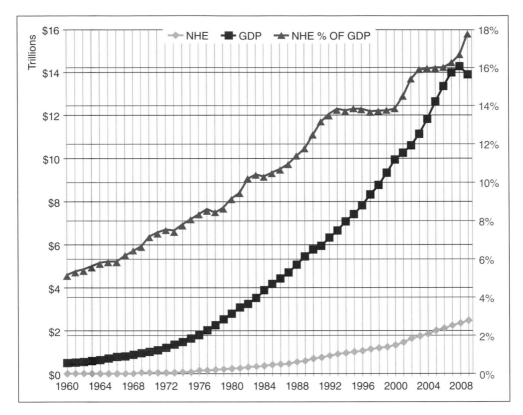

grams. Figure 12.4 displays the relationship among private and government spending sources as a percentage of total national health care spending.

High total health care spending does not guarantee favorable outcomes, largely due to high administrative expenses inherent in the private sector, inefficiencies, and other waste within the health care system—and due to differing individual health levels and the impact of genetics and the environment. Notle and McKee (2008) reinforce that although the United States spends more than any other country on health care, forty-five million Americans have no health care coverage and infant mortality is comparatively higher than for other industrialized nations. Fuchs (2010) also emphasizes

Figure 12.4   Private and Government Health Care Spending
Source: Baker, 2011.

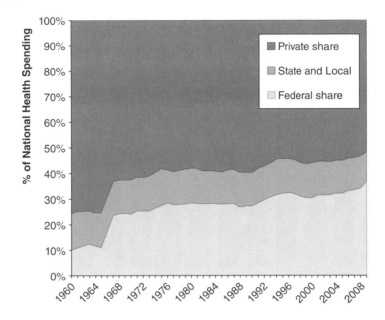

the dramatic increase in federal and state governments' share of personal health expenditures, from more than 20 percent in 1960 to approximately 45 percent in 2007. The gap between what the United States spends on health care versus the expenditures of the next-highest spender is substantial: the United State spends 50 percent more for heath care than the next-highest spender. In fact, we spend twice as much on health care as the average country in the Organisation for Economic Co-operation and Development (OECD), according to Fuchs (2010). Figure 12.5 compares the United States' $7,538 in per capita health care spending with the expenditures of other select countries.

As shown in Figure 12.6, the United States has also widely outpaced other selected countries in terms of the growth in health expenditures.

Based on current trends, health care spending is expected to increase to approximately $4 trillion by 2015, excluding any economic impact of reform or other measures to bend or flatten the trend line. Even one-time savings and any new cost containment measures over the period may only slightly

Figure 12.5 Total Health Expenditures per Capita, United States and Selected Countries, 2008

Source: Organisation for Economic Co-operation and Development (OECD), 2010, as cited in Kaiser Family Foundation (KFF), 2011.

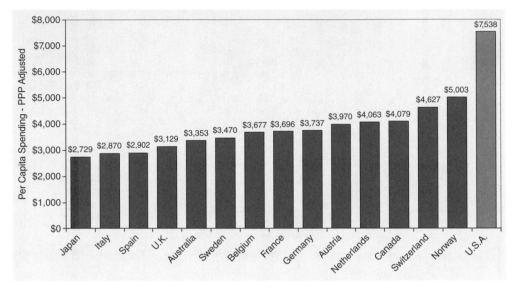

Note: Data from Australia and Japan are from 2007. Figures for Belgium, Canada, the Netherlands, Norway, and Switzerland are OECD estimates.

reduce total health care spending. Figure 12.7 demonstrates an anticipated trend in national health expenditures over a ten-year period from 2005 through 2015. The chart assumes three scenarios: status quo or baseline, a trend based on the current health care system; one-time savings, which theoretically could occur as a result of a shift to a government-run, single-payer plan with immediate, up-front savings due to a reduction in administrative expenses; and additional cost containment or other measures designed to slow the trend by creating efficiencies, improving the quality of care and outcomes, and enhancing health levels (Fuchs, 2009).

As explained previously, America spends, on average, twice as much as other industrialized nations on health care, but it does not have outcomes twice as good. As the trends suggest, the current system cannot continue to bear the financial burden of health care financing and delivery. Medical inflation, more elderly individuals, and an increased volume of chronic diseases all add to the rampant costs (Pettingill, 2009). Fuchs and Emanuel

Figure 12.6   Growth in Total Health Expenditures per Capita, United States and Selected Countries, 1970–2008
Source: OECD, 2010, as cited in KFF, 2011.

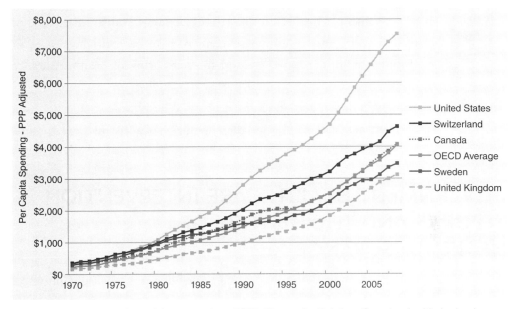

Note: Data from Australia and Japan are from 2007. Figures for Belgium, Canada, the Netherlands, Norway, and Switzerland are OECD estimates.

Figure 12.7   Growth in National Health Expenditures Under Various Scenarios
Source: Source data from Borger et al., 2006, as cited in Davis et al., 2007, p. 11.

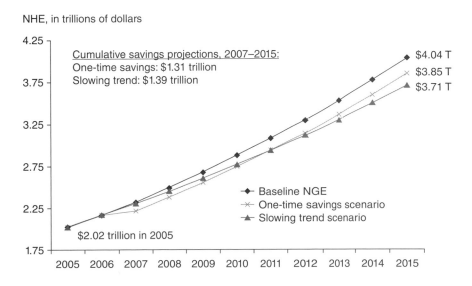

(2005) refer to the large number of uninsured Americans, rapidly rising health expenditures, and significant medical inflation rates—along with inefficiencies including excessive administrative costs and medical errors—as the "palpable symptoms of our 'sick health care system'" (p. 1399). The American values of equality of opportunity combined with the exercise of personal freedom and consumer sovereignty have been driving forces in determining health care coverage and the purchasing of health insurance and health services. In a capitalist society those values are paramount, and accordingly in the United States the delivery of health care should be based on sound economic principles and the assumption of a free market economy.

GOVERNMENT HEALTH CARE INTERVENTION EFFORTS AND THE HISTORY OF HEALTH INSURANCE

For decades the topic of health care reform—and more specifically "universal coverage," the most commonly advocated form of which is single-payer national health insurance—has been a public health policy issue heatedly debated from Main Street America to Pennsylvania Avenue. As far back as 1945, Harry S. Truman began promoting national health insurance for all Americans shortly after assuming the presidency. President John F. Kennedy also made health care for social security beneficiaries a priority during his administration, and finally President Lyndon B. Johnson signed Medicare into law on June 30, 1965, with Truman at his side at the Truman Presidential Library (Cutler, 2010). Still, significant changes in the financing and delivery of health care, and in levels of access to health care, have not yet occurred, and the cost of health care continues to escalate at rates significantly greater than inflation. In the latter half of the last century, per capita health care spending in the United States increased sixfold while national out-of-pocket expenses for consumers fell by 50 percent (Finkelstein, 2007).

Government policy and intervention as well as public and private sector health insurance have facilitated the dramatic growth of the existing health care infrastructure and the services available as well as the rapid construction and establishment of new health care organizations. A historical look at the roots of third-party payer and government funding sources provides an important perspective on the broad impact that health policy, market forces, and insurance have had on the expansion of the health care industry and the related expenditures in the United States. A review of the public sector health care financing and intervention mechanisms will be presented first.

As Moran (2005) describes, the U.S. government focused on expanding the health care infrastructure by stimulating the growth of health care facilities and services after World War II. The **Hill-Burton Act** of 1946 provided a commitment by the federal government to the renovation of existing hospitals and the construction of new facilities. The **Health Professionals Education Act** of 1963 committed resources to expand the supply of professional services. The stimulus probably exceeded the government's growth expectations. By the early 1970s Congress created Professional Standards Review Organizations through the 1972 Social Security Amendments, and by 1974 Congress mandated the use of **certificates of need** for new health care facilities to constrain the growth in health services and infrastructure expansion (Moran, 2005).

While intervention was rapidly stimulating facility and health services supply as just described, the government also began providing insurance to its federal employees in the 1950s. Also, the **Kerr-Mills Act** of 1960 formalized the practice of financing health care for welfare recipients. The adoption of Medicare and Medicaid in 1965 created a government payer as the primary health care financier in the United States, with the government making generous payments for hospital visits and physician services (Moran, 2005). This financing mechanism, which provided for the reimbursement of costs plus a markup, failed to create any incentive for the provider community to be efficient and cost effective, and in reality had the reverse effect of rewarding institutions with higher cost structures and service volumes.

Finkelstein (2007) estimates based on her research that prior to the implementation of Medicare, only 25 percent of the elderly had private sector insurance from third-party payers like Blue Cross and Blue Shield. Upon the enactment of Medicare, however, 100 percent of the elderly had immediate and covered access to health care, which influenced broader use of the health care system. Despite the government's attempt to put the brakes on the stimulus created by the Hill-Burton Act, its expenditures for health care through its public sector Medicare and Medicaid insurance programs rose at a dramatic 10 to 20 percent annual rate in the 1970s, which in and of itself fueled expansion of the health care system (Moran, 2005).

Efforts to control supply proved futile. To contain rapidly growing health expenditures, the federal government in the 1990s implemented reimbursement fee schedules. Through tight provisions in the 1997 Balanced Budget Act, the implementation of comprehensive unit price controls actually produced for the short term a reduction in Medicare expenditures in the few years that followed. However, unit price controls are only part of the equation, and an inability to manage the volume of procedures and to effectively implement medical consumption and preventative measures have rendered us unable to contain costs in the long run (Moran, 2005). O'Neill and O'Neill (2007) note that although a strained Medicare trust fund now regulates provider fees, it has not attempted to control physicians' incomes, and under the current system providers may be incentivized to increase procedures to offset fee controls or even refuse to serve Medicare patients because of the current reimbursement fee schedules.

While government resources were flowing into the health care system, the private sector employers and third-party payers also began expanding their participation in fueling health care system growth. Fronstin (2001) explains that private sector, **employer-based health insurance** experienced substantial growth during World War II, after the National War Labor Board froze wages and businesses used health care benefits as a tool to retain existing employees and to recruit new hires in a tight labor market. Because labor unions supported these benefits and the National Labor War Board ruled that employer contributions to the cost of insurance were not considered wages, employer-based health insurance coverage tripled during the war (Weir, Orloff, & Skopal, 1988). In 1954 the Internal Revenue Code clarified both the exemption of employer-paid health care benefits from employee wages and the tax deductibility of these premium payments as a business expense (Fronstin, 2001). Although subsequent to World War II most industrialized nations provided some form of government-provided health care coverage, employment-based insurance provided by third-party payers became the most common form of health care coverage in the United States.

According to Moran (2005), during the 1970s and 1980s private plan sponsor strategies were based on economics. In 1974 the enactment of the **Employee Retirement Income Security Act (ERISA)** provided for the conversion of employer-sponsored health plans to self-funded plans, which were exempted from state regulation. Under this conversion strategy, healthier workers exited the fully funded group insurance segment, leaving a much riskier insured pool and driving up premiums for small employer group sponsors and individuals. Reforms designed in part to halt the erosion of the group insurance segment contributed to the enactment of the **Health Insurance Portability and Accountability Act (HIPAA)** of 1996 (Moran, 2005).

As health care costs and the respective health insurance premiums increased at double-digit rates during the 1980s, plan sponsors also leveraged an alternative approach to managing costs by moving their covered employees into managed care plans. According to Fronstin (2001), from 1992 to 1999 enrollment in traditional indemnity plans decreased from 52 percent to 11 percent, whereas enrollment in managed care plans increased from 48 percent to 89 percent. As a result of the transition to managed care, health care cost inflation decreased in the early years as measures for strict prospective medical consumption review and a required shift of certain types of care from costly inpatient facilities to outpatient environments were implemented. Prospective medical consumption review provides for evaluation and approval or disallowance of medical procedures in advance, whereas retrospective review provides for an evaluation after the care has been administered. The move toward managed care in the United States has not been without controversy. According to Fronstin (2001), members of managed care plans with gatekeepers that have the authority to approve or disallow medical procedures reported that they were 75 percent satisfied, as compared to 82.5 percent among members of other employer-based health plans.

Current trends in health car have migrated toward the concepts of **accountable care** and a patient-centered approach to preventative care and curative medical procedures, whereby individuals are charged with having an active role in influencing favorable outcomes. Not dissimilar to these former accountability approaches, consumer-directed plans that allow employees to customize their benefits and give them choice among plan designs have become more popular in the private sector. Accordingly, under this consumer-directed scenario the employee has choice and assumes an active role in designing a plan that fits his or her particular requirements. At the same time, employers continue to shift the health insurance cost burden from the business to the workforce by increasing employees' required contributions toward the cost of insurance premiums or by adopting high-deductible plans. Finally, some employers operating in our challenging economic climate with high unemployment may conclude that health care benefits are neither affordable at any price nor required to attract or retain employees.

CHARACTERISTICS OF HEALTH CARE FINANCE

Ever since World War II, health care financing has really been about the insurance mechanism, which has driven both supply and demand in the marketplace as resources poured into the health care system. Reimbursements based on volume rather than outcomes offered incentives for an increased number of procedures, and insured plan members typically lacked material incentives to ration services paid for by the government or a third-party payer. In addition, concentrated interests have preferred and benefited from the status quo, and have therefore spent significant financial and political capital to maintain the current system.

As previously discussed, the delivery of health care in the United States is supported by two main financing systems: third-party payers, whose insurance is primarily purchased by employers, and public sector insurance systems like Medicare and Medicaid, which support the aged and poor and are not employment based (Moran, 2005). These funding sources create most of the financing for health care, with 70 percent of the expenditures coming from government and third-party payer insurance. Figure 12.8 shows the originating sources of the money paid into the health care system.

Figure 12.8   The Nation's Health Dollar, Calendar Year 2009: Where It Came From
Source: CMS, 2009.

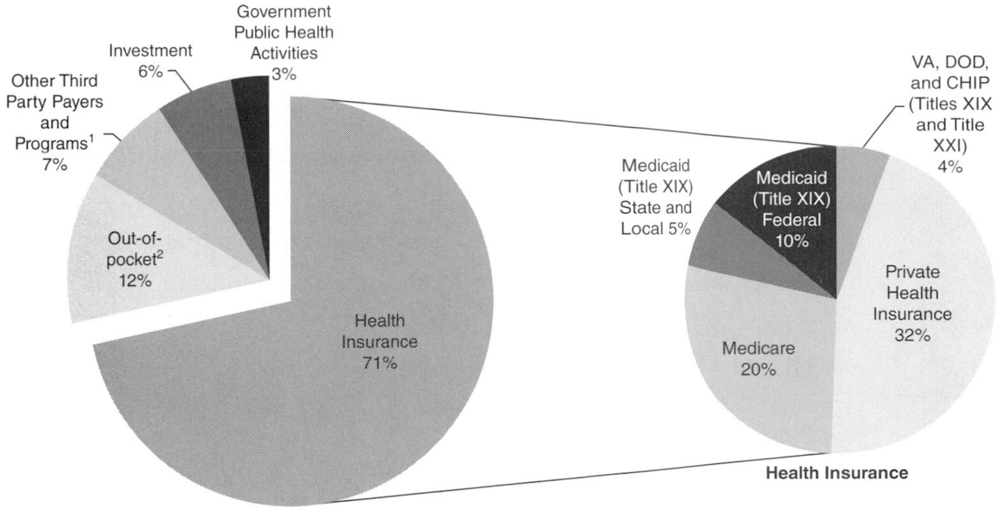

[1]Includes work site health care, other private revenues, the Indian Health Service, worker's compensation, general assistance, maternal and child health, vocational rehabilitation, the Substance Abuse and Mental Health Services Administration, school health, and other federal and state local programs.
[2]Includes co-pays, deductibles, and any amounts not covered by health insurance.
Note: Sum of pieces may not equal 100% due to rounding.

Organizations that deliver health services have engaged in an upstream approach, whereby issues are dealt with after they have happened, and providers have historically been paid and incentivized based on the volume and types of curative procedures rather than on proactive and preventative measures and outcomes. Accordingly, low access levels and high costs have become symptoms of the underlying problem with health care delivery in this country: poor health levels caused by practicing high-risk behaviors.

Government payment deficiencies in Medicare and Medicaid reimbursements, and inadequate procedural reimbursements from third-party payers, often lead to upcoding or gaming the system by the provider community, which has been rewarded based on the volume of procedures rather than the quality of care. Funding stream shortfalls over the past decade have placed additional pressure on providers to streamline operations. Furthermore, entrenched third-party payers with robust networks and significant membership are able to negotiate steep discounts while aggressively managing care, which has caused further funding pressures in the provider community.

Spirited discussion has ensued concerning the importance of preventative measures, personal accountability for health, and reimbursement approaches that reward outcomes rather than the volume of procedures. However, actions typically speak louder than words, and a commitment to fund or reimburse prevention efforts and outcomes must occur to incentivize the health care industry to focus more strongly on these important areas that have a potential to bend the cost trend by improving health levels in the long run.

The substantial increase in the cost of health care and the cost of insurance for those fortunate enough to have coverage; the inherent inefficiencies in a fragmented system of health care delivery; and a staggering number of uninsured Americans, estimated at one in six, have prompted heated and widespread debate. As a result Congress and the Obama administration charged ahead with the controversial passage of the Patient Protection and Affordable Care Act, which became law on March 23, 2010, and which was amended shortly thereafter by the Health Care and Education Reconciliation Act.

Reform measures emphasize a phasing in of changes in the health care system's financing arm, with sweeping modifications that will have an impact on third-party payers while expanding coverage to an estimated thirty-two million Americans by 2014. Health care reform establishes mandated health insurance while eliminating screening for preexisting conditions, removing annual and lifetime coverage limits, establishing a floor on medical loss ratios (medical care costs divided by insurance premium revenue), and creating health insurance exchanges designed to promote price competition and greater choice.

New, more effective solutions must be developed to address the mismatch of demand and supply in the current health care system. Chronic diseases are pervasive, and creating a more efficient, collaborative, and accountable approach to *managing* care in the current system requires unique leadership skill sets. Gone are the days of a single leader in charge of operational and administrative restructuring designed to create efficiencies and reduce expenses. A team approach to cost containment and operational efficiency may serve as a critical element in well-managed health care organizations, particularly given ongoing funding and reimbursement pressures.

Shifting the dynamics of the provider structure and "forcing" integration among the component parts of health care organizations, facilitating accountable care, and incorporating physician and support staff input and buy-in will provide the foundation for coordinated and quality care. Moving toward a coordinated and collaborative care environment is paramount for current stabilization and future sustained growth in the health care arena.

FINANCIAL CHALLENGES CONFRONTING PROVIDERS, THIRD-PARTY PAYERS, AND PATIENTS

As the cost of care continues to escalate at annual rates greater than inflation, third-party payers struggle with programs designed to contain expenses and even shift costs to patients through high-deductible plans and by more aggressively managing care. Providers also struggle with balancing cost containment and achieving quality outcomes. A major contributor to increased health care costs includes the deployment of new advanced technology, according to Darling (2010). Unlike in other industries in which new technology typically replaces old technology, in health care technology is often introduced incrementally, meaning additional services are provided (Darling). Darling also points out that a lack of standardization among third-party payers in reporting and tracking medical care costs and an inadequate use of electronic medical records contribute to much higher administrative costs in the United States as compared to other industrialized nations.

Patient behavioral factors, such as obesity and smoking; clinical factors, such as defensive medicine and preventable hospital readmissions; and finally operational issues, such as inefficient claims processing and the ineffective use of technology, all contribute to waste and excess spending within the health care system (Darling, 2010). Collaboration among providers, payers, patients, and the government is required to implement change aimed at creating efficiencies and improved outcomes within the health care system.

High-risk behaviors may be more likely to change when the government commits more meaningful funding to public health initiatives to educate the public and reinforce healthy living, and when more community-level intervention programs are designed to reduce high-risk behaviors that lead to chronic diseases. By way of example, studies have shown that two interventions in California, instituting a cigarette tax and banning smoking in public places, significantly reduced cigarette smoking. The reduction in this high-risk behavior resulted in decreased heart disease and lung cancer in the state (Chernichovsky & Leibowitz, 2010).

According to Chernichovsky and Leibowitz (2010), an integrated health care organization must foster coordination among stakeholders, formulate policies that promote appropriate incentives designed to create efficiencies, encourage choice among and responsiveness to patients, and institute financial discipline and cost containment measures. A key component to an integration process that delivers more favorable outcomes is a greater leveraging of the primary care physician (PCP) and deploying of the patient-centered medical home approach, which provides care that is comprehensive, coordinated, and compassionate (Rushton, 2009). The patient-centered model of health care delivery, whereby primary care and the active involvement of the patient and his or her family coalesce, along with evidence-based approaches, have begun to evolve in the health care marketplace. However, because patient-centered approaches are in their infancy, their total impact on cost containment and improved outcomes has not yet been fully evaluated (Rittenhouse & Shortell, 2009). Rather than accepting the purely paternal approach exercised by the physicians of the past, the patients of today continue to take a more active role in the management of their health, and in modern medicine open communication and collaboration among patients and their treating physicians help health care organizations coordinate care and deliver effective treatment and curative results. Again, the PCP plays a critical role in this coordination process by representing a single source in charge of both directing and managing care and reducing duplicative and unnecessary care. However, health care financiers, largely the third-party and government payers, have rewarded providers with robust reimbursements based on the volume of procedures and specialized testing and treatments, creating a decline in PCPs in the United States. According to Mirabito and Berry (2010), a payment and incentive system must recognize the benefits of the PCP and the patient-centered medical home approach, which is designed to promote quality and improved outcomes and to increase value for health care spending. Value-based purchasing and payment arrangements by third-party payers require new reimbursement methods that complement traditional fee-for-service structures. The optimal reimbursement structure will motivate the provider community to offer enhanced services aimed at prevention, education, better management of chronic diseases, and improved patient satisfaction and outcomes.

In addition, cost shifting from the third-party payer to the consumer through higher co-pays and higher deductibles is intended to reduce the cost to the employer of group health plans. This cost shifting also creates a financial incentive for the end-user patient to take a more accountable role in the health care process. Gone are the days of a carte blanche approach to health care by the consumer, who will probably contribute a greater portion of the cost of the care.

Although the challenges and solutions just described in theory should create efficiencies and contain costs for providers and third-party payers while improving outcomes for patients, in reality many providers, such as hospitals, operate with thin or even negative margins and are faced with Medicare and Medicaid reimbursements that fail to cover the cost of services. Further, bills for services rendered that become uncollectible and the provision of charity care to patients who are uninsured or unable to afford treatment exacerbate an already challenging fiscal environment. With increased competition from large, national, multihospital systems with access to capital, and given low rates of return on liquid investments and a reduction in contributions to nonprofit health care facilities during the recession and postrecession period, community and regional health care facilities are facing serious challenges that may not be cured by even the most astute financial executive.

According to Davis and Robinson (2010), a decline in the demand for hospital beds, which has been a result of increased use of outpatient facilities and costs that are rising faster than reimbursement rates, has created significant pressure on the financial viability of providers. In addition, the consolidation of health care facilities has been a growing trend, and independent facilities are finding it difficult to compete with multihospital systems (Davis & Robinson). Finally, also creating financial uncertainty for providers is health care reform, under which health insurance coverage will be provided to thirty-two million Americans who are currently uninsured. An increase in health insurance coverage will decrease uncompensated and charity care, but providers also anticipate reduced reimbursement rates. The U.S. health care system, which is already strained, may face additional challenges, and the expanded medical consumption may not offset decreased reimbursement rates (Davis & Robinson). In the end, although health care reform may create winners and losers among stakeholders, such reform should be about the controlled and focused enforcement of a system that delivers better access and care to all Americans.

COST-EFFECTIVENESS AND REFORM

According to the Centers for Disease Control and Prevention (CDC, 1999a), "Since 1990, the average lifespan of the persons in the United States has lengthened by > 30 years; 25 years of this gain are attributable to advances in public health" (as cited in CDC, 1999b, p. 1481). Far-reaching public health achievements from 1900 to 1999 have to do with the use of vaccinations to eradicate a host of infectious diseases as well as

> motor vehicle safety; safer workplaces; the control of infectious diseases [through] improved sanitation; improved food handling; [increased] access to family planning; [the] fluoridation of drinking water; recognition of tobacco use as a health hazard [and the launch of antismoking campaigns]; [the improved health of mothers and babies and the decline in infant mortality]; and the decline in deaths from coronary heart disease and stroke. (CDC, 1999a, pp. 241–243)

Public health activities in communities have also been a driving force in elevating the health status of the U.S. population, and a local-level approach to health education and prevention efforts provides flexible and deliberate strategies and methods to address unique health issues within a community (Witmer, Seifer, Finocchio, Leslie, & O'Neil, 1995).

Americans are healthier than they were a century ago, and they are living longer. They also have higher expectations and demand better products and more responsive services. In today's world, consumers can bid for, buy, compare, and order any product they desire and have it shipped to their doorstep 24/7. When patients visit health care professionals, they are surrounded by the latest scanners, laboratory equipment, surgical robots, and medical advancements, yet basic data, such as medical records, often reside with primary care physicians and sit in colored folders on dog-eared paper. That this information may not be readily available to other critical users of such data, such as specialists or even pharmacists, underscores the challenges of a disjointed health care system.

A perverse financing system that has fostered significant growth in the health care sector has also created inherent inefficiencies. Means-tested Medicaid and Medicare insurance, which covers 30 percent of the population (Fuchs & Emanuel, 2005), provides for administrative costs that are lower than those of private sector insurance (Marmor et al., 2009). Often, as in the case of Medicaid, means-tested insurance requires the costly process of determining eligibility, encourages cheating with respect to income reporting, and generates discontinuities of coverage as recipients move into and out of eligibility. Fuchs and Emanuel (2005) have described Medicare as a program providing an open-ended entitlement that does not consider the costs of technologies relative to their benefits. Its fee-for-service approach to reimbursement is fundamentally flawed, rewarding providers for generating volume over value (albeit at lower reimbursement rates than those of third-party payers), rather than providing incentives to physicians and patients for cost containment, managing medical consumption, and rewarding positive outcomes on a relative basis (Feldstein, 2007). It has been predicted that by 2019 the Medicare Hospital Insurance Trust Fund will be depleted (CMS, 2005). Medicare and Medicaid are major players in the financing of health care, and Fuchs and Emanuel (2005) have concluded that without a material increase in taxes or a decrease in the health care spending trend, Medicare is headed for insolvency.

In addition to flaws in the financing system, a lack of innovation with respect to information technology has stifled efficiencies. Despite the ability of larger institutions and large group practices to invest in innovative information technology platforms, most physicians operate in a small practice environment with limited resources, and the costs associated with electronic medical records (EMRs) outweigh their benefits. Furthermore, other quality control issues and a lack of standardization in and knowledge of expert-recommended procedures and best practices among providers has been observed in the health care system (Fuchs & Emanuel, 2005).

A lack of attention by industry leaders and physicians to the value of cost-benefit analysis presents another problem. Fuchs and Emanuel (2005) have claimed that most physicians may evaluate the benefits as compared to the risks of a course of action. However, they may not have a clear understanding of the costs involved, and they may not consider costs when their intervention is based on delivering the best possible care. Furthermore, the financing of health care generally has failed to provide physicians with the incentives to deliver cost-effective care.

The physician-centered health care system in the United States has been structured to react to acute and chronic care requirements. Historically it has not been largely designed to address wellness or chronic disease management in a proactive manner. Collaboration among the fragmented provider and third-party payer systems in an environment often riddled with customer disengagement must occur today rather than tomorrow. The health care industry has been challenged with the task of targeting and using limited resources to continuously improve outcomes. Advances in medical technology have arguably played a significant role in the reduction of mortality rates and increased life expectancy. However, a focus on preventative care, on health outcomes rather than the volume of services, and on new ways to leverage limited resources will become critical in elevating the health status of the population through the creation of a more responsive and cohesive health care system.

Improved technology, which bridges information gaps among health care stakeholders; a shift toward consumer accountability; and the revamping of health care financing systems dominated by government and third-party payers are critical in creating efficiencies in the health care system.

Public opinion has established that the status quo as it relates to health care—and the costs associated with health care—is no longer a viable course. Health care leaders in turn are set to address a call for action by the government in light of failures in a free market economy to correct health care access and cost containment problems. When individuals are confronted with change they may experience fear and skepticism. Accordingly, to accomplish sweeping reform, mind-sets must adjust and become open to change, objections must be addressed, and specific details describing the practical outcomes associated with the change must be properly conveyed. Therefore, support and buy-in from Main Street America are required to facilitate any successful reform process. Fuchs (2009) argues, however, that "there should be no settling for appearance over substance. Any reform plan not controversial is certain to be inconsequential" (p. 964).

Comprehensive tax reform may be the driving force to implement, sustain, and strengthen the health care system. Tax reform has the ability both to finance the delivery of health services and to contain costs. Sessions and Lee (2008) advocate the following fundamental changes, which leverage taxes to drive health care reform: simple and transparent tax revenue streams designated for health care financing, coupled with public disclosure of total health care costs and an elimination of fragmented health care financing. It is important that an equitable plan be structured, whereby the vast majority of Americans pay into and benefit from the program. For example, Medicare beneficiaries, with strong lobbying power, are incentivized to maximize benefits without any regard for costs. Although benefit cuts do have an impact on Medicare recipients, any enhancements to Medicare are funded by others. Finally, Fuchs and Emanuel (2005) argue that a value-added tax may be leveraged to fund universal health coverage for the currently uninsured, to be paid for with vouchers.

Other reforms target long-term cost containment and improved outcomes. Hyman (2009) suggests incorporating into reform efforts a change in reimbursement that includes payment for integrated health care teams focused on lifestyle-based treatment of chronic diseases and reimbursement for wellness initiatives; improved food policy in school and community environments, and the encouragement of health by prohibiting foods that are known to promote obesity and disease therein; imposed limits on unhealthy food advertising; an improved flow of information by linking medical records electronically and eliminating fragmentation in the health care system; and the creation of an Office of Wellness to promote good health and provide public education designed to improve behaviors and individual health levels. The importance of the last of these initiatives has been underscored by Pettingill (2009), who argues that access is not enough and reinforces the value of health promotion: "Studies suggest that access to health care improves health 10% of the time. Personal health behaviors, environment factors and genetics impact 90% of the health status" (p. 18). Accordingly, individual behavior rather than acute treatment by physicians is a key driver of cost containment and better health.

Pettingill (2009) also recommends incentivizing providers for prevention efforts and chronic disease management; ensuring the connectivity of electronic medical records; administrative simplification and the reduction of wasteful bureaucratic measures; and the provision of catastrophic coverage for children and underserved populations.

The model of health care delivery crafted by primary care organizations in 2007 called the **patient-centered medical home (PCMH)** has been gaining traction. Macinko, Starfield, and Shi (2007) contend that primary care is the foundation of the PCMH model, and that decades of research demonstrate improved outcomes and lower costs associated with primary care. The primary care physician essentially manages health issues ranging from preventative care to the treatment of acute and chronic illnesses across the patient's life span. Rittenhouse and Shortell (2009) submit that the health care system historically has been organized with the physician at the core. The PCMH model places the patients at the center, and urges each patient and his or her family to participate actively using decision-making tools and readily available information. In addition, evidence-based treatments and metrics and innovative, information-technology-supported means to measure performance are also included as important components of the model. Finally, the PCMH model recommends a payment structure that combines fee-for-service and pay-for-performance payments, with compensation for care coordination and integrated management and for the use of innovative technology and quality target achievements.

With significant reductions in reimbursements and a shifting away from a fee-for-service philosophy toward outcome-based compensation by government and third-party payers, the stakes for corporate managers and physicians become more closely aligned in the health care system. The administration, physicians, and support staff must work closely together in garnering efficiencies while exceeding the expectations of their consumers. To achieve coordination of care, clinical connectivity must occur, and the nonphysician business executive must engage and include manageable task forces of physicians in the decision-making process. In health care, then, the ability to establish strong executive and physician relationships serves as a key core competency for the transformational leader. Physician input and buy-in in an organization dedicated to the mission and vision of the leader, combined with the application of appropriate technology platforms with an associated return on investment, serve as a recipe designed to position the evolving health care organization for future success.

The physician community has typically been hesitant to widely accept the use of standards of care and specific evidence-based rules in the process of treatment. Coordination of care will become mainstream as health care organizations become better integrated, and the deployment of relevant best practices and standards of care will become a requirement by the health care financiers—government and third-party payers—in an outcome-based environment. The use of guaranteed checklists and "warranties" on postoperative procedures and treatments begins to shift the burden of risk from the payer to the provider. Although physicians may be reluctant to find ways to work with payers, a shift in philosophy toward accountable care models suggests that inevitably the provider community will be required to acquiesce to an outcome-based payment platform. Therefore, health care organizations and their leaders must take the necessary steps now to produce the best outcomes for tomorrow.

Under an accountable care approach in an integrated health care organization, third-party payers deliver greater compensation up front to the provider, unlike in the traditional fee-for-service model, but the physician and the entire integrated provider structure must absorb future risks and associated costs for poor health outcomes. This shift in accountability from payer to provider is designed to motivate efficiency while underscoring the importance of achieving the best possible outcomes through the financing mechanism. Such a shift cannot be supported with a nonintegrated decision-making platform, whereby the physicians are excluded from the process and have no stake in maximizing profits and minimizing unnecessary costs and nonreimbursable procedures.

The health care and health insurance reform legislation of 2010 aims to provide additional incentives for organizations to merge and vertically integrate. Although conventional wisdom has yet to explore the issue, coordination of care, a shift toward accountable care, and vertical integration may have an impact on consumer choice and increase monopolistic behavior in the health care arena.

Pundits may engage in robust debate over antitrust concerns stemming from further consolidation of the provider market as well as the economic impact of a lack of choice, less competition, and a push toward more coordinated and collaborative care among both payers and providers. It is important to note that margins in the health care system will continue to be strained. Medical care cost floors and the monitored and regulated underwriting profits among health insurers will force providers to become more efficient and produce the same outputs at a reduced cost. However, a coordinated care approach appears to provide one of the best solutions for greater efficiencies and outcomes in an industry plagued by the symptoms of high costs and access issues resulting from poor health levels.

SUMMARY

Sound business and operational policy should be grounded in economic practices that align with the organization's mission. The primary driver in the growth of national health expenditures in the United States has been public and private sector insurance: the main financing vehicles. Explosive growth occurred as a result of a financing system that increased access to the health care system and offered payment incentives based on the volume of procedures. At the same time, the consumers of health services had little motivation to regulate their use of the health care system when their government or third-party payer financed the cost of the health services.

The challenges in the health care sector are not expected to lessen as the financiers of health services continue to apply strict medical consumption review, cost control measures, and reimbursement pressures on providers to reduce medical inflation. In addition, an increase in chronic diseases, the expanded number of insured Americans that will result from the current health care reform legislation, the aging physical plants of providers, and rapidly changing technology necessitate substantial investments in the infrastructure and talent pool of health care organizations across the country. These investments, although needed, will become more difficult to support due to resource constraints. Providers will find themselves realigning budgets and available financial resources to pay for the broad reforms among insurers. Because of our aging population, more and more baby boomers will be migrating to Medicare, whose reimbursements provide a reduced revenue stream for all providers when compared to reimbursements from third-party payers, thereby generating significant financial shortfalls in the industry. Health care organizations and their leaders in conjunction with frontline employees will need to find new revenue streams and move toward accountable, coordinated, quality care. *Health care will in effect require a shift from volume to value.*

Bringing a greater number of Americans into the private health care market will drive health insurers to compete for new members, and greater out-of-pocket costs for employees, especially those opting to purchase additional coverage beyond required minimums, will make all consumers more sensitive to price. Increased access to health care by all Americans, improved efficiencies, continued innovation, and higher-quality care that includes coordinated and proactive health measures will not by themselves help contain escalating costs. Americans must embrace wellness and proactively manage their health. Physicians cannot force patients to improve behaviors, particularly after years of poor habits. Education and prevention must start early, during the formative years of an individual's life, and any proponents of reform as well as health care financiers should consider a more substantial investment in public health and wellness initiatives designed to facilitate healthy behaviors and enhanced health levels among members of the general population.

Finally, the consolidation of facilities may be appropriate to wring out expenses and create a more efficient health care marketplace. Even though antitrust concerns over consolidation in the health care industry may surface, in the end reform should be about controlled and focused efforts to deliver better care at a more affordable price to all Americans.

KEY TERMS

accountable care

certificates of need

consumerism

Employee Retirement Income Security Act (ERISA)

employer-based health insurance

Health Insurance Portability and Accountability Act (HIPAA)

Health Professionals Education Act

Hill Burton Act

Kerr-Mills Act

Medicaid

Medicare

patient-centered medical home (PCMH)

REVIEW QUESTIONS

1. How might a profit motive conflict with a mission of providing access and affordable, quality care to patients in a health care organization? Can a profit motive and this mission coexist?

2. What is a likely outcome for organizations that fail to evolve, operate efficiently, and exceed consumer expectations in a competitive environment?

3. What were some of the ways in which government intervention fueled growth in health care in the post–World War II era?

4. What have been the cost drivers of the explosive growth in U.S. health expenditures?

5. Who are the primary financiers of health services?

6. Explain why providers and consumers of health services have not been incentivized to conserve resources within the health care system.

13

Ethics, the Law, and Doing Good

Tina Marie Evans

LEARNING OBJECTIVES

- Explain ethics as it applies to health care
- Recognize the importance of studying ethics as part of managerial training
- Clearly articulate how the central principles of ethics apply to today's health care manager
- Describe the dimensions of autonomy and justice as they relate to health services
- Summarize the importance of nonmaleficence and beneficence as they relate to patient and staff satisfaction

Depending on whom you ask and what their level of access to care is, you'll receive a wide variety of opinions and comments on our current health care system. Society continues to demand high levels of quality health care as costs rise and resources are increasingly limited. Today we have greater opportunities than ever to diagnose and treat injuries and illnesses, and medical technology is improving at a rapid pace. These many wonderful advances in technology have extended the human life span and delayed death for many patients—but the current state of our economy combined with rapid and progressive advances in technology have made this a very challenging time for ethics and ethical decision making. Weber (2001) sums up the rationale for the study of ethics at the management level by stating, "Health care ethics is not just about decisions made at the bedside. It is also about decisions made in executive offices and in boardrooms" (book cover).

Let's begin with a baseline definition of the term. **Ethics** refers to a system of principles and values that is centered on doing good and avoiding evil in terms of our duties and obligations to both others and ourselves. Ethics is concerned with standards of behavior in terms of right and wrong that exceed the basic requirements of the law (Judson, Harrison, & Hicks, 2006). A functional way to think about ethics in health care management is to consider it as a way to examine or study moral behaviors, and also their consequences. Purtilo and Criss (2005) add that ethics is a way to evaluate moral problems methodically, using reflection to analyze a situation. This reflection, if given time and proper attention, should lead you to the resolution of the situation through appropriate action.

So what is the role of the health care manager in the ethical puzzle? How do we create an environment of integrity and trust for our employees and patients? Where do we turn when confronting an ethical dilemma— especially when the correct path seems so unclear? Morrison (2011) explains that although managers do not directly provide health services, conduct the research, or design the technologies that are used in the clinical setting, they are nonetheless critical to the success of all of those functions because they control and set the tone for the environment in which each takes place. In addition to gaining a solid understanding of system functions, finance, human resources management, and leadership, it is essential that both health care managers and physician and nonphysician care providers develop a clear understanding of personal and professional ethics, and use this understanding as the basis on which to build a relationship with patients, employees, the organization, and the larger community. Ethical dilemmas arise when managers and clinicians are pulled in two different directions by competing courses of action, such as those stemming from differing philosophies, inconsistent duties, or a poorly defined personal sense of right versus wrong. Add in the emotional dimension that is inherent in health care, and you can easily see how ethical issues can lead to conflict and heated discussions. Whether in times of dire emergency or when receiving routine care, those who come to your facility for care assume that you are dependably grounded in ethical behavior and practice, and it is your responsibility not to let them down.

In this chapter the foundational concepts of health care ethics will be presented and explained to help guide you in understanding basic ethical practice in health care management. These concepts and suggested applications will prepare you well with the tools you will need to make solid managerial decisions that are ethically appropriate according to your own standards as well as those of your organization and society at large. Health care organizations are made up of a variety of people with a variety of ethical standards, so the establishment of baseline expectations and ethical standards for staff will also be discussed. The practical applications and suggestions that are given are helpful starting points, and can be adapted to fit your particular organization and needs.

ETHICS IN THE WORLD OF HEALTH CARE

Before we start our journey down the road of ethics in health care management, let's get everyone on the same page with a strong explanation of the term previously defined. According to Darr (2005), ethics is more than simply obeying the law. The law is the minimum that is acceptable by the standards of society in terms of our actions or behaviors, but ethics goes much deeper than this. It is theoretically possible for one to obey the law but at the same time to not be ethical. You may be able to think of instances in which the law has not been broken but ethics violations have occurred. Darr stresses the point that there is a dynamic between the law and ethics, as each affects and is affected by the other. Much of regulatory law and tort law is actually based on the standards of practice that the professions have chosen to set for themselves (Ahronheim, Moreno, and Zuckerman, 2000).

The managers and practitioners who consistently practice according to the standards and limitations that are set by their respective fields, who make a good faith effort to understand and obey the law, and who rely on their conscience for guidance in terms of right and wrong are well on their way down the ethically correct path. Managers must recognize each of their ethical duties as leaders, and strive to turn those ideals into reality.

Ethical issues have arisen over time not only because of substantive controversial issues that are inherent in health care but also because of shifts in the manner and location of the provision of health services, how such care is paid for, and how organizations are structured. Ahronheim et al. (2000) note that these factors have obviously sparked the need for changes to policies and procedures, and have also caused ethical conflicts and tensions to surface within health care organizations. A significant responsibility of management is to create and then orient all staff to an ethical climate that is consistent with both the mission of the organization and the expectations of the employees and patients. Managers must educate themselves and keep themselves updated in the discipline of ethics so that the ethical climate is current and well understood by all, and so that there is a clear process in place to resolve any ethical conflicts or tensions that inevitably arise.

Timko (2001) tells us that as the field of health care ethics has developed, four main principles "have come to dominate the discipline" (p. 1). They are autonomy, nonmaleficence, beneficence, and justice. Knowledge of each of these principles provides a solid base for ethical correctness in our dynamic and interactive health care environment. When principles such as these come into conflict, as commonly happens, the outcome is likely to be an ethical dilemma. With many stakeholders present in the health care system—managers, care providers, individual patients, families of patients, and the larger community—it is not an uncommon event to see clashes in values. In fact, many hospital accreditors and some external regulators now require ethical values to be consistently examined, monitored, and addressed—especially in the areas of physician integrity, the confidentiality of information, conflicts of interest, and research ethics.

The ethical dilemmas that will challenge you in your career will not always be black and white—sometimes the grey is very deep and distressing.

The principles that follow in the next few pages should be used to guide your consideration of those who come to your door seeking health services in light of varied financial and insurance resources; these principles should also help you as you examine the various intangibles, such as loyalty and trust, that are important in the provision of health care. So many factors must be considered—mission, vision, values, trust, human dignity, service to the community, and so on—so how do managers make the difficult decisions that will inevitably land on their desk? With so many people relying on you for ethically and legally correct decision making, let's begin our review of the key principles that should guide your work.

AUTONOMY

The first of the four central principles of ethics that will be discussed in this chapter is **autonomy,** which relates back to its Greek definition of self-rule and self-determination (Beauchamp & Childress, 2009). Autonomy assumes that a person has the capability to make his or her own decisions, and that this person is free from the control of others. In addition, the principle of autonomy provides the right to hold viewpoints that may not be in agreement with those of others. This gives patients the option to agree or disagree with the views of their care providers—to either comply with their suggested instructions or not—without penalty. In the clinical setting, patients must also be allowed to exercise their free will in either signing or refusing to sign consent forms for medical testing or treatment. Because the patient has the right to choose what happens to his or her body, care providers have the ethical duty to obtain consent for testing and treatment—but only after the recommended actions are thoroughly explained to the patient at a level that he or she can understand.

Beauchamp and Childress (2009) suggest a model for us to use in fulfilling this informed consent dimension of autonomy. They tell us informed consent requires patients' competence to understand what is explained to them as well as their voluntariness in the act of making their decision. Most adults are considered competent to make their own decisions, but provisions are made for situations in which health care involves children, the mentally ill, and patients who have an altered mental status from trauma or substance abuse. As noted previously, true informed consent also requires the care provider to provide the patient with honest and complete information concerning the risks and benefits of both accepting and refusing the recommended care. This information must also include any possible alternative care plans that would be valid for the patient to consider, whether they are covered services or not. A patient who does not receive complete information from a care provider is at risk of making a choice that may not be consistent with his or her personal wishes and values.

Finally, informed consent as part of autonomy requires that the patient be in agreement with the treatment plan, and the patient must give his or her authorization to proceed with the recommended care. This authorization, as explained by Timko (2001), is "essentially a permission, and as such does not require the health care provider to perform certain actions; it merely entitles them to do so" (p. 19).

It is a worthwhile practice for managers to randomly check on the process of obtaining consent and also to monitor the types of communication that are used by staff members, whether they are verbal messages or patient handouts. Patient satisfaction with explanations they were given concerning their medical status and the intended plan of care can also be evaluated in patient satisfaction surveys using questions directed toward communication. Managers are ethically obliged to rectify any deficiencies found in patient satisfaction surveys pertaining to consent and patient education. Every effort must be made to ensure that a patient clearly understands his or her medical situation and the proposed plan of care before any choices are made.

Because attaining informed consent is an ethical duty, we must do all we can to ensure that staff are aware of this concept and avoid situations in which coercion may play into consent. If a patient feels coerced into treatment or participation in a research study by a care provider who is threatening dreadful consequences or is overly aggressive, autonomous consent is not a possibility. Failure to respect patient autonomy can be viewed as negligence, and can lead to accusations of malpractice. Another portion of the manager's role is to ensure that all patient consent forms are written at the appropriate level, avoiding any terminology that a patient would not understand. The readability of all patient educational materials and handouts should be reviewed, with all materials set between the sixth- and eighth-grade reading levels. It is essential that managers stay up to date on all applicable federal and state legal mandates (such as changes to HIPAA), and that they ensure that correct procedures are followed in consistently using and correctly and confidentially storing the consent forms. External accreditors are likely to require random checks of the use and content of consent forms as well as the procedures for storing them, so it is advisable not to wait until just prior to a site visit or quality assurance review to ensure that your facility is in line with the requirements of the law and the external accreditors.

True autonomy also involves the obligations of truth-telling and fidelity. Whether in health care or outside of the field, human interactions are based on the assumption of truth as the basis of trust. Therefore, patients, care providers, and managers must work from the perspective that honesty is the norm rather than the exception. The confidence that comes with this trust is central to good relationships in all categories. By virtue of their powerful administrative position, managers have the ethical responsibility of truth-telling. Lying (whether intentionally or by omission) has destroyed the careers of many managers—and it is known that a lack of trust will lead to decreased employee performance, resentment, and retention issues. Dosick (2000) also warns us that dishonesty causes a loss of integrity, and may lead to the loss of your position.

Along the same lines, **fidelity** as a portion of autonomy refers to the keeping of your promises and holding true to your word. This has been a long-standing dimension in management: managers want promises to them to be kept by others, and they should in turn keep the promises they make. Fidelity is an expectation in health care and the larger community, and you must therefore be aware of what you say and what you promise. Managers should also be cautioned that in some situations silence may be viewed as agreement, and some may trust in your consent via silence. Have the courage to voice your thoughts and set the record straight, whether verbally or by written communication. Either way, be clear about where you stand, and don't give others the opportunity to make assumptions.

Because mission statements guide health care organizations, such a statement can also be viewed as containing promises that will be kept to others who seek health care at your facility. Does your mission statement reflect your passion for quality service and ethical behavior? Managers must take the time to periodically review the mission statement that guides their organization, and consider whether such a statement is still appropriate over time. Staff must be trained and updated as needed to ensure that they understand the mission and how the promises to those who seek care will be fulfilled. Setting the tone that honesty is what you give and what you expect will create a working environment that promotes truth.

Autonomy may seem like a simplistic principle, but ethical situations that challenge the ability of a manager and his or her staff to respect autonomy are all too common in today's health care environment. Your organization and your community are counting on you to rise to these challenges and do what must be done to preserve the right of autonomy. Periodic reviews of mission statements and continuing education efforts aimed toward ethical practice are needed, as is direct staff observation and evaluation in light of the dimensions of autonomy.

NONMALEFICENCE AND BENEFICENCE

In our current health care system these two principles are viewed as inseparable partners, and are central to trust-based care. **Nonmaleficence** is best explained by the Latin phrase *primum non nocere*—"first, do no harm." Most managers and care providers view this as a primary consideration, because an ethical and legal duty clearly exists in medicine to avoid harming others (Beauchamp & Childress, 2009). Care providers must consider whether the benefits that are likely to be conferred as a result of their recommended care will outweigh any suffering that may be caused along the way. In other words, the potential benefits of the care should be balanced against the potential harm. If the benefits outweigh the harm, the care is probably ethical. Nonmaleficence is a frequent assertion in medical malpractice cases, so it must be given the attention that it deserves to protect patients from harm, care providers from disciplinary actions including the loss of a license or credential, and also the organization from financial loss.

Morrison (2011) explains that nonmaleficence does not only apply to care providers. Managers must have policies in place to address the safety of all, as well as to protect the patient's physical health and dignity. Infection control policies and appropriate environmental practices are common standards used to avoid harm. The application of this principle is not just restricted to the treatment of patients; it applies to the treatment of staff as well. An additional responsibility of managers is to

> provide a working environment that is safe and does not harm your employees. Such an environment allows for discussion of concerns without fear of reprisal. It should also be an environment where values are respected and employees can do their best work on behalf of the patients they serve. (Morrison, p. 49)

Appreciating the diversity of your staff and patients while honoring their individual values and beliefs will go a long way in creating a culture of inclusion.

The partner principle of nonmaleficence is **beneficence.** Beneficence includes acting for the good or benefit of the patient, and on good values. Pellegrino and Thomasma (1988) argue that beneficence must go beyond the negative principle of "doing no harm" to also include a focus on addressing each component that makes up the complex concept of a patient's "good." They argue that medicine is neither a science nor an art, but rather a practice that gives rise to ethical standards. If these standards are violated, then good medicine is violated as well.

Therefore, care providers who pledge to do no harm must strive to create a positive balance of good over potential harm. The focus of your facility should be on meeting the obligation to create good by contributing to optimal health for your patients and community. Patients assume that care providers are there for their benefit, and that these providers will always do all that is possible to heal with kindness. Yes, seems egotistical, but it's true.

Isn't that how you think when you approach providers for your own care? You wouldn't assume that your care providers would not do all they can to heal you—the common assumption is that care providers will do all that is possible to give you the best outcome.

Staff issues may arise when a manager does not proactively work to create and maintain a culture of beneficence. Such a culture must be both encouraged and reinforced from the top down. Morrison (2011) explains that beneficence is not just between the care providers and patients; this principle must include your staff as well. If patients are shown active beneficence and staff members are not, **compassion deficit** may occur. It can be very emotionally draining for care providers to give of themselves in a spirit of active beneficence day in and day out—and we must recognize that this spirit of giving is not always rewarded. Managers who work more "in the trenches" are at risk of experiencing compassion deficit as well. Tong (2007) reminds us that the business of health care puts people in the position to see patients and families at their highest levels of grief and despair, and seeing this pain and suffering is an inherent part of working in health care. Care must be taken to provide and manage services with compassion but also to help staff as well as yourself to retain balance, manage stress, and avoid personal and professional burnout.

Ongoing stressful circumstances, such as those commonly experienced by workers who have regular contact with the very ill and injured, can lead health care workers to feel that they are of little value and importance to the organization, and this may hamper their motivation to perform well in the workplace. Managers must be aware of how administrative behaviors and attitudes help prevent compassion deficit, and must work to keep employees feeling valued. One of the ways that you can prevent compassion deficit is to remember to praise your employees at all levels, rather than simply assuming that it's their job to do everything well. Dye (2000) notes that practicing respect and remembering to praise the work of your staff will help foster a climate of caring. Small acts of kindness, such as hosting occasional group lunches for all staff in the department or frequently using the words "thank you," not only will honor the worth of the employees but also will save you time and trouble in dealing with low morale (or worse, constant recruitment and rehiring). Always use your administrative power in a manner that respects staff and promotes positivity and self-esteem.

JUSTICE

As we begin to study **justice** in terms of health care ethics, let's start with its definition. Justice refers to doing what is perceived to be deserved or fair in a given situation. However, each health care organization will usually create its own definition as a guide for providing fair treatment to patients. How should we go about providing health services to the various sectors of society—and what is our responsibility to see that services are extended fairly regardless of patients' ability to pay? What is our social justice responsibility to our community and to those who do not have access to care? It is so challenging to balance the needs of patients with those of the stockholders and payers, so the managerial duty to decide what your organization's role is in caring for all patients in a just manner is not one to take lightly. How will the organization provide care and balance its financial responsibilities? Will the care that is provided be different based on patients' ability to pay, and how do we allocate scarce health care goods and services in our health care setting? Justice is not an easy concept to implement consistently in today's health care environment. The complexities of mission and margin along with technological advances and widely varying levels of access to care make justice a struggle for managers. Clearly, remaining compassionate while maintaining an acceptable bottom line is an ongoing test of managerial skill.

Community assessment in terms of risk potential is an important first step (Pearson, Sabin, & Emanuel, 2003). The organization's administration must be aware of the surrounding community's health status and the amount of available resources—and also what future trends and changes are likely. Will you balance the number of Medicare, Medicaid, and uninsured patients against your well-insured patients to ensure profit, or will your organization focus more on the ethical side of care provision and allow access to all regardless of their ability to pay? Who will provide for the indigent in your community—how can they be best served? There is no one formula to help you balance your margin, mission, and ethical image. Such decisions are influenced by the managers of each organization, and you must be prepared to help in this regard.

Boyle, DuBose, Ellingson, Guinn, and McCurdy (2001) acknowledge that although it may be tempting to exclude Medicaid or uninsured patients, this strategy will not serve you well when it comes to your image in the eyes of the community. If you are knowledgeable of the surrounding community's health and social status, you will save yourself time in setting up appropriate education programs early on and also dealing with the ethical issues surrounding the decisions that will need to be made on the way to achieving balance. The income loss from low-paying and nonpaying patients can be minimized by an accurate assessment of needs, strong outreach efforts, and partnering with other community agencies (Pearson et al., 2003).

Justice in terms of providing health services while keeping a facility's doors open is only one of a manager's concerns, because the concept also extends to dealings with staff. Building and maintaining the image of a fair and just administrator is necessary for success, as how you choose to present yourself will go a long way in shaping the staff's perceptions of you. Your actions (or inaction) also set the tone for this portion of the work environment. Managers who exhibit a sense of justice will take the creation and periodic review of policies and procedures very seriously. Are the documents clearly written and fair to all? Have you consulted various staff members for their thoughts and suggestions? Insight into how policies and procedures look from the viewpoints of others can give you additional information and also foster the building of trust with your staff members. In addition, it is only fair that all staff members be made clearly aware of what is expected of them in their respective positions, and that any changes to those expectations be communicated to them in a timely manner.

Managerial decision making is another area in which justice concerns exist. When a difficult decision must be made, how do you approach it? Have you gathered all of the facts, clarified all of the points, and taken the time (if possible) to consider the alternatives and the short- and long-term impacts and consequences of the decision? Finally, are you in a calm mood that lends itself to sound decision making? If not, refrain from stating your decision until the tension passes.

Justice also comes into play when dealing with employee discipline. Formal discipline must be consistent from case to case to preserve the perception of just treatment and keep employee morale intact (Boyle et al., 2001). If you consistently treat staff in a fair way, they are more likely to treat each other fairly—but if iniquity is perceived (whether it is true or not), the atmosphere in the office will certainly change in a negative way. In addition, the working environment must be free of all types of discrimination and harassment, regardless of an employee's status. If violations of stated policies occur, suitable sanctions should be applied and documented. The staff will only take policies and procedures as seriously as they see you taking them, so it is essential that employee discipline be applied consistently and fairly across the board. Each decision you make is a building block of your legacy, so acting with fairness toward both staff and patients is a daily necessity.

MORALITY

As it relates to health care management, **morality** refers to the everyday behaviors that allow us to live successfully with one another (Purtilo & Criss, 2005). This includes our duties (things we are required to do) and our values (things we treasure). Beauchamp and Childress (2009) explain that morality is usually learned as one grows up and recognizes the norms of right and wrong in social conduct; it is a form of agreement for the good of the social order. On a personal level, these norms consist of duties and values that you hold independent of others in your various social or work groups. These duties and values allow people to live in a peaceful society, because they form the reasonable expectations people place on one another. As part of growing up, a moral person will realize that he or she shouldn't lie, steal things, cause harm to others, damage others' property, and so on. Edge and Groves (1999) describe how this "broad understanding of what is right and wrong in human conduct is taught to us by our families, religion, national culture, and legal structure" (p. 70), and is handed down from generation to generation, with evolution and reinterpretation happening over time.

Frankl (1971) provides us with another dimension of morality by adding the concepts of choice and responsibility. He reminds us that each of our choices comes with inherent responsibility for that choice, and Tauber (2005) adds that we remain responsible for all potential effects of our choices—including those we cannot predict. As a manager, you will be required to make the best moral choices that you can in the situations with which you are presented, and you must take responsibility for them. This is consistent with the need to practice as a moral agent for your organization and your community (Darr, 2005). To fulfill this role, you must make personal and professional choices that have a clear foundation in ethics.

Moral integrity is not genetically programmed; rather it is developed over time through education, life experiences, self-assessments, and informed decision making. It is clear that moral practice demands a clear commitment to personal growth and lifelong learning. Johnson (2009) suggests that we work to develop the personal virtues and characteristics that moral leaders possess, which include courage, integrity, humility, reverence, optimism, and a sense of justice. He believes that these are more than just qualities; they are critical components of one's inner life and behaviors. Beauchamp and Childress (2009) add conscientiousness, trustworthiness, fidelity, gratitude, lovingness, and kindness to the list of virtuous character traits. Negative traits, such as a spirit of malice, dishonesty, a lack of integrity, and cruelty, "are universally recognized as substantial moral defects" (p. 176). Many of the positive traits contribute toward the concept of professionalism, which is a must in health care practice and administration. Nwomeh and Caniano (2011) remind us of not only the critical importance of professionalism but also the value of an apology, a simple "I'm sorry," when the situation warrants. Johnson (2009) also recommends that we identify moral role models for ourselves who can serve as examples as we practice morality in our position. These mentors can be sounding boards, consultants, and living examples of how to act when situations become morally challenging. It is also recommended that you read and reflect on the actions of known moral leaders, as well as evaluate case studies that have a moral dimension, to help in developing your sense of morality and preparing you to make good decisions when action is needed.

At times, conflicts between personal morality and the law will occur. An example of such would be the conflict between requirements to offer abortion services and the beliefs of health care practitioners or managers who feel it is immoral to do so. A challenge such as this clash of the law versus personal morality may be difficult, but with careful practice one can learn to abide by the law while respecting the tenets of his or her own personal morality—even if this requires a change in one's setting. The administrative role makes these decisions very challenging, but by paying consistent attention to your choices and the consequent responsibility for them, you will do well in building your legacy as a manager of integrity. Gilbert (2007) discusses morality and personal integrity in terms of one's legacy, mindfulness, and choice. Your employees as well as your superiors will be closely watching what you do (and, in some cases, don't do), and will form their opinions of you based on these observations. It is advisable to evaluate moral situations ahead of time as much as possible to help develop your moral senses, and also to evaluate your biases and develop your own system of decision making. The choices that you make as a manager must be consistent with your personal values. If they are not, you will have a hard time finding personal peace at the end of the day.

Your personal values (whether spoken or unspoken) must also match your actions. Gilbert (2007) reminds us that ethical managers "own" their choices and actions and do not push them off on others. He also cautions managers against making quick decisions that may seem good in the short term but may have tragic long-term consequences. Taking the time to make a calm, level-headed decision when all the facts have been gathered is a fine way to start. However, if you realize that you've failed to make the best moral decision, you must use that as a learning opportunity to avoid making the same error in future situations. What moral lesson can you find in that experience? Use that lesson to create good out of a negative situation. It also helps to think of your career as a path that will allow you to truly make a difference, and not just as something you have to do day-to-day. Your legacy is built step-by-step, slowly over time. How do you want your supervisors and employees to remember you and your work?

So what can we do as managers to affect the morality of those around us? Hoffman and Podgurski (2008) and Dye (2000) recommend that both current and future employees be evaluated for their moral integrity. Do they fit well with the moral environment of your organization? Using the typical interview questions with regard to morality will only take you so far in evaluating new employees. These authors recommend that managers ask candidates how they have specifically handled ethical situations in the past, and perhaps present the candidates with ethics-based case studies to respond to and discuss. This should be done in keeping with your goal of hiring only persons of integrity who will mirror your moral qualities and lessen the chances of moral disruption in your organization. Case study discussions can also be used to check the moral compass of your current employees, and they constitute a valuable learning experience that will help build the moral integrity of your staff. In fact, moral conduct should be a dimension of staff performance evaluations on a regular basis. You can't work to alleviate problems of which you aren't aware, so carefully designed and routinely implemented evaluations are highly recommended.

Because moral development occurs over time, it is possible for stresses, burnout, and negative dynamics to erode the integrity of staff members. Gilbert (2007) warns that ethical erosion can happen within an organization as employees slowly slip away from positive moral values, and that these eroded values can become more commonly accepted in place of the once moral and positive values. Staff morality should be monitored consistently because even "good" managers can be tempted to misuse the power that comes with their role by negativity (Dye, 2000). Ethical erosion can occur through a series of small choices rather than in one large event, so we must be mindful of the moral perceptions and consequences of our small decisions as well. Johnson (2009) encourages us, however, by noting that it does become easier to discriminate between good and bad moral choices as our moral character is built up and reinforced over time.

Griffith (1993) holds managers as "moral beacons" (p. 278) for their subordinates and the larger community. You, as a health care manager, are the model for the actions you expect from your staff, and it is your behavior that will set the tone in regard to what is and is not acceptable. In other words, don't hide your pledge to do what is morally correct—let your moral convictions be known, and enjoy the benefits that come with being an ethical manager. Griffith also recommends that you manage your staff in a way that fosters integrity by designing policies and procedures that encourage good decisions. It is also essential to keep in mind, however, that your behavior will always speak louder than any policies you create.

Because ethical issues will undoubtedly arise during your tenure, there must be recognized ways for staff members to report breaches of morality by others, and they must not feel threatened by punishment for reporting such troubles. If you make it known that the reporting of issues will be taken seriously and that reports will be researched and acted on when necessary, you will have a strong checkpoint in place for staff to help you police the moral environment of your organization. Simple methods of accountability will help maintain vigilance in creating and maintaining a climate of moral integrity for all parties. Being consistently true to your personal values and morals is not easy, but it is necessary to be a success in the eyes of all.

CODES OF ETHICS

As a health care manager, you will regularly face situations in which the path toward ethical decision making is unclear, and in these cases you will need to access resources that are available to help you make your decisions. The American Medical Association adopted its first code of ethics in 1847, with many organizations to follow in subsequent years (Walter & Klein, 2003). A code of ethics is a tool that can provide a greater level of guidance and wisdom based on the theories and principles of ethics, and on the experiences of ethical professional leaders (Morrison, 2011). Worthley (1999) reminds us that professional codes of ethics are more than just simple words—they are designed to help regulate your actions. An understanding of what your profession expects of you can guide your problem solving and decision making. Darr (2005) sums up the function of codes of ethics well by stating that they are there to help managers who "want to do the right thing, but need help determining what it is" (p. 62). Codes of ethics can and do change over time as updates are needed, so periodically reviewing them for yourself as well as keeping your staff apprised of any changes must be part of the continuing education plan.

Codes of ethics not only assist us in defining our ethical positions but also serve as a level of protection from lawsuits and the increasing demands of external accrediting and regulating bodies (Johnson, 2009). By knowing your professional obligations and the behaviors that are expected, you may possibly avert legal problems. Codes of ethics also help in preventing ethical dilemmas by defining boundaries for acceptable behaviors in your setting, which in turn will make it easier to communicate expectations to your staff. It is therefore necessary that you not only know the code of ethics that governs your profession but also focus on living your professional life by its guiding contents.

The American College of Healthcare Executives (*American College*, 2011) provides a specific and well-organized code that is meant to delineate standards of ethical conduct for managers in their professional relationships. A portion of the preamble to the ACHE *Code of Ethics* tells us, "Healthcare executives have an obligation to act in ways that will merit the trust, confidence and respect of healthcare professionals and the general public. Therefore, healthcare executives should lead lives that embody an exemplary system of values and ethics." The ACHE *Code of Ethics* divides the responsibilities of health care managers into six logical segments. The first five of these include a manager's responsibilities to the profession, to patients or others served, to the organization, to the employees, and to the community and society. The sixth segment explains the duty for an affiliate to report violations of the code. In addition, a varied selection of policy statements are linked to the ACHE Web site to provide managers with some extra assistance in areas that are known to be ethically challenging.

The ACHE *Code of Ethics* and the codes that govern some of the clinical professions are only beneficial if you are aware of their contents and make a conscious effort to incorporate their guiding principles into your daily work. Posting the appropriate and most recent copies of codes in prominent places where staff can read and also be visually reminded of them can have a positive influence on behavior. Seeing ethical codes posted in prominent locations also serves as a reassurance to patients and families, and such postings show your commitment to an environment of integrity.

ETHICS COMMITTEES

Since the mid-1960s there has been a great increase in the number of ethics committees formed by hospitals, hospice programs, nursing homes, and home health agencies. In 1995 the Joint Commission on Accreditation of Healthcare Organizations, now simply The Joint Commission, specifically demanded clear evidence that all hospitals have in place mechanisms for resolving dilemmas in an ethical manner. Judson et al. (2006) explain that although managers may be able to resolve the majority of issues that arise by using their personal sense of moral values, the presence of an ethics committee is a golden resource in the more ambiguous cases. Hospital or other health care facility ethics committees usually comprise physicians, nurses, clergy members, the CEO (or his or her delegate), social workers, and an attorney. Although you may not be directly involved with your organization's ethics committee, it is important to be aware of its role and functions.

Boyle et al. (2001) tell us how ethics committees, as integral resources in health care settings, typically have three functions: education, policy development and review, and patient case consultation. In terms of education, ethics committees commonly offer in-service sessions on specific and timely ethical topics, changing requirements, or technology-related scenarios. Such sessions are usually open to all stakeholders in the organization— including both the medical and administrative staff and also the community at large. By their visibility, such education programs take on a vital role in demonstrating the organization's commitment to ethical behavior, adding to ethical awareness, and sparking dialogue concerning relevant issues.

The policy development and review role of an ethics committee is usually activated at the request of the organization's CEO or another member of upper-level management. In this capacity the committee members act as consultants to structure appropriate policy on recurrent issues, or issues arising from newly created technologies. For example, Morrison (2011) identifies advance directives, withholding treatment, withdrawing treatment, informed consent, and organ procurement as some of the ongoing issues that may trigger the need to convene the ethics committee for policy development and review. Macklin (1993) adds that creating policies pertaining to the care and treatment of AIDS patients, and policies in regard to the care of Jehovah's Witnesses who refuse blood transfusions, are common work items at ethics committee meetings. She explains that ethics committees may also be charged with creating or reviewing policies related to the allocation of resources, and also the preservation of the mission and vision of the organization. Policies on community outreach services, fundraising efforts, and charitable contributions also fall within the purview of ethics committees (Monagle & West, 2009). Regardless of the topic they are addressing, ethics committees strive to create and maintain policies that are fair to all who will be affected by them.

The third function of an ethics committee is patient case consultation. When an ethically difficult case is referred to the committee, the members meet to review it. The committee helps clarify the issue at hand and elucidate the medical facts of the case, then evaluates the possible alternatives to resolve the situation (Judson et al., 2006). Hall (2000) states that definite progress has been made, as ethics consultations are now widely known about and available to both care providers and patients. Depending on the health care facility, some members of the committee will rotate on an on-call schedule for handling emergent cases. Anyone involved in the patient's case may request the assistance of the ethics committee—even the patient or the patient's family. Lachman (2009) speaks from her experience serving on two ethics committees, stating that most conflicts occur between the care provider and the patient's family—so one who serves on an ethics committee must be a skilled mediator. Some situations may need only an informal review (meaning that the concerned individual or individuals simply pose questions to the ethics committee members for advice); however, other cases require a full case review, whereby all members are present to follow the organization's formal procedure in giving input and making recommendations on the patient case. Note that the outcome here is a recommendation.

The recommendations of ethics committees are not binding, but rather serve as ethically sound advice to those who seek it.

One final point concerning ethics committees is that they are not to be viewed as your organization's "ethics police" who look for care providers and staff who commit unethical acts. The responsibility to create and maintain an environment of ethical correctness and morality still falls to the health care manager, which underscores the importance of working early on to set the proper tone in regard to what behaviors are expected and the consequences of stepping off the prescribed path.

DISCRIMINATION ISSUES IN HEALTH CARE

The concept of justice also carries forward into the discussion of discrimination issues in health care. We have come a long way in studying the areas in which discrimination exists and have taken some steps to eliminate it, yet we continue to have concern for those whose social condition marginalizes them and leaves them vulnerable to discrimination. Boyle et al. (2001) note that our concerns should still be with the "poor, the uninsured and underinsured, children, single parents and the elderly; those with incurable disease and chemical dependency; and racial minorities, immigrants and refugees" (p. 213). The ACHE *Code of Ethics* also makes specific mention of the health care manager's responsibility for this problem, stating that the manager must "avoid practicing or facilitating discrimination and institute safeguards to prevent discriminatory organizational practices" (*American College*, 2011).

As a manager, you will have a central role in evaluating and studying the needs of your local community, and in deciding what your organization's obligations are in terms of balancing the provision of covered and charity services. Stepanikova and Cook (2008) remind us of the right of everyone to receive health care that is nondiscriminatory. This includes those with physical or mental disabilities, who must be treated as unique persons with the right to the same health care as everyone else (Boyle et al., 2001).

In today's health care environment, managers are challenged to ensure that the organization will make money while keeping the community happy by taking care of the sick and injured who show up on the organization's doorstep—regardless of their ability to pay. A positive community image of the organization is essential, so being totally profit motivated will probably cause the community to see the facility as unethical and insensitive. So how do you work to keep a good profit margin and also stay true to your social justice responsibilities? A realistic assessment of the balance of delivering ethics-based, quality health services and turning a profit to enable organizational survival is a good starting place.

A serious look at the mission of your organization is one of the initial steps in such an assessment. The mission is a powerful statement that should guide the decisions made and the functions performed. Morrison (2011) explains that this can only happen when the mission "is clearly and operationally defined, well understood by all and used consistently by all levels of decision-making" (p. 183). The mission should include reference to the delivery of quality health services within the structure of the community's need for them (Boyle et al., 2001). Managers must ensure that the organization's mission is well supported by appropriate staff, equipment, supplies, and departmental budgets. Good financial planning will allow for the mission to be upheld and the needs of the community to be addressed.

The mission must be more than a simple statement on paper that hangs on the wall in a pretty frame. It is necessary to put the mission into action and demonstrate to all that the mission is lived and visible in the actions of employees. An organization cannot have different standards of care when dealing with those who are insured or financially capable of paying for services versus those who cannot pay for some or all of the services they receive. The organizational budget that is put into place is best thought of as both a financial and an ethics statement. Does the budget allow for adequate staffing and equipment, and provide some allocations for funding community needs? Are you meeting your obligation to be a good steward of these resources? Are you treating the organization's resources with the same level of protection that you would give your own?

The organization's image in the eyes of the community is something to be studied both at present and periodically over time. Organizations that are so profit driven that they struggle with discrimination in the delivery of health services are risking damage to their community image. Patients who may feel discriminated against are quick to spread the word about how they were treated by a care provider or facility. One study described how social isolation and exclusion as a result of stigma and age discrimination cause serious inequalities in access to health care, referrals, and treatment (Davies, 2011). These inequalities were noted as mostly prevalent among elders who suffer from mental health issues as well as persons from black and minority ethnic backgrounds. One recommendation from this study is to work toward a greater involvement of these populations in health promotion and community-based health services. Treating those in a lesser position well is not just something that is done to keep a positive image; it is the ethically correct thing to do. Anyone can end up in a disadvantaged position in society at any time—all it takes is the unexpected loss of a job, a divorce, a death, a serious car accident, and so on, and it may be you or I who must seek charity health services.

There are other actions that we can take to help prevent discrimination and bias in health care. A recent study by Stepanikova and Cook (2008) found that good communication between doctors and patients seemed to protect against racial and ethnic bias in the health care environment. Good communication was associated with a 71 percent decrease in the chance of a patient's reporting racial or ethnic discrimination during a health care visit. This finding suggests that it is the breakdown in communication between the physician and the patient that may lead to the patient's perceiving racial or ethnic bias—regardless of the quality of care that was given to him or her. This underscores the importance of good verbal and nonverbal communication, and also the need to respect a patient's right to know the facts surrounding his or her situation.

Therefore, managers should address and reinforce the topic of communication with all levels of staff to ensure that their communication is adequate for patient understanding. This may include using ancillary personnel, such as physician assistants or nurses, to help with explanations; consistently providing patient educational handouts that are written at a level that patients can understand (again, between sixth- and eighth-grade reading levels); and employing the services of an interpreter of foreign languages or

American Sign Language when necessary. It is also wise to bring up and reinforce with staff members the idea that assumptions should never be made concerning a patient's individual values or preferences based on his or her cultural background. Ahronheim et al. (2000) believe that differing philosophies and medical preferences that are linked to culture may be kept in mind, but that these should not be presumed to apply in the case of every patient from a particular cultural background. Managers who know and understand the basis of cultural competence, combined with staff members who consistently take the time to understand how a patient's culture plays into the plan of care, will enhance the overall patient experience and raise the likelihood that the patient will adhere to the treatment plan.

Finally, in addition to allocating budgetary resources to community health care needs, managers ought to encourage their staff members to serve as volunteers at community health events. These events are wonderful opportunities to make contact with the local community. Before sending employees to such events, it is wise to first study where deficits may exist in local health services, or which segment in your community is most in need so you can tailor the information and services offered at the event. Specifically, you should be aware of where the gaps are in local care, and also if there is a possibility of grant funding from local, regional, or national agencies or the government to address such gaps. Groups of staff members can be delegated to design, market, and run community health fairs and other outreach activities that have been defined as beneficial to the specific community population your organization serves. Sandel (2009) observes that "if a just society requires a strong sense of community, it must find a way to cultivate in citizens a concern for the whole, a dedication to the common good" (p. 263). Many employees enjoy service activities and giving something back to the community in which they live. Encouraging volunteerism is one way to cultivate a strong sense of community as well as an organizational tie to the community at large. The people of the community will benefit by getting the health advice or services that are needed, and you can promote your organization's image and public relations in a positive and compassionate way by putting your competent and friendly employees out in contact with the people.

TECHNOLOGY AND ETHICS

In recent years, the advent of a wealth of new medical technologies has changed the direction of testing and treatment. Artificial organs, genetic therapies and genetically engineered drugs, functional magnetic resonance imaging and functional computed tomography scans, sensor chips to monitor tumors, stem cells used to heal arterial and neurological damage, and Bluetooth devices for monitoring blood pressure and blood sugar are just a few of the many that have saved lives in times of crisis and extended the lives of many others. With the promise of each new technology that is approved and released comes the ethical challenge of deciding who should be the recipients of the technology, and under what conditions. Competition within the health care system for scarce resources is already high in some areas, and steady increases in life expectancy have resulted in a higher number of persons seeking care.

Unfortunately, with every new technology comes a steep price. Much research and development goes into each of these new additions, and the costs are then passed on to the health care organizations and their prospective consumers of the needed health services. Although many clinicians are uncomfortable with including financial considerations in determining the definition of appropriate care, most health care managers as well as insurance companies see it as necessary to take cost control into account (Weber, 2001). According to Weber,

> Cost control is an ethical value, not just a practical requirement, but it is not the only ethical value at stake in most decisions. The skilled ethical manager knows how to balance considerations of cost with considerations of quality, risk, patient needs, patient preferences, clinician integrity, etc. (p. 24)

Should these other considerations take priority over cost savings? What is the proper balance between the cost and these other considerations in patient care? Health care managers must be well versed in each new technology and trend that presents itself, having taken the time to study existing information so that they are prepared when approached for decisions on technology that has an impact on care.

The current setting in which health care managers function includes a limited amount of available health care resources as well as the need for careful stewardship of those resources. Some of the newly marketed technologies have solid research behind their outcomes and effectiveness, as the trend of evidence-based medicine continues. However, some technologies are so new that the outcomes haven't been studied enough to show whether or not they truly add benefit to a patient's care. A committee appointed by the Institute of Medicine (2008) that recently studied this issue concluded that our current health care system is "plagued by overuse, underuse, and misuse" (p. 1) of health services, and that there is an urgent need to "know what works" in terms of what is effective in clinical practice. This clearly highlights the need for an ongoing commitment to research—both from the researchers themselves and from the managers in charge of supplying budgetary support. We have a duty to continue to perform and support quality studies that will help clarify the questions that surround our decision making.

Weber (2001) believes that meeting our community's health care needs calls for a conservative approach to the use of resources, arguing that a foundational requirement of ethical stewardship of resources is to choose to provide a less costly treatment unless there is "substantial evidence that a more costly intervention is likely to yield a superior outcome" (p. 29). Using that line of thinking, a manager may choose to question whether there is a sufficient added benefit associated with the more costly treatment. Some managers believe that providing only the best to patients is the correct choice, whereas others feel that using the least expensive treatment that works well is the way to go. Depending on the location of and community demographics near your facility, you may play a role in influencing your organization to adopt and use new technologies. However, you may also have or eventually take a position in a location where keeping a close eye on costs is vital to keeping the facility's doors open. Weber (2001) feels that patients aren't done a disservice when they are given "good, competent medical care" (p. 25) instead of a more expensive option that may be only marginally better. Recognizing cost as a necessary consideration in establishing what health services are most appropriate is critical if there is to be a fair and just allocation of resources in times of scarcity. New medical technology holds great promise for the future of health care delivery, so keep looking for the newest advances that may benefit those in your setting, and research their risks and benefits carefully. Keeping up with the latest professional conference information and credible journal research, joining professional listservs, and also listening to the ideas and input of staff members are highly advisable.

New technology also leads to managerial dilemmas in terms of end-of-life care. Nonmaleficence is challenged when advanced technology plays into the issues that involve withholding or withdrawing life support as well as death-with-dignity decisions made to avoid potential further harm to the patient (Morrison, 2011). Your responsibility as a manager with respect to technology and end-of-life care is to ensure that your facility has clear and current advance directive policies in place and that your employees are well educated and updated about their responsibilities in consistently following those policies. Protecting the dignity of the patient while providing honest and accurate information are keys to meeting ethical responsibilities in making these decisions.

As mentioned previously, depending on the location where you are or will be working, technology may also force you to make difficult decisions about the rationing of care. Whether it is a question of allocating scarce resources in general or of the applicability of a new medical technology to the case of a specific patient, remember that this is a valid reason to seek the advice of your organization's ethics committee. Especially in uncharted territory, such as when considering the adoption and use of a new technology, the advice of an ethics committee or professional ethics consultant is critical in forming new policies and deciding the role of the new technology with regard to individual patient cases.

The last topic related to medical technology and ethics that I'd like to address in this chapter is the advent of electronic medical records (EMRs). EMRs are meant to be complete compilations of all patient information and encounters that will allow the streamlining and automation of information gathering. They should increase patient safety by facilitating the use of evidence-based support for decisions, enabling quality assurance checks, and assisting in the consistent reporting of all outcomes. They not only make information portable but also provide opportunities for rapid learning and the examination of large data sets that may confer the benefit of quick knowledge development and application at various stages of health care delivery. The Institute of Medicine's 2010 workshop summary on evidence-based practice suggests that EMRs may give us a deeper and faster understanding of how diverse patient populations respond to treatments. The data contained in EMRs, if a process is developed to use such data in an ethically responsible and confidential way for the purpose of research, could yield a diamond mine of evidence that is greatly needed to find out the best and most cost-effective ways to provide care for patients in a short amount of time. See Figure 13.1 concerning trends on the adoption of EMRs by office-based physicians.

As a manager, you have the ethical duty to make responsible decisions concerning the purchase of new technologies. Morrison (2011) suggests that

Figure 13.1   Percentage of Office-Based Physicians Using Electronic Medical Records, United States, 2001–2009 and Preliminary 2010–2011
Source: Hsiao, Hing, Socey, & Cai, 2011, p. 1.

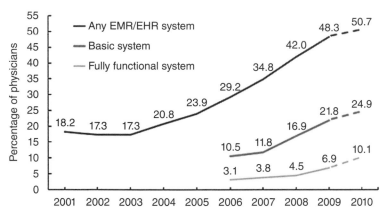

Note: EMR/EHR is an electronic medical record/electronic health record. "Any EMR/EHR system" is a medical or health record system that is all or partially electronic (excluding systems solely for billing). Data for 2001–2007 are from the in-person National Ambulatory Medical Care Survey (NAMCS). Data for 2008–2009 are from combined files (in-person NAMCS and mail survey). Data for 2010–2011 are preliminary estimates (dashed lines) based on the mail survey only. Estimates through 2009 include additional physicians sampled from community health centers. Estimates of basic systems prior to 2006 could not be computed because some items were not collected in the survey. Data include nonfederal, office-based physicians and exclude radiologists, anesthesiologists, and pathologists.

you should take the time to read information supplied by multiple sources and should always rely on more than just the information that is provided by the vendor of the technology. That way you will compile a variety of opinions and truly work toward an understanding of what you are purchasing (or choosing not to purchase). What are the maintenance costs? What is the expected life of the technology, and when will it need to be replaced? How much staff training will be involved, and at what cost? Morrison assures us that putting time and effort into this understanding in an attempt to make the best possible decision not only demonstrates good stewardship of resources but also makes financial sense: you are limiting excessive spending and potential waste while keeping the patient's best interest in mind.

The growing popularity of EMRs also puts additional pressure on health care managers to ensure that quality assurance processes are in place and that proper data management and coordination are standard. A lack of coordination among health care managers can lead to quality gaps and errors, which yield unintended results and unsatisfactory patient treatment outcomes. Choosing the best EMR system, deciding on the personnel in charge of EMRs, and determining how to train employees in the use of EMRs are not decisions to be taken lightly—or made quickly.

SUMMARY

Knowledge of each of the foundational principles of ethics (autonomy, nonmaleficence, beneficence, and justice) provides a solid base for ethical correctness in our dynamic and interactive health care environment. At times it will not be easy to uphold these principles or to ensure that all staff are consistently abiding by them as well.

Always keep in mind the power of your administrative position over your staff and your role in creating and maintaining an ethical working environment. Clear policies and procedures that match your organization's mission and values should be developed, reviewed on an ongoing basis, and communicated to all stakeholders. Never underestimate the importance of communication—between care providers and patients or managers and staff, whether written or verbal. As a manager, you must communicate so that your followers understand what the law requires, what your accreditors require, what the applicable codes of ethics require, and what the organization expects in terms of ethical correctness. Staff training specifically in regard to ethics upon their entry into the organization, and also periodic updates to such training, are crucial. Be transparent about the behaviors that are encouraged, and also those that will not be tolerated. Remember that staff want to be treated with the same level of respect and fairness that your organization demands they give to patients. Staff will value you for keeping this in mind, and you'll probably have fewer morale and retention issues to handle in the long run.

When in a difficult situation, always take time to think before you act. If a situation is heated, walk away and cool down. Be sure to think about how your actions will be perceived by others before you take them. Gather all the information that is needed to make a sound, ethically correct decision that is true to your values. Consider all of the alternatives carefully, as well as the likely short- and long-term consequences of each of your decisions. Never hesitate to turn to your ethics committee for their recommendations on a situation, or for help in policy formulation and revision. Ethics committees are also there to serve managers, not just the care providers, patients, and families. Seek out their expertise when a situation is difficult, unclear, or unprecedented—either they will reaffirm your thinking, or they may unveil an alternate path that you might not have been considering.

Never forget the importance of being a lifelong learner. Laws are modified, codes of ethics are updated, professional policy statements are revised, and you have to be aware of what changes are coming to be able to handle them well. You must ensure your own competence and that of your staff. Moral practice demands a clear commitment to personal growth and lifelong learning. Included in this is keeping close tabs on your organization's role in providing covered as well as charity and social justice services to the surrounding community. Community demographics shift over time, and you'll want to keep abreast of those changes. Likewise, take the time to evaluate and reevaluate your organization's image in the eyes of the community, learn how your organization or department is viewed by others, and see what lessons can be taken from that information. Having a strong community presence of volunteers sends a clear message that your organization truly cares about the overall health status of the community.

Clearly, balancing the business of health care with compassion is a difficult task, so the cultivation of an ethically proper working environment comes down to you—and your words must match your actions. You are the role model and example for those who report to you, and, believe me, they are watching your every move. Even small ethical slips here and there can do a large amount of damage to your image or, worse yet, end your career. Be willing to put your reputation behind the moral position you choose to take. Uphold your profession's code of ethics, honor your organization's mission, and always stay true to your conscience and personal values. Your legacy is on the line with every decision you make and action you take—how do you want to be remembered?

KEY TERMS

autonomy

beneficence

compassion deficit

ethics

fidelity.

justice

morality

nonmaleficence

REVIEW QUESTIONS

1. What are the key issues for managers with respect to autonomy?

2. What does it mean to be a just manager to your staff?

3. How can professional codes of ethics help guide difficult decision making?

4. What are the functions of a health care organization's ethics committee?

5. What are the management issues in regard to new medical technology?

6. What are some specific ways you can prepare yourself to be an ethical health care manager?

14

A Look into the Future of Health Services

Bernard J. Healey

LEARNING OBJECTIVES

- Understand the future managerial problems in the health care industry

- Become aware of the need for greater accountability concerning the use of scarce health care resources

- Understand the value of better management in the health care industry

- Recognize the value of health care managers' developing leadership skills in managing health care facilities

- Be able to explain the importance of culture in acquiring and retaining talent in a health care organization

Health care delivery in our country is on the verge of monumental change that will disrupt every health care professional and facility in our country. There will also be great challenges to be faced by those responsible for managing this reforming system of health care. To prepare for these changes, health care organizations will have to change, managers will change, and employees will be changed forever. This book was written to help those responsible for managing the largest industry in the United States learn how to become better managers. A secondary purpose of this text is to help managers and employees in health care delivery understand the challenges they will face in the very near future and what they will need to do to respond to them. Health care managers and followers will require the development of new skill sets to be successful in the coming years.

One of the most used definitions of management found in the literature centers on getting things done through people. Applying this definition to health care would yield a definition of delivering health services to people by people. The way health services are delivered to consumers is changing at a very rapid rate, a trend that will continue and escalate into the foreseeable future. The health care sector of our economy is attracting all types of competitors that are competing for the right to deliver health services to consumers who are much better informed than they were in the past. This competition from outside forces is demanding better management of health care facilities and the people who deliver health services to consumers. Health care managers must deepen their understanding of leadership and the appropriate uses of power and influence. These changes are necessary to enable health care facilities to respond immediately to the challenges issued by their competitors and their consumers. These new demands will require health care managers to constantly learn and grow in their chosen profession.

Health care facilities and their managers must become acutely aware that they exist for the benefit of their patients. These patients—the consumers—are demanding successful outcomes from their health care purchases, which they measure in terms of good health and excellent services from health care professionals. The future in health care delivery is going to require the health care manager to become obsessed with the quality of the services that are provided by his or her health care facility. In fact, health care managers will have to spend the vast majority of their time working on quality improvement in the delivery of health services to consumers. This is going to require the health care manager to lead individuals and manage things.

The first thing that all health care managers need to realize is that they cannot deliver quality health services on a continuous basis without the help of a dedicated team of health care employees. This focus on **continuous quality improvement** will also require the health care manager to move away from bureaucratic management practices. Gittell (2009) points out that many of our cost and quality problems in health care delivery are found deep in the work process itself. To solve these problems the manager has to be able to move away from bureaucratic rules and regulations to find a new means of ensuring quality. The manager will need to learn how to motivate employees to become obsessed, just as he or she is, with delivering quality services as part of a team process. He or she will, therefore, have to spend a great deal of time in team development.

Gittell (2009) also argues that individuals working in our current health care system demonstrate far too little cooperation in the pursuit of quality and need to develop better teamwork in their work process. Those who are attempting to lead their health care organization through the many challenges of health care reform must start their journey by recognizing the importance of their employees who actually deliver the services. Health services are the result of many health care professionals' working to produce **positive outcomes** for their patients. To achieve this goal of delivering a quality experience for the recipients of this care, they must work together. Teamwork—the ability to function effectively as a team—is what separates the winners from the losers in health care delivery. The health care manager has to become an active part of the team-based work process. He or she must also recognize the real challenges that health care managers will face as the delivery of health services changes to meet the demands of the consumer. Health care managers must learn to become less rigid in their chosen approach to managing people.

Health care facilities and their managers have to learn how to adapt to their situation. Harford (2011) argues that successful **adaptation** requires them to experiment with new ways of accomplishing the goals of the organization. When attempting to adapt to rapid change, there will be some successes and many failures. This adaptation cannot be done at the top of the organization, so it must be driven by empowered lower-level employees.

This is so very true in regard to the problems that confront health care institutions in today's turbulent environment. Adaptation is the key to successful resolution of these problems, but it must be allowed to happen immediately at the lowest level of the organizational structure and build from there.

The real secret to organizational success in this adaptation process, based on the first step of trying new things, is to include the customer in the process of deciding what the organization should offer that is new. For an organization in any industry, the decision to offer new products or services should always be driven by the desire to provide an outstanding customer experience. This process can be more successful if an organization asks for advice from its current customers and then delivers to them what they desire. Many of the top businesses in the world today have successfully enlisted the consumer in cocreating their new products or services.

This is an excellent strategy for health care facilities faced with the formidable task of lowering costs while improving the quality of their services. Because the services they offer are consumed by patients and delivered by employees, it seems logical to enlist both of these groups in defining and delivering improved services. Chesbrough (2011) points out that the best way to involve the consumer is to stop treating him or her as passive in the innovation process surrounding the services he or she receives from the health care organization. In fact, the consumer needs to be heavily involved. To be able to then respond to the requests of the consumer, all of the health care employees have to be empowered to deliver to the consumer the services he or she has requested.

ECONOMIC ISSUES IN HEALTH CARE

The most important goal in health care delivery must become to achieve high **value** for consumers while simultaneously reducing the monetary costs associated with high-quality health care. Porter (2010) points out that value in health care is defined based on the outcomes that occur for the dollars spent on those outcomes. For health care managers to improve the value of health services, they need to concentrate all of their efforts on outcomes rather than activities. If this is true, why are we paying so many providers for activities rather than for the health outcomes achieved by their efforts? This is a very important question that needs to be answered by the managers of scarce health care resources. Financial incentives will have to be put in place to improve the outcomes associated with the delivery of health services.

Another way to reduce the costs associated with the delivery of health services is to improve **productivity.** This is where better management of scarce health care resources comes into play. The health care manager has to take the lead in an effort by the health care organization to improve productivity, which in turn will usually reduce the cost of providing these health services. There is tremendous waste in our current health care system that needs to be eliminated if we are serious about reforming health care in our country. Health care employees know where this waste is found, and they also know how it can be reduced or eliminated. Therefore, health care managers must learn how to involve employees in the process of improving productivity as well as the bottom line for their health care facility. The purpose of this last chapter is to discuss the major challenges facing health care managers as they attempt to reengineer their health care organization, transforming it into a successful, high-velocity organization. This reengineering process will require an emphasis on leadership, culture, innovation, trust building, and the establishment of the organization's brand and reputation.

REENGINEERING HEALTH CARE DELIVERY

We have moved from a relatively simple health care system, one with very few treatments until the discovery of antibiotics in the 1930s, to an unbelievably complicated system of tests and medical procedures that attempt, it seems, even to cure death. With the development of new technology and growing complexity, the system changed and became much more error prone along the way. There are many errors that range from problems in the delivery of health care to the lack of caring for patients entirely. These problems associated with the delivery of health services to consumers in the United

States are in the process of being fixed by the various players in health care organizations.

There have been numerous papers and texts written about reengineering health care in the last several years. To accomplish the goals of any reengineering project, radically different management processes must first be developed. According to Champy and Greenspun (2010), there are many processes in health care delivery that can and should be redesigned to improve the quality, safety, and convenience—and ultimately the cost—of delivering health services to consumers. The problem has been that because health care facilities were usually reimbursed for this work, they continued to perform valueless and sometimes dangerous medical processes to get paid. To become competitive and survive in the turbulent environment, health care facilities and the people they employ are going to have to change how they operate. The starting point for this reengineering effort involves redesigning not only the work process but also the practices of those who do the work in health care delivery.

It is a well-known fact that during times of change the evaluation of employees becomes critical to helping them understand what is expected of them in the new work process. This is the major responsibility of the health care manager, and it requires a great deal of attention if the health care facility is really serious about continuous quality improvement. Lombardi (2001) argues that the most important component of successful performance appraisal is appropriate documentation, particularly when these evaluations are needed to aid employees in understanding what constitutes quality patient care and how such care can be improved. Because quality in health services is ultimately determined by the consumer of these services, it is very important that health care managers spend more time with consumers to discover what quality means. These should be the areas of concern for the manager when evaluating his or her employees. The customer is very concerned about improving his or her outcome by visiting a health care facility without encountering a medical error or hospital-acquired infection.

One aspect in health care delivery that requires immediate change is the current epidemic of medical errors in many health care facilities throughout the country. The Institute of Medicine (IOM, 1999) released a study revealing that as many as ninety-eight thousand of the thirty-three million individuals hospitalized each year die, and many more receive hospital-acquired infections because of poor-quality health care while hospitalized.

We must assume that health care workers do not deliberately injure their patients. Most who enter the health care employment sector do so because they want to help other people, not to hurt them or cause their death. That so many medical errors occur suggests that the health care system must be reengineered to eliminate these unnecessary errors. We must therefore devote time to understanding from a system perspective how the errors occur. We then need to empower our employees to help in the process. Because health services are provided primarily by individuals, the solution to the problem of medical errors is a very human one.

The IOM (1999) points out that 60 percent of events that could harm patients in the emergency room are the result of human errors. A closer examination revealed that many of these events were the result of "human intervention errors," such as not recording the time when medications were administered or failing to plug in a medical device. These errors represent a system breakdown involving human errors that affect patients. This problem can only be resolved by health care workers' resolving to work as a team and demanding zero medical errors and secondary infections within their facility. This is an unbelievable challenge for the staff, but it can be met with leadership, teamwork, and innovation in the process of providing care.

Spear (2009) argues that the old approaches to health care delivery must be changed to more sophisticated approaches that improve when problems are discovered. This is exactly the strategy that needs to be followed when dealing with the problem areas that are known to frequently result in medical errors. This feat can only be achieved when all of the health care staff stop working around the problem of medical errors and redesign the work process as soon as problems are discovered. Spear asserts that medical facilities should use the same process followed by Paul O'Neill at Alcoa when that company faced an epidemic of safety issues. As discussed in earlier chapters, the process instituted by Alcoa represented a reengineering effort that included the immediate reporting of safety issues (within twenty-four hours) to senior managers, including the CEO. Safety problems were to be swarmed at the time and place where they occurred, the work process was then to be redesigned to eliminate these issues, and the results of this effort were to be immediately shared with the entire organization. To eliminate the dangers of health care delivery there will need to be a change in the culture of the health care facility, which will require empowerment and a team approach from health care practitioners, insurance companies, health care managers, and consumers, all of whom must demand effective and error-free medical care.

Once we are successful in keeping our patients safe from medical errors, we can then begin to reengineer our staff to keep patients happy and satisfied with their experience at the health care facility. This same process of swarming problem areas can be used with all types of issues pertaining to the quality of care. Once the issue is identified and a solution formulated by those who deliver services, the process can be reengineered to eliminate the problem.

The empowerment of workers and teams in health care delivery requires team members not only to apply their expertise to resolve errors at the moment they occur but also to share the event with team members; further, team members must accept that they are accountable for each other's individual actions. This will require considerable trust and confidence among team members and their immediate supervisors.

According to Dlugacz (2010), we have slowly been moving from a treatment-focused approach to a patient-focused approach to the delivery of health care in an attempt to bring the patient and his or her family into the health care delivery process. Many successful health care organizations are asking what the patient wants rather than concentrating on what the organization wants to offer. This is the way it is done in the business world, in which the consumer determines who is and is not successful by voting for the provider of choice with his or her purchases.

Dlugacz (2010) points out that the key to patient-focused care is effective communication between the one providing care and the consumer of this care. Patients have been expressing a desire to be involved in making decisions concerning their health care. They want a better understanding of what their health status is, why medical procedures are being done, what risks are associated with all of the tests being ordered, and what they should be doing to regain their health.

Another area in need of immediate change and reengineering is the epidemic of chronic diseases—and our lack of attention to, and ignorance about, this problem. Our health care system has faced and survived several disease epidemics over its many years of existence. These diseases were infectious diseases, better known as communicable diseases because they were spread from person to person. These diseases were also characterized by short incubation periods and the ability to be cured with antibiotics.

Today, however, our health care system is being forced to cope with chronic diseases, such as heart disease, diabetes, and many forms of cancer, that result from lifestyle choices. The relatively new epidemic of chronic diseases poses significant challenges for our health care system and the managers of the scarce resources available to deal with these diseases. We need to change our attitude of allowing disease to develop and then trying to cure the incurable. The focus needs to be on prevention rather than on the cure of disease.

According to Halvorson (2009), we need to have a culture of health that includes an agenda for the improvement of the health of the population. Managers and employees will have to begin their journey into culture building by spending a great deal of time focusing on the epidemic of chronic diseases, which can be reduced in incidence and prevalence only by the expansion of health education programs throughout the United States. By including prevention programs for chronic diseases, a health care facility can gain a competitive advantage in an industry searching for answers to escalating costs and diminishing outcomes in the delivery of health services.

The majority of health care organizations have been moved from the protection of monopoly power to the very dangerous environment of competition. Many health care facilities are fighting for their very survival as they face the realities of competing for customers, which is indeed new territory for most businesses that provide health services to Americans. These health care facilities have to gain business skills in a very short period of time, and the new knowledge acquired has to be shared and accepted by all members of the health care team. Many of the proactive health care organizations have already developed these business skills and have become convinced that they work. These health care facilities are very serious about winning the battle for superiority in health care delivery.

According to Spear (2009), a **competitive advantage** is created when organizations become excellent at consistently managing uncertainty in their work process. Health care reform has created this uncertainty. It seems as though overnight the entire health care arena has been transformed into an extremely competitive environment with nowhere for the weak organizations to hide. These entities must become **high-velocity organizations.** Spear (2009, pp. 22–27) argues that the most important capabilities of high-velocity organizations are

> *Capability 1:* Specifying design to capture existing knowledge and building in tests to reveal problems
>
> *Capability 2:* Swarming and solving problems to build new knowledge
>
> *Capability 3:* Sharing new knowledge throughout the organization
>
> *Capability 4:* Leading by developing capabilities 1, 2, and 3

These capabilities have not been present and encouraged in health care organizations because their implementation would require organizational change along with a great deal of expense. Improving quality in health care delivery therefore requires health care facilities to make a very serious effort in developing these capabilities. It is very important to keep in mind that health care involves the delivery of services by people to people and usually entails a team approach to the entire delivery process—and this is what makes organizational design and redesign so difficult. When you attempt to reengineer health care delivery, you must understand that all of the team players have to be included in the redesign process. Everyone involved in changing the system of health care delivery will also need a great deal of training. This requires change and commitment from the top to the bottom of the health care facility.

Health care organizations have become very complex in both their structure and their work process. The team has really become the focus of the delivery of health care, incorporating many separate disciplines that need to work together in focusing on patient outcomes. Because there is such a high degree of interconnectedness in the delivery of many health services, special attention must be paid to the design of the work process.

The success of most high-velocity organizations is found in how individual managers and employees look at their organization. These individuals are capable of considering the work process as a whole system that consists of smaller subsystems designed to deliver a product or service to a final consumer. They do not see a number of separate pieces but rather a number of equally important pieces of a final process that exhibits quality as ultimately determined by the consumer. This is so very true in the process of delivering health services to a highly demanding and better-informed health care consumer. The media and the consumer are calling for transparency in the delivery of health services, a process that requires tremendous attention if it is to be improved. The greater use of advanced technology can help managers achieve this important goal.

In fact, Champy and Greenspun (2010) argue that a very large part of health care delivery today involves the use of sophisticated technology. This is certainly true, but it must be understood that technology in health care is only an adjunct or enabler of the delivery of services. The human component is still the most important to giving the consumer a quality experience. This human part of the process is determined by the human interactions among a team of professionals responsible for delivering care to a certain patient on a given day.

Greater use of technology along with motivated employees in high-velocity organizations will be very useful in helping develop solutions for two of the most important problem areas found in our health care system, medical errors and poor quality in health care delivery. One very important aspect of quality has to do with the fact that our health care system allows individuals with chronic diseases to go on and develop the complications from these diseases later in life. Both of these problems—medical errors and poor quality—are found in far too many health care facilities, and both result from process design flaws. To make the necessary changes in the design of health care organizations, managers and the employees who actually deliver the services to the consumer need to establish a unity of purpose. This shared purpose is the real key to fixing process design flaws and creating high-velocity organizations in health care. It is going to take universal commitment to leadership; employee empowerment; a thick, positive culture; and innovation in the delivery of health services. For example, Alcoa's emphasis on worker safety led to many additional improvements in product design and quality.

According to Spear (2009), focusing on safety problems at Alcoa revealed problems of process ignorance, which means that not all employees were able to understand the entire production process. Spear asserts that similar process ignorance can also be found in other organizational problems, such as those pertaining to quality. A large number of health care facilities still do not recognize the importance of the consumer in the determination of whether or not the health care delivery process in fact yields a quality experience. Lombardi and Schermerhorn (2007) argue that process reengineering includes seeking input from patients, fostering teamwork, and improving efficiency with a goal of redesigning health care delivery to better meet the needs and expectations of patients. The reengineering process also attempts to reduce the cost of health care delivery by increasing the efficiency of organizational operations. This is most easily accomplished by the health care manager and his or her team's concentrating on the elimination of wasted efforts. If a mistake is made, whether in the form of a medical error or a break in quality, it is evident that either the service was delivered incompletely or the process of delivering that service was misunderstood. This should never happen, and if it does it should be treated as a critical incident that requires immediate attention. The key is not to waste valuable time blaming individuals for the incident but to begin immediately to search for the cause, eliminate the error, and learn from the event. Spear (2009) points out that individuals in high-velocity organizations learn from and educate each other in a number of ways, such as by gleaning new information that is uncovered by swarming an incident or problem, discovering the cause, and then sharing it with everyone.

Champy and Greenspun (2010) argue that the reengineering process in health care must begin small and concentrate on a few areas. Then, once success is proven, this process can be expanded to encompass other areas as the success of the reengineering process in one part of health care facility becomes desired by other parts. It seems that success is capable of breeding additional success throughout the organization.

The long-term improvement of our health care system will require information systems, team-based care, and disease management programs (Lee & Mongan, 2009). It is argued that these three components will provide solutions to the many challenges health care organizations face throughout our country. If properly implemented, these components can help eliminate medical errors and improve the quality of health care delivery, while at the same time reducing the costs associated with health care. In fact, these components are already in place in many high-velocity organizations that are delivering excellent health care in our country—all health care managers need to do is learn from the health care facilities that have dealt successfully with major challenges and then begin the reengineering process in their own facility. Duplicating these success stories will require tremendous change in the vast majority of health care organizations in our country. This change, in the form of organizational reengineering efforts, is only possible with strong leadership and a culture that upholds the idea that to become the best at what you do, you have to develop a low tolerance for ambiguity in the work process and a desire not to work around problems but to solve them. In other words, the culture must support the required change.

THE ROLE OF LEADERSHIP IN REENGINEERING HEALTH CARE

There is no question that any major reengineering effort requires managers' constant involvement. This is especially true in the improvement of health services, which encompasses complicated issues of finance and medicine, multiple professions, and many ethical dilemmas. The organization's managers have the ultimate responsibility of shaping the work process and how services are delivered.

A reengineering effort in any industry requires the manager to come forth to begin this change process, provide the required training to make the process work, and then evaluate the success or failure of the reengineering effort. These individuals will need to provide transformational leadership that is capable of uniting all health care employees in the delivery of quality health services. There needs to be tremendous cooperation among all employees and agreement concerning the goals of the change process, which should be viewed as a learning experience for those directly involved in—and those responsible for managing—the delivery of health services. The vast majority of health care workers want to improve how they deliver health services but feel powerless to begin the change process. However, these employees now seem ready to respond to leadership that is designing the new world of health care.

Health care reform resulting from either legislation or market forces is demanding that health care facilities throughout our country implement and embrace transformational leadership to remain relevant. This leadership style cannot only be espoused by the leaders at the top of the health care facility, but rather must become part of health care managers and all lower-level employees. The process of delivering quality health services to customers requires that all employees develop and use leadership skills to be successful in the reengineering effort. This is not to say that we do not require managerial skills in delivering health services. Managers will always be needed in a health care facility, but the managers along with the other people responsible for delivering health services will all need to be leaders. The skills of a health care leader are necessary for the successful health care organization to go beyond the organizational mission to the development and implementation of a compelling vision. This long-term vision will require employees to willingly follow, not just to respond to the power wielded by the organization. All employees also must develop interpersonal skills to contribute to the constant improvement of health services as they communicate with customers, managers, and each other.

The health care manager is indeed going to be challenged as health care facilities rise and fall in facing the challenges and changes inherent in health care system reform. The changes, which have never been so important, are occurring with greater intensity on a daily basis. According to Goldsmith (2011), the major challenge to health care facilities involves reconstructing themselves to maximize their efficiency and effectiveness. They have to do this while minimizing stress and dissatisfaction among employees and consumers. This incredible task is going to require the power of leadership, which will need to be available from all employees who have been truly empowered by their superiors. This is why developing leadership skills must become a required component of the training of every health care employee.

Most health care employees are accustomed to working in a bureaucratic, top-down, hierarchical organization. However, a bureaucratic organizational structure does not work very well in uncertain times, rendering a health care organization unable to respond rapidly to the rapidly changing health care environment. This organizational structure must be flattened for a health care facility to meet consumers' demand for high-quality health services.

Health care managers need to recognize that their health care facility must prepare its employees not only to understand the value of change but also to exploit it. This is why true empowerment of all employees is an absolute requirement to be able to respond to the new consumer of health services. Further, to properly assume the responsibilities that come with empowerment, these employees must also develop and employ their leadership skills. By learning how to lead, employees are better prepared to accept and use empowerment to better serve their customers.

According to Wiseman and McKeown (2010), micromanagers control every aspect of work assignments, thereby forcing employees to wait for the manager to tell them what to do and when to do it. In their recent book *Multipliers* they discuss how the management techniques of a micromanager create free rider employees who sit back and wait for the boss to tell them how to complete their work. This is exactly what has happened in most health care facilities in our country. The health care sector of our economy has created numerous micromanagers who do not allow their employees to learn how to lead. These employees are prevented from trying new things, making mistakes, and learning from those mistakes.

For health care employees to become truly empowered to better serve their customers, they cannot be micromanaged. They have to be allowed to anticipate the needs and wants of their customers and to take the initiative to deliver that which the customer desires. They also need to receive the proper training in how to accept empowerment and must continue to develop both personally and professionally. The empowerment of workers, and the consequent development of leaders throughout the health care organization, result directly from the vision of the organization as well as the type of culture the organization has developed and nurtured.

THE IMPORTANCE OF ORGANIZATIONAL CULTURE IN REENGINEERING HEALTH CARE

As already argued, to make any reengineering effort work, the culture that is present in the organization must support the effort of changing the work process. The culture is capable of providing the ingredients that are so very important in organizational change, and in fact it has become one of the most important determinants of the success or failure of an organization over the long run.

A thick, positive, patient-centered culture devoted to the attainment of the vision of the health care facility must be developed and nurtured if the quality of health services and the outcomes associated with those services are to be improved. According to Connors and Smith (2011), organizations often have little time to make necessary changes once the need for these becomes apparent. This becomes even more serious when an organization does not want to change, and the leaders of the organization do not really understand the value of culture in the change process. Unfortunately, even today many health care facilities have not even considered the need for radical change in the ways in which they deliver services to their customers.

The manager is the key to culture building in a health care facility. It is sad that most health care managers in bureaucratic health care organizations have not gained a better understanding of the value of the organization's culture in making necessary change happen. Often they have not done so because they were too busy managing through power and control. It is therefore extremely important that the health care manager understand the value of culture and the role that it plays in enabling an organization to respond to the challenges of health care reform. In fact, the vast majority of successful managers believe that nurturing the organization's culture is one of the most important functions they perform on a daily basis (Schein, 2004).

According to Schein (2004), culture is the result of learning by a group concerning how things should be done in an organization. This learning process continues over a long period of time as employees come to know by trial and error what the organization considers valuable. This understanding of organizational values usually results from daily interactions between managers and employees as they go about their business of delivering quality health services to customers. The culture of the organization is a living and breathing component of an organization, whether or not the organization is successful. The successful business has a thick, positive culture directed toward serving the customer, whereas the unsuccessful businesses exhibits the opposite cultural components. An organization's culture simply becomes "the way things are done around here," and it can be positive or negative depending on the past experiences of the organization. If things are not going well, it is up to the team leader or manager to aid in the process of changing the culture. To improve the quality of health services, the health care manager has to learn through leadership skill development how to facilitate such change.

Schein (2004) points out that one of the most important duties of managers is to help create and manage the culture of an organization. This responsibility may include destroying and then rebuilding a culture that has become dysfunctional. Health care organizations do not have a great deal of time to change the existing culture in an attempt to deal with the challenges they face in responding to health care reform. Health care managers must therefore begin to develop and implement a culture of innovation in their health care organization. Stevenson and Kaafarani (2011) point out that everyone in this type of organization knows his or her role in the innovation process.

A culture of innovation is defined by how its people are treated. A bureaucratic organization does not provide the environment that is conducive to innovation, usually because there are rules and regulations in place that block the creativity of employees. This is where the successful health care manager needs to understand the value of the organization's most important resource, its people. The employees are central to an innovation-based culture, whereby health care teams use the skills and abilities of each employee to better serve their customers. Branson (2011) argues that innovation requires not only that very simple questions be asked by managers but also that the employees are given the resources and power to answer these questions. For example, Google attracts bright employees and then lets them use 20 percent of their time at work to explore any project that interests them. This is one example of a very successful company that gives its employees ownership of their work and workplace. Ownership is crucial in any effort to continually motivate talented individuals to learn and grow personally and professionally.

This culture of innovation is exactly what is required to solve the difficult problems facing the majority of health care organizations today. The health care manager needs to make use of the tremendous human resources available within the health care organization to discover the problems, break them down into their simplest components, and then solve them. This process has to become part of the culture of the modern health care organization—a culture that not only empowers employees but also encourages innovation in problem solving with no fear of failure.

CONSUMER EMPOWERMENT

A major component of the new world of health care reform is that health care organizations will have to become accountable for the use of scarce resources. There are several ways to make these organizations more transparent in regard to both the cost and the quality of the health services they deliver. A popular way to achieve this transparency is through the use of publicly available report cards on health care facilities throughout the country. These cards include information about cost and quality issues for a given health care organization and can be used by consumers when choosing a health care provider.

This empowerment of consumers is going to place an even greater emphasis on the production of value in health care for all providers of health services. This in turn will force health care managers to spend more time motivating workers toward quality improvement to stand up to the competition. The consumer of health services has always been a passive recipient of health care. This is rapidly changing with the introduction of electronic medical records, allowing the consumer a larger role in the health care process. The changing relationship between the health care consumer and the various providers of health services is going to require new processes in the delivery of care. According to Lombardi (2001), there is a real need for the use of imagination and ingenuity in the health care workplace. Lombardi's I-Formula, shown in Figure 14.1, represents a comprehensive approach to the development of creativity, which will entail new processes and problem solving in the workplace. This formula represents an excellent approach for health care facilities to take in dealing with the two major challenges of improving outcomes and increasing efficiency facing them in the next several years. It offers the health care manager a unique means of defining these challenges and developing a strategy to turn these problems into opportunities—and to turn the health care entity into a high-velocity organization.

The starting point for the I-Formula is a need, which should be determined by the consumer of health services. The need phase usually represents a tremendous opportunity for health care managers to determine exactly what the consumer wants in the health care experience, when he or she wants it, and how he or she wants it delivered. This need, as outlined by the consumer and the employees of the health care organization, can be looked at as an idea for how to deliver better-quality health care. One need that has already been identified by consumers is to receive safe and courteous health services.

The second phase of the formula involves the design of a plan to accomplish the goal that was set forth in the need phase of the formula. This design phase can be looked at as a time for creativity and innovation. The employees, with the help of their manager, will attempt to apply their expertise to develop an appropriate response to the need that was previously uncovered.

Figure 14.1   I-Formula: Conceptual Overview
Source: Lombardi, 2001, p. 242. Reprinted with permission of John Wiley & Sons, Inc.

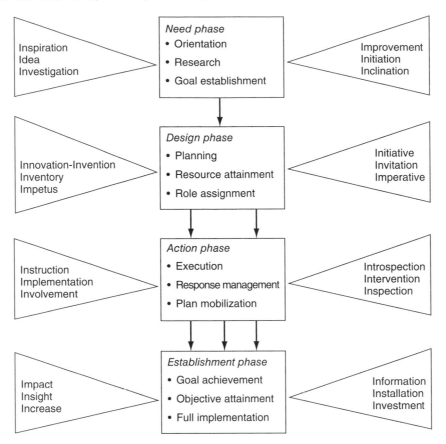

This phase is best handled with empowered and motivated employees who are determined to solve the problem posed in the need phase. The health care manager must understand that it is the employees who are capable of eliminating medical errors, improving the quality of the services delivered, and also reducing the costs associated with the delivery of these services by eliminating waste.

The third phase in this process involves the implementation of the action plan to meet the needs of the consumer. This action phase is usually going to require change in the work process that will involve most of the employees in the health care facility. This very important part of the I-Formula requires the health care manager to instruct his or her followers about their part in the change process. This is the most difficult part of the I-Formula because of the bureaucratic nature of health care organizations, which allows power to reside at the top. The health care manager must empower his or her employees to solve the problems in health care delivery as they occur and immediately share the solutions with everyone in the organization.

The final phase in this process involves the establishment of a strategy centered on long-term change for the organization. In this establishment phase the health care manager helps the employees understand that the change and improvement process will never end. The organization will only remain competitive if it develops a culture that continues to seek out and rapidly exploit opportunities for improvement. It is going to be a difficult task to motivate employees to improve when they believe that they are already the best. They have to realize that every time they improve it must be looked at as a learning process bringing them one step closer to greater improvement.

Unfortunately, many successful organizations begin to believe that they do not need to keep improving when they have beaten back their competition and become recognized as the best in their particular field. They seem incapable at this point in their growth phase of understanding that there is always a product life cycle, which means that at some time they will enter a maturity phase and then a decline phase in their expansion. They are not then prepared to deal with their competition by innovating and creating new services to again enter a growth phase in their product life cycle.

INNOVATION IN HEALTH CARE DELIVERY

To improve health care delivery, health care facilities need to respond to consumer demands for new ways of delivering health services. It is a well-known fact in most organizations that creativity and innovation cannot occur unless the climate is right. The right climate for innovation is usually one in which empowered employees are freed from normal responsibilities so they can be creative in the workplace. Bureaucratic management will have to be eliminated and replaced with an empowered workforce capable of instantly responding to consumer demands. The health care manager is going to be responsible for instilling the spirit of creativity and innovation in his or her employees to meet these new demands. It is an undeniable fact that the higher you move in an organization, the more removed you become from where the action is. This means that the manager who recognizes the need for innovation in health care delivery must figure out a way to connect with those close to the action—employees and customers—to discover what customers really want.

According to Stevenson and Kaafarani (2011), there are four levels of innovation: transformational, marketplace, category, and operational. Although all of these levels are important to every industry, the operational level of innovation is probably the most important for health care facilities during this time of rapid change and intense competition. This type of innovation concentrates on changing the organizational structure and the various processes that are required in the delivery of products and services to the customer. In the case of health services, this will necessitate the empowerment of those who deliver the services to improve the entire process of delivery—and therefore the customer experience—because of their expert insight into what the health care consumer really wants.

True innovation requires convincing individuals that they can accomplish things that they never knew were possible (Stevenson & Kaafarani, 2011). It requires the health care manager to open up his or her people to new discoveries of what can be accomplished in an open organization. These employees will thus be allowed to grow and develop on a daily basis, which in turn enables the health care organization to grow beyond anything that could previously have been imagined.

Stevenson and Kaafarani (2011) point out that there are four different styles of leadership, which correspond to the four levels of innovation just discussed, when it comes to the culture that supports creativity and innovation in the workplace. They include transformational leadership, category leadership, marketplace leadership, and operational leadership. The operational leader exhibits the characteristics that are vital to innovating and improving the quality of health care delivery. This leadership style brings rational thought to the process of innovation in the workplace. This is the way health care facilities must proceed as they attempt to reduce costs and improve the quality of the services delivered. Rational thinking makes it very evident that because much of what is done in health care places the patient at risk for medical errors, cutting back on the delivery of excessive medical care will reduce costs while increasing quality.

The health care manager functioning as the operational leader spends a great deal of time and energy discovering ways of solving complex problems, which is necessary for the elimination of medical errors and for stopping the spread of infections in health care facilities. Operational leaders also help build a strong culture that is dedicated to peak operational efficiency, which also includes improved quality at a reduced cost. For this style of leadership to be successful, a culture of innovation must be developed and nurtured that is fully dedicated to quality health care delivery. This is really what most health care employees and patients want from their health care facility.

This culture produces a team approach to problem solving that is vital to delivering consistent, quality health services with limited resources while always trying to improve the process. The health care manager has to lead this culture of innovation while allowing the staff to continue to learn and use new skills without working through layers of bureaucracy. The manager has to create an environment in which all members of the health care team respect each other and are eager to support and help their team members develop and grow. This culture recognizes that to achieve personal success, health care professionals need to be able to achieve success as a team.

In his new book *Prescription for Excellence: Leadership Lessons for Creating a World-Class Customer Experience from UCLA Health System*, Joseph Michelli (2011) discusses four areas of success that are critical to any business enterprise. These areas include "growing while maintaining quality, inspiring innovation while generating cohesion, balancing technological advances with humanity and achieving recognition and respect for extraordinary accomplishments" (p. 6). The first of these seems to hold particular significance for health care facilities that are attempting to grow in size to obtain economies of scale and reduce costs without losing a focus on quality. This becomes a very difficult task because many facilities have been unable to clearly define what quality means to their customers.

THE IMPORTANCE OF TRUST, BRAND, AND REPUTATION

In recent years it seems that the one thing that has been predictive of long-term success in organizations is a combination of trust, brand, and reputation. These are certainly the most important components for continued success found in organizations that provide services, especially health services. Consumer trust, brand loyalty, and the reputation of the organization are critical when an individual is making a decision to purchase health services that may very well determine his or her quality of life. The health care manager has to appreciate the significance of this fact and dedicate a great deal of time in tending to the never-ending process of improving trust, brand, and reputation.

As already discussed, there is a need to become consumer focused in the delivery of health services. This is where the development of trust, brand, and reputation comes into play. You cannot buy these ingredients, you have to earn them; and you have to recognize that one mistake can turn them against your health care facility. Trust and reputation have to be managed actively, and this responsibility will only increase in the future as consumers continue to exert their purchasing power (Diermeier, 2011). This is certainly the case in health care delivery as health care reform efforts change the way health care is delivered. Diermeier argues that the most important factors for an organization in maintaining the trust of its employees, customers, and community are transparency, expertise, commitment, and empathy. Trust, brand, and reputation are vital for a health care facility's growth and very survival in the unprotected world of competition. The health care manager is responsible for helping his or her employees excel at cultivating these factors by providing them with resources and appropriate training.

Transparency involves being honest with stakeholders at all times, especially when the health of patients is involved. Expertise is quite simply found in the fact that employees of the health care facility know what they are doing and are very capable of solving health care problems for their patients and the community. Commitment requires the involvement of managers and employees in attending to the issues that are most important to patients and community members. This factor becomes essential when the health care organization is facing a crisis situation, such as that caused by a medical error or an outbreak of illness within the health care facility. The last factor of great importance in building trust in the organization has to do with empathy, which must be present whenever a manager or employee addresses a problem in a health care facility. It involves a sincere expression of sorrow when things go wrong in the delivery of health services.

Branson (2011) points out that a brand is quite capable of communicating what benefits the product or service has to offer the consumer. The brand becomes a guarantee of what you can expect from the product or service based on previous purchases by different consumers. Maintaining a brand is highly important for the health care facility because word of mouth from previous purchasers of the same service can make or break the organization. This is demonstrated by many successful companies on a daily basis. For example, Southwest Airlines has included customer service as one of its top goals for the entire organization.

According to Blanchard and Barrett (2011), "Southwest Airlines has the following goals: to be the employer of choice, the provider of choice, and the investment of choice" (p. 30). Southwest Airlines depends heavily on trust and the reputation of the organization to be successful in the achievement of these goals. This company believes that its employees are its most important component. By treating employees with respect and earning their trust, Southwest Airlines ensures that these employees will then treat their customers with the same respect, thereby keeping customers' business. This in turn will ultimately produce the profits necessary to keep the investors happy.

Diermeier (2011) points out that the management of the organization's reputation needs to be incorporated into the company's strategy, organization, and culture. This daunting task needs to become one of the health care manager's major responsibilities. The reputation of the health care organization is so very important in attracting employees, customers, and investors because it is capable of separating the premier providers of health care from the rest of the providers. In fact, having a good reputation is quite often the major reason why a health care facility's market share increases.

OTHER SIGNIFICANT FORCES FACING THE HEALTH CARE MANAGER

The health care manager is obliged to confront many additional forces as we move through this new turbulent era of health care reform. There are employee challenges, along with significant environmental factors that are resulting in rapid, daily change. Several of these employee forces are covered in a book titled *The 2020 Workplace: How Innovative Companies Attract, Develop, and Keep Tomorrow's Employees Today* (Meister & Willyerd, 2010). The major forces covered in this text are shifting demographics; the growing importance of knowledge workers, who produce value through problem solving using creative skills; expanding information technology; and a culture of connectivity. Other areas of change covered in this book are medical tourism, which involves traveling to other countries for medical procedures that are less expensive there; issues surrounding end-of-life care; changing government regulations; and the globalization of the workforce. The most significant forces that will affect future health care managers seem to revolve around technology and people issues.

The Information Technology Revolution in Health Care Delivery

Our country is experiencing a revolution in information technology. There are significant costs involved in the increased use of technology in health care delivery, but most health care facilities believe that these are far outweighed by the benefits of expanding the use of information technology. Information technology offers the potential to improve outcomes, safety, and productivity in the delivery of health services, and therefore the quality of care. It seems self-evident that the efficient use of patient information by health care practitioners not only can make these professionals more efficient in their diagnosis and treatment of their patients but also can improve patient safety. If this is true, then expansion of the use of information technology may very well be the solution to a number of our most pressing problems.

Many of us who teach in the field of health services and research health care issues have usually defined the major problems in health care to be cost, access, health levels, and, recently, quality issues in the delivery of these very special services. In recent years many of us who study health care for a living have found that the primary problem has become insufficient information about health and health care delivery. This becomes evident when we consider the current epidemic of chronic diseases along with their very dangerous complications, useless and dangerous testing and medical procedures, along with the escalating problem of medical errors and hospital-acquired infections. These three preventable areas of concern are responsible for an extremely large percentage of the costs associated with health care delivery in our country. The one common solution to these expensive and often deadly problems is the rapid dissemination of quality information to both the consumers and providers of health services.

The major reason for adopting information technology for use in health care delivery is to improve the quality of patient care. Even though much more research, including cost-benefit analysis, is needed, the expansion of the use of information technology by both patients and providers of health care seems to be very promising as we all respond to the demands for reform. Some uses of information technology that benefit health care providers include electronic medical records, computerized physician order entry, bar coding, clinical decision support systems, and picture archiving and communication systems. There are many more available and proposed uses of information technology to improve patient care in our health care facilities.

Most consumers of health services are also going to benefit from the information technology revolution in the health care sector of our economy. Some improvements for the consumer are the availability of electronic patient records; electronic scheduling of appointments; electronic prescribing of prescriptions; e-mail access to physicians for simple advice; and, most important, the availability of reliable medical information about various medical conditions, including prevention information. Another area of potential benefit for consumers, especially if a patient has multiple chronic diseases, is the ability of information to be shared rapidly among multiple providers. This will also be useful when the patient is prescribed multiple drugs, which may be causing dangerous medical events.

There are also some very important drawbacks to the expansion of information technology in health care delivery. The first of these is, of course, the cost of purchasing and maintaining information technology tools for the health care facility or physician office. There will also be the necessity of expensive training programs in the use of new technology as well as the problem of resistance on the part of managers and employees to the change required to begin using this technology.

Another possible pitfall of the extensive use of information technology in health care was recently pointed out in the *New York Times*. An article titled "As Doctors Use More Devices, Potential for Distraction Grows" (Richtel, 2011) expressed concern in regard to the potential for health care employees to become distracted by information technology applications when they are delivering patient care. The article gave examples of several reports of health care providers talking on their cell phone and even sending text messages during very serious surgeries and other medical procedures.

People Issues

The most important component of the delivery of quality health services is the people delivering these services. There are numerous changes in the workforce whose members deliver health care in medical facilities throughout our country. How a manager handles these changes will be critical to his or her success or failure in overseeing the delivery of quality services to consumers. Meister and Willyerd (2010) argue that our country is faced with shifting workforce demographics, the emergence of knowledge workers, growing diversity, and a connective and participative workforce that produces our products and services. This changing workforce will present many challenges and opportunities for the health care manager, who must consider these various people issues as he or she attempts to forge a thick, positive culture capable of improving organizational output and the quality of the services the health care facility delivers.

SUMMARY

Health care managers must expand their understanding of leadership and of how to wield power and influence appropriately so that health care organizations can respond in a timely fashion to challenges posed by both competitors and consumers. Health care managers require new skills to learn and grow continually, and to respond to future challenges. These serious challenges for managers include the need to be proactive, to supply leadership and empowerment to their employees, to manage cultural change, to foster creativity and innovation among staff members, and to prepare their people for difficult economic issues and the epidemic of chronic diseases.

The entire health care industry is engaged in a massive reengineering effort that is designed both to reduce costs and to improve the quality of the services delivered. This unbelievable task is going to demand the best from everyone working in health care delivery. This effort will not succeed with the same old strategies and ways of doing business that have failed in the past. Health care workers need to unleash their creativity and innovation. This effort will also require a new type of health care manager who is dedicated to changing the way health care is delivered in our country.

Health care managers also should recognize the importance of trust, brand, and reputation to the long-term success of their organization. These organizational components are crucial in attracting employees, becoming the provider of choice, and ultimately becoming the investor of choice. They will all be mandatory for organizational success as we move into a very different world of health care delivery.

KEY TERMS

adaptation

competitive advantage

continuous quality improvement

high-velocity organizations

positive outcomes

productivity

value

REVIEW QUESTIONS

1. What is the most important health care management issue that needs to be confronted during the next few years? Explain.

2. To improve quality in health care delivery, health care facilities need to concentrate on changing their culture. What role does the health care manager play in the cultural change process?

3. How can a leader foster the development of creativity and innovation in the delivery of health services? Explain.

4. Explain the most important capabilities of high-velocity organizations. What role do these capabilities play in finding solutions to the major problems found in the delivery of health services today?

CHAPTER 1

Berry, L. L., & Seltman, K. D. (2008). *Management lessons from Mayo Clinic: Inside one of the world's most admired service organizations.* New York: McGraw-Hill.

Black, J., & Miller, D. (2008). *The Toyota way to healthcare excellence: Increase efficiency and improve quality with lean.* Chicago: Health Administration Press.

Buchbinder, S. B., & Shanks, N. H. (2007). *Introduction to health care management.* Burlington, MA: Jones & Bartlett.

Callahan, D. (2009). *Taming the beloved beast: How medical technology costs are destroying our health care system.* Princeton, NJ: Princeton University Press.

Champy, J., & Greenspun, H. (2010). *A manifesto for radically rethinking health care delivery.* Upper Saddle River, NJ: Pearson Education.

Chassin, M. R., Loeb, J. M., Schmaltz, S. P., & Wachter, R. M. (2010). Accountability measures—using measurement to promote quality improvement. *New England Journal of Medicine, 363,* 683–688. Retrieved from www.nejm.org/doi/full/10.1056/NEJMsb1002320

Collins, J. (2009). *How the mighty fall and why some companies never give in.* New York: HarperCollins.

Dlugacz, Y. D. (2010). *Value-based health care: Linking finance and quality.* Burlington, MA: Jones & Bartlett.

Drucker, P. F. (2010). *The practice of management.* New York: HarperCollins.

Dye, C. F. (2010). *Leadership in healthcare: Essential values and skills* (2nd ed.). Chicago: Health Administration Press.

Fottler, M. D., Ford, R. C., & Heaton, C. P. (2010). *Achieving service excellence: Strategies for healthcare* (2nd ed.). Chicago: Health Administration Press.

Fuchs, V. R. (1998). *Who shall live? Health, economics, and social choice* (Vol. 3, Expanded ed.). Hackensack, NJ: World Scientific.

Fuchs, V. R. (2009). Health reform: Getting the essentials right. *Health Affairs, 28,* 180–183.

Gittell, J. (2009). *High performance healthcare: Using the power of relationships to achieve quality, efficiency and resilience.* New York: McGraw-Hill.

Goldsmith, J. (2010). Healthcare IT's unfulfilled promise: What we've got here is failure to communicate. In Society for Healthcare Strategy and Market Development (Ed.), *Futurescan 2010: Healthcare trends and implications 2010–2015* (pp. 32–35). Chicago: Health Care Administration Press.

Griffith, J. R., & White, K. R. (2007). *The well-managed health care organization* (6th ed.). Chicago: Health Administration Press.

Halvorson, G. C. (2007). *Health care reform now: A prescription for change.* San Francisco: Jossey-Bass.

Halvorson, G. C. (2009). *Health care will not reform itself.* New York: CRC Press.

Hammer, M. (2007, April 1). The process audit. *Harvard Business Review*, *85*, 111–123.

Hsieh, T. (2010). *Delivering happiness: A path to profits, passion, and purpose*. New York: Business Plus.

Hwang, J., & Christensen, C. M. (2008). Disruptive innovation in health care delivery: A framework for business-model innovation. *Health Affairs*, *27*, 1329–1335.

Jacobson, G. A. (2007). *CRS report for Congress: Comparative clinical effectiveness and cost-effectiveness research; Background, history, and overview*. Retrieved from http://aging.senate.gov/crs/medicare6.pdf

Kaiser Family Foundation & Health Research & Educational Trust. (2010). *Employer health benefits: 2010 annual survey*. Retrieved from http://ehbs.kff.org/pdf/2010/8085.pdf

Langabeer, J. R. (2008). *Health care operations management: A quantitative approach to business and logistics*. Burlington, MA: Jones & Bartlett.

Lombardi, D. N. (2001). *Handbook for the new health care manager: Practical strategies for the real world*. San Francisco: Jossey-Bass.

Love, A., & Cugnon, M. (2009). *The purpose linked organization: How passionate leaders inspire winning teams and great results*. New York: McGraw-Hill.

Maxwell, J. C. (2004). *Today matters: 12 daily practices to guarantee tomorrow's success*. New York: Hachette Book Group.

Moon, Y. (2010). *Different: Escaping the competitive herd*. New York: Crown Business.

Mushlin, A., & Ghomrawi, H. (2010). Comparative effectiveness research: A cornerstone of healthcare reform. *Transactions of the American Clinical and Climatological Association*, *121*, 141–155.

Nussbaum, A., Tirrell, M., Wechsler, P., & Randall, T. (2010, March 24). Obamacare's Cost Scalpel. *Bloomberg Businessweek*. Retrieved from www.businessweek.com/magazine/content/10_14/b4172064340424.htm

Oberlander, J., & White, J. (2009). Systemwide cost control—the missing link in health care reform. *New England Journal of Medicine, 361,* 1131–1133.

Orszag, P. R., & Emanuel, E. J. (2010). Health care reform and cost control. *New England Journal of Medicine, 363,* 601–603.

Rae-Dupree, J. (2009, February 1). Disruptive innovation, applied to health care. *New York Times.* Retrieved from www.nytimes.com/2009/02/01/business/01unbox.html.

Remington, P. L., Brownson, R. C., & Wegner, M. V. (2010). *Chronic disease epidemiology and control* (3rd ed.). Washington DC: American Public Health Association.

Senge, P. M. (2006). *The fifth discipline: The art and practice of the learning organization.* Doubleday: New York.

Shenkar, O. (2010). *Copycats: How smart companies use imitation to gain a strategic edge.* Boston: Harvard Business Press.

Shi, L., & Singh, D. A. (2010). *Essentials of the U.S. health care system* (2nd ed.). Burlington, MA: Jones & Bartlett.

Shortell, S. M. (2010). Delivery system reform: Accountable care organizations and patient-centered medical homes. In Society for Healthcare Strategy and Market Development (Ed.), *Futurescan 2010: Healthcare trends and implications 2010–2015* (pp. 16–20). Chicago: Health Administration Press.

Spear, S. J. (2009). *Chasing the rabbit: How market leaders outdistance the competition and how great companies can catch up and win.* New York: McGraw-Hill.

Swayne, L. E., Duncan, J., & Ginter, P. M. (2008). *Strategic management of health care organizations* (6th ed.). San Francisco: Jossey-Bass.

Zenger, J. H., Folkman, J. R., & Edinger, S. K. (2009). *The inspiring leader: Unlocking the secrets of how extraordinary leaders motivate.* New York: McGraw-Hill.

CHAPTER 2

Abelson, R., & Singer, N. (2010). Pharmacists take larger role on health team. *New York Times*. Retrieved from www.nytimes.com/2010/08/14pharmacist.html

Atchison, T., & Carlson, G. (2009). *Leading healthcare cultures: How human capital drives financial performance*. Chicago: Health Administration Press.

Barton, P. L. (2010). *Understanding the U.S. health services system* (4th ed.). Chicago: Health Administration Press.

Beeret, A. (2009). *Leadership and change management*. Thousand Oaks, CA: Sage.

Berry, L. L., & Seltman, K. D. (2008). *Management lessons from Mayo Clinic: Inside one of the world's most admired service organizations*. New York: McGraw-Hill.

Blanchard, K. (2010). *Leading at a higher level*. Upper Saddle River, NJ: FT Press.

Borgatti, S. (1996). Bureaucracy. Retrieved from www.analytictech.com/mb201/bureau.htm

Branham, L., & Hirschfeld, M. (2010). *Re-engage*. New York: McGraw-Hill Professional.

Champy, J., & Greenspun, H. (2010). *Reengineering health care: A manifesto for radically rethinking health care delivery*. Upper Saddle River, NJ: Pearson Education.

Christensen, C. M., Grossman, J. H., & Hwang, J. (2009). *The innovator's prescription: A disruptive solution for health care*. New York: McGraw-Hill.

Dlugacz, Y. D. (2010). *Value-based health care: Linking finance and quality*. San Francisco: Jossey-Bass.

Dyck, B., & Neubert, M. (2009). *Management: Current practices and new directions*. Boston: Houghton Mifflin Harcourt.

Fottler, M. D., Ford, R. C., & Heaton, C. P. (2010). *Achieving service excellence: Strategies for healthcare* (2nd ed.). Chicago: Health Administration Press.

Gittell, J. H. (2009). *High performance healthcare: Using the power of relationships to achieve quality, efficiency and resilience.* New York: McGraw-Hill.

Goldsmith, S. B. (2011). *Principles of health care management: Foundations for a changing health care system* (2nd ed.). Burlington, MA: Jones & Bartlett.

Halvorson, G. C. (2009). *Health care will not reform itself.* New York: CRC Press.

Hamel, G. (2007). *The future of management.* Boston: Harvard Business Press.

Hammer, M. (2007, April 1). The process audit. *Harvard Business Review, 85,* 111–123.

Hammer, M., & Champy, J. (2003). *Reengineering the corporation: A manifesto for business revolution.* New York: HarperCollins.

Institute of Medicine. (2001). *Crossing the quality chasm: A new health system for the 21st century.* Washington DC: National Academies Press.

Institute of Medicine. (2003). *The future of the public's health in the 21st century.* Washington DC: National Academies Press.

Johnson, S. W. (2005). Characteristics of effective health care managers. *Health Care Manager, 24,* 124–128.

Kovner, A. R., Fine, D. J., & D'Aqila, R. (2009). *Evidence-based management in healthcare.* Chicago: Health Administration Press.

Lee, T. H., & Mongan, J. J. (2009). *Chaos and organization in health care.* Cambridge, MA: MIT Press.

Lepak, D., & Gowan, M. (2010). *Human resource management: Managing employees for competitive advantage.* Upper Saddle River, NJ: Prentice Hall.

Lombardi, D. M., & Schermerhorn, J. R., Jr. (2007). *Health care management: Tools and techniques for managing in a health care environment.* Hoboken, NJ: Wiley.

MacGillis, A. (2010, August 15). Are bigger health-care networks better or just creating a monopoly? *Washington Post.* Retrieved from www.washingtonpost.com/wp-dyn/content/article/2010/08/15/AR2010081503201_pf.html

Maslow, A. (1998). *Toward a psychology of being* (3rd ed.). Hoboken, NJ: Wiley.

McGregor, D. (1957). The human side of enterprise. *Management Review,* *46*(11), 22–28, 89–92.

Muzio, E. (2010). *Make work great: Supercharge your team, reinvent the culture, and gain influence—one person at a time.* New York: McGraw-Hill Professional.

Pyzdek, T., & Keller, P. (2010). *The Six Sigma handbook* (3rd ed.). New York: McGraw-Hill.

Schermerhorn, J. R., Jr. (2010). *Exploring management* (2nd ed.). Hoboken, NJ: Wiley.

Shi, L., & Singh, D. A. (2010). *Essentials of the U.S. health care system.* Burlington, MA: Jones & Bartlett.

Shortell, S. M., & Kaluzny, A. D. (2006). *Health care management: Organization design and behavior* (5th ed.). Clifton Park, NY: Delmar Cengage Learning.

Summer, D. C. (2011). *Lean Six Sigma: Process improvement tools and techniques.* Upper Saddle River, NJ: Pearson Education.

Swayne, L. E., Duncan, J., & Ginter, P. (2008). *Strategic management of health care organizations* (6th ed.). San Francisco: Jossey-Bass.

Taylor, F. W. (n.d.). The principles of scientific management. Retrieved from www.marxists.org/reference/subject/economics/taylor/principles/index.htm

Thomas, R. K. (2010). *Marketing health services* (2nd ed.). Chicago: Health Administration Press.

Williams, S., & Torrens, P. (2008). *Introduction to health services* (7th ed.). Clifton Park, NY: Delmar Cengage Learning.

CHAPTER 3

Crabtree, A. D., & DeBusk, G. K. (2008). The effects of adopting the balanced scorecard on shareholder returns. *Advances in Accounting, 24*(1), 8–15.

Drucker, P. F. (1974). *Management: Tasks, responsibilities, practice.* New York: Harper & Row.

Hodge, B. J., Anthony, W. P., & Gales, L. M. (2003). *Organization theory: A strategic approach* (6th ed.). Upper Saddle River, NJ: Prentice Hall.

Kaplan, R. S., & Norton, D. P. (2000). *The strategy focused organization.* Boston: Harvard Business Press.

Miles, R. E., & Snow, C. C. (1978). *Organizational strategy, structure, and process.* New York: McGraw-Hill.

Niven, P. R. (2008). *Balanced scorecard step-by-step for government and nonprofit agencies* (2nd ed.). Hoboken, NJ: Wiley.

Olden, P. C., Roggenkamp, S. D., & Luke, R. D. (2002). A post-1990s assessment of strategic hospital alliances and their marketplace orientations: Time to refocus. *Health Care Management Review, 27*(2), 33–49.

Porter, M. E. (1980). *Competitive strategy.* New York: Free Press.

Porter, M. E. (2008). *On competition* (Updated and expanded ed.). Boston: Harvard Business Press.

Porter, M. E., & Teisberg, E. O. (2004, June 1). Redefining competition in health care. *Harvard Business Review, 82,* 64–76.

Swayne, L. E., Duncan, W. J., & Ginter, P. M. (2008). *Strategic management of health care organizations* (6th ed.). Hoboken, NJ: Wiley.

Thompson, A. A., Jr., Gamble, J. E., & Strickland, A. J., III. (2008). *Crafting and executing strategy: The quest for competitive advantage; Concepts and cases* (17th ed.). New York: McGraw-Hill/Irwin.

CHAPTER 4

Altman, D. E., Clancy, C., & Blendon, R. J. (2004). Improving patient safety—five years after the IOM report. *New England Journal of Medicine, 351,* 2041–2043. doi:10.1056/NEJMp048243

Barnard, C. I. (1938). *The functions of the executive.* Cambridge, MA: Harvard University Press.

Barrett, D. J. (2011). *Leadership communication* (3rd ed.). New York: McGraw-Hill.

Berry, L. L., & Seltman, K. D. (2008). *Management lessons from Mayo Clinic: Inside one of the world's most admired service organizations.* New York: McGraw-Hill.

Blanchard, K. (2009). *Leading at a higher level.* Upper Saddle River, NJ: FT Press.

Bolden, R., Hawkins, B., Gosling, J., & Taylor, S. (2011). *Exploring leadership: Individual, organizational and societal perspectives.* New York: Oxford University Press.

Brownlee, S. (2007). *Overtreated: Why too much medicine is making us sicker and poorer.* New York: Bloomsbury USA.

Buchbinder, S. B., & Shanks, N. H. (2007). *Introduction to health care management.* Burlington, MA: Jones & Bartlett.

Burns, J. M. (1978). *Leadership.* New York: Harper & Row.

Champy, J., & Greenspun, H. (2010). *Reengineering health care: A manifesto for radically rethinking health care delivery.* Upper Saddle River, NJ: Pearson Education.

Dolan, T. C. (2010, September/October). Leadership skills for healthcare reform. *Healthcare Executive, 25,* 6.

DuBrin, A. J. (2007). *Leadership: Research findings, practice, and skills* (5th ed.). Boston: Houghton Mifflin.

Duhigg, C. (2012). *The power of habit: Why we do what we do in life and business*. New York: Random House.

Dye, C., & Garman, A. N. (2006). *Exceptional leadership: 16 critical competencies for healthcare executives*. Chicago: Health Administration Press.

Emanuel, E. J. (2008). *Healthcare, guaranteed: A simple, secure solution for America*. New York: Public Affairs.

Fiedler, F. E. (1967). *A theory of leadership effectiveness*. New York: McGraw-Hill.

Fottler, M. D., Ford, R. C., & Heaton, C. P. (2010). *Achieving service excellence: Strategies for healthcare* (2nd ed.). Chicago: Health Administration Press.

Greenleaf, R. K. (1996). *On becoming a servant-leader: The private writings of Robert K. Greenleaf* (D. M. Frick & L. C. Spears, Eds.). San Francisco: Jossey-Bass.

Hamel, G. (2007). *The future of management*. Boston: Harvard Business Press.

Hesselbein, F., & Shrader, A. (2008). *Leader to leader: Enduring insights on leadership*. San Francisco: Jossey-Bass.

Hickman, G. R. (1998). *Leading organizations: Perspectives for a new era*. Thousand Oaks, CA: Sage.

Institute of Medicine (IOM). (1999). *To err is human*. Washington DC: National Academies Press.

Kenney, C. (2008). *Best practice: How the new quality movement is transforming medicine*. New York: Public Affairs.

Kotter, J., & Heskett, J. (1992). *Corporate culture and performance*. New York: Free Press.

Ledlow, G. R., & Coppola, N. (2011). *Leadership for health care professionals: Theory, skills, and applications*. Burlington, MA: Jones & Bartlett.

Lighter, D. E. (2011). *Advanced performance improvement in health care principles and methods.* Burlington, MA: Jones & Bartlett.

Lombardi, D. M., & Schermerhorn, J. R., Jr. (2007). *Health care management: Tools and techniques for managing in a health care environment.* Hoboken, NJ: Wiley.

Lussier, R. N., & Achua, C. F. (2010). *Leadership: Theory, application and skill development* (4th ed.). Mason, OH: South-Western.

Malandro, L. (2009). *Fearless leadership: How to overcome behavioral blind spots and transform your organization.* New York: McGraw-Hill.

McGregor, D. (1960). *The human side of enterprise.* New York: McGraw-Hill.

Northouse, P. G. (2010). *Leadership: Theory and practice* (5th ed.). Thousand Oaks, CA: Sage.

Pierce, J. L., & Newstrom, J. W. (2008). *Leaders and the leadership process: Readings, self-assessments and applications* (5th ed.). New York: McGraw-Hill.

Rice, C. (2007). Four priorities: Build bonds with stakeholders. *Leadership Excellence, 24*(3), 15.

Sanders, D. J. (2008). *Built to serve: How to drive the bottom line with people-first practices.* New York: McGraw-Hill.

Schein, E. H. (2004). *Organizational culture and leadership* (3rd ed.). San Francisco: Jossey-Bass.

Senge, P. (2006). *The fifth discipline: The art and practice of the learning organization.* New York: Random House.

Sultz, H. A., & Young, K. M. (2011). *Health care in the USA: Understanding its organization and delivery* (7th ed.). Burlington, MA: Jones & Bartlett.

Thompson, M. (2009). *The organizational champion: How to develop passionate change agents at every level.* New York: McGraw-Hill.

Toussaint, J. (2010). *On the mend.* Cambridge, MA: Lean Enterprise Institute.

Trompenaars, F., & Voerman, E. (2010). *Servant leadership across cultures.* New York: McGraw-Hill.

Yukl, G. A. (1989). *Leadership in organizations* (2nd ed.). Upper Saddle River, NJ: Prentice Hall.

Zenger, J. H., Folkman, J. R., & Edinger, S. K. (2009). *The inspiring leader: Unlocking the secrets of how extraordinary leaders motivate.* New York: McGraw-Hill.

CHAPTER 5

Bennis, W. (2009). *On becoming a leader.* New York: Perseus Book Group.

Bennis, W., Goleman, D., & O'Toole, J. (2008). *Transparency: How leaders create a culture of candor.* San Francisco: Jossey-Bass.

Cameron, K. S., & Quinn, R. E. (2011). *Diagnosing and changing organizational culture: Based on the competing values framework.* San Francisco: Jossey-Bass.

Champy, J., & Greenspun, H. (2010). *Reengineering health care: A manifesto for radically rethinking health care delivery.* Upper Saddle River, NJ: Pearson Education.

Chesbrough, H. (2011). *Open service innovation: Rethinking your business to grow and compete in a new era.* San Francisco: Jossey-Bass.

Christensen, C. M., Grossman, J. H., & Hwang, J. (2009). *The innovator's prescription: A disruptive solution for health care.* New York: McGraw-Hill.

Conant, D., & Norgaard, M. (2011). *Touch points: Creating powerful leadership connections in the smallest of moments.* San Francisco: Jossey-Bass.

Conway, S., & Steward, F. (2009). *Managing and shaping innovation.* New York: Oxford University Press.

Dyer, J., Gregersen, H., & Christensen, C. M. (2011). *The innovator's DNA: Mastering the five skills of disruptive innovators.* Boston: Harvard Business Press.

Fullan, M. (2011). *Change leader: Learning to do what matters most*. San Francisco: Jossey-Bass.

Gallo, C. (2011). *The innovation secrets of Steve Jobs: Insanely different principles for breakthrough success*. New York: McGraw-Hill.

Hamel, G. (2007). *The future of management*. Boston: Harvard Business Press.

Holstein, W. J. (2011). *The next American economy*. New York: Walker.

Hwang, J., & Christensen, C. M. (2008). Disruptive innovation in health care delivery: A framework for business-model innovation. *Health Affairs, 27*, 1329–1335.

Institute of Medicine. (2003). *The future of the public's health in the 21st century*. Washington DC: National Academies Press.

Locke, E., & Latham, G. (1984). *Goal setting: A motivational technique that works*. Englewood Cliffs, NJ: Prentice Hall.

Lombardi, D. N. (2001). *Handbook for the new health care manager* (2nd ed.). San Francisco: Jossey-Bass.

Lombardi, D. M., & Schermerhorn, J. R., Jr. (2007). *Health care management: Tools and techniques for managing in a health care environment*. Hoboken, NJ: Wiley.

Marciano, P. L. (2010). *Carrots and sticks don't work: Build a culture of employee engagement with the principle of respect*. New York: McGraw-Hill.

Michelli, J. A. (2011). *Prescription for excellence: Leadership lessons for creating a world-class customer experience from UCLA Health System*. New York: McGraw-Hill.

Pink, D. H. (2009). *Drive: The surprising truth about what motivates us*. New York: Riverhead Books.

CHAPTER 6

Anderson, D., & Anderson, L. (2010). *Beyond change management: How to achieve breakthrough results through conscious change leadership*. San Francisco: Pfeiffer.

Becker, E. F., & Wortmann, J. (2009). *Mastering communication at work: How to lead, manage, and influence*. New York: McGraw-Hill.

Berry, L. L., & Seltman, K. D. (2008). *Management lessons from Mayo Clinic: Inside one of the world's most admired service organizations*. New York: McGraw-Hill.

Burchell, M., & Robin, J. (2011). *The great workplace: How to build it, how to keep it, and why it matters*. San Francisco: Jossey-Bass.

Champy, J., & Greenspun, H. (2010). *Reengineering health care: A manifesto for radically rethinking health care delivery*. Upper Saddle River, NJ: Pearson Education.

Connors, R., & Smith, T. (2011). *Change the culture, change the game*. New York: Penguin Group.

Conway, S., & Steward, F. (2009). *Managing and shaping innovation*. New York: Oxford University Press.

Duhigg, C. (2012). *The power of habit: Why we do what we do in life and business*. New York: Random House.

Emanuel, E. J. (2008). *Healthcare, guaranteed: A simple, secure solution for America*. New York: Public Affairs.

Gittell, J. (2009). *High performance healthcare: Using the power of relationships to achieve quality, efficiency and resilience*. New York: McGraw-Hill.

Hamm, J. (2012). *Unusually excellent: The necessary nine skills required for the practice of great leadership*. San Francisco: Jossey-Bass.

Institute of Medicine (IOM). (1999). *To err is human*. Washington DC: National Academies Press.

Kouzes, J., & Posner, B. (2010). *The truth about leadership: The no-fads, heart-of-the-matter facts you need to know*. San Francisco: Jossey-Bass.

Lee, T., & Mongan, J. (2009). *Chaos and organization in health care*. Cambridge: MIT Press.

Leinwand, P., & Mainardi, C. (2010). *The essential advantage: How to win with a capabilities-driven strategy*. Boston: Harvard Business Press.

Li, C. (2010). *Open leadership: How social technology can transform the way you lead*. San Francisco: Jossey-Bass.

Lombardi, D. M., & Schermerhorn, J. R., Jr. (2007). *Health care management: Tools and techniques for managing in a health care environment*. Hoboken, NJ: Wiley.

Pink, D. H. (2009). *Drive: The surprising truth about what motivates us*. New York: Riverhead Books.

Porter, M. E. (2010, December 6). What is value in health care? *New England Journal of Medicine, 363,* 2477–2481.

Sarver, K. (2010). Medicare hospital patients face 25% chance of adverse event. *American Medical News.* Retrieved from www.ama-assn.org/amednews/2010/12/06/gvsc1206.htm

Schein, E. H. (2004). *Organizational culture and leadership* (3rd ed.). San Francisco: Jossey-Bass.

Schimpff, S. (2012). *The future of health care delivery: Why it must change and how it will affect you*. Washington DC: Potomac Books.

Senge, P. M. (2006). *The fifth discipline: The art and practice of the learning organization*. New York: Doubleday.

Szollose, B. (2011). *Liquid leadership: From Woodstock to Wikipedia*. Austin, TX: Greenleaf.

Tracy, B. (2010). *How the best leaders lead*. New York: American Management Association.

Wennberg, J. E. (2010). *Tracking medicine: A researcher's quest to understand health care*. New York: Oxford University Press.

Zenger, J. H., Folkman, J. R., & Edinger, S. K. (2009). *The inspiring leader: Unlocking the secrets of how extraordinary leaders motivate*. New York: McGraw-Hill Professional.

CHAPTER 7

Avakian, L. (2011). Retrieved from www.hhnmag.com

Barsukiewicz, C. K., Raffel, M. W., & Raffel, N. K. (2010). *The U.S. health system: Origins and functions* (6th ed.). Clifton Park, NY: Delmar Cengage Learning.

Champy, J., & Greenspun, H. (2010). *Reengineering health care: A manifesto for radically rethinking health care delivery.* Upper Saddle River, NJ: Pearson Education.

Council on Ethical and Judicial Affairs. (2008). Section 1.02: The relation of law and ethics. In *Code of medical ethics of the American Medical Association* (2008–2009 ed.). Chicago: American Medical Association.

Falcone, R. E., & Satiani, B. (2008). Physician as hospital chief executive officer. *Vascular and Endovascular Surgery, 42,* 88–94.

Feldstein, P. J. (2012). *Health economics* (7th ed.). Clifton Park, NY: Delmar Cengage Learning.

Huff, C. (2010, April). Are your docs management ready? *Hospitals and Health Networks.* Retrieved from http://www.hhnmag.com/hhnmag_app/jsp/articledisplay.jsp?dcrpath=HHNMAG/Article/data/04APR2010/1004HHN_Coverstory&domain=HHNMAG

Leatt, P. (1994). Physicians in health care management *in* Physicians as managers: Roles and future challenges. *Canadian Medical Association Journal, 150*(2), 171–176.

Lee, T. H., & Mongan, J. J. (2009). *Chaos and organization in health care.* Cambridge, MA: MIT Press.

Lombardi, D. N. (2001). *Handbook for the new health care manager* (2nd ed.). San Francisco: Jossey-Bass.

Schwartz, R., Pogge, C., Gilles, S., & Halsinger, J. (2000). Programs for the development of physician leaders: A curriculum process in its infancy. *Academic Medicine, 75,* 133–140.

CHAPTER 8

Aversa, J. (2010, January 5). Americans' job satisfaction falls to record low. Retrieved from http://news.yahoo.com/s/ap/20100105/ap_on_bi_ge/us_unhappy_workers/print

Bohlander, G., & Snell, S. (2010). *Managing human resources* (15th ed.). Mason, OH: South-Western.

Bureau of Labor Statistics. (2011, January). Union members summary. Retrieved from http://data.bls.gov/cgi-bin/print.pl/news.release/union2.nr0.htm

Carver, L., & Candela, L. (2008). Attaining organizational commitment across different generations of nurses. *Journal of Nursing Management, 16,* 984–991.

Cohn, K. H., Bethancourt, B., & Simington, M. (2009). The lifelong iterative process of physician retention. *Journal of Healthcare Management, 54,* 220–226.

Cozzetto, D. A., & Pedeliski, T. B. (1997). Privacy and the workplace: Technology and public employment. *Public Personnel Management, 26,* 515–527.

Drew, M., & Garrahan, K. (2005). Whistleblower protection for nurses and other health care professionals. *Journal of Nursing Law, 10,* 79–87.

Flynn, W. J., Mathis, R. L., & Jackson, J. H. (2007). *Healthcare human resource management* (2nd ed.). Mason, OH: Thomson/South-Western.

Hill, T. (2010, February). Whistleblowing: The patient or the paycheck? *Kansas Nurse, 85*(2), 4–8.

Kossman, S., & Scheidenhelm, S. (2008). Nurses' perceptions of the impact of electronic health records on work and patient outcomes. *CIN: Computers, Informatics, Nursing, 26,* 69–77.

Labor law: Nursing home RN's, LPN's are supervisors, use independent judgment to direct, discipline other employees. (2006, June). *Legal Eagle Eye Newsletter for the Nursing Profession,* p. 8.

Lewis, T. B., & Dambeck, A. B. (2005). Restrictive covenants in a physician's employment agreement: The New Jersey example. *Employee Relations Law Journal, 31*(3), 12–27.

Linzer, M., Konrad, T. R., Douglas, J., McMurray, J. E., Pathman, D. E., Williams, E. S., et al. (2000). Managed care, time pressure and physician job satisfaction: Results from the physician worklife study. *Journal of General Internal Medicine, 15,* 441–450.

Lyncheski, J. E., & Garrett, L. L. (2006, August). Update on DOL's regulations for employee exemption. *Nursing Home Magazine,* pp. 40–43.

Moushon, M. A., & Asher, G. E. (2007). Preventing wrongful discharge: Know your facts. *Nursing Management, 38*(6), 18, 20, 22, 62.

Muchinsky, P. M. (2009). *Psychology applied to work* (9th ed.). Summerfield, NC: Hypergraphic.

National Labor Relations Board (NLRB). (2011a). Employer/union rights and obligations. Retrieved from www.nlrb.gov/rights-we-protect/employerunion-rights-obligations

National Labor Relations Board (NLRB). (2011b). Rights we protect. Retrieved from www.nlrb.gov/rights-we-protect

National Labor Relations Board (NLRB). (2011c). What we do. Retrieved from www.nlrb.gov/what-we-do

National Labor Relations Board (NLRB). (2011d). Who we are. Retrieved from www.nlrb.gov/who-we-are

Noe, R. A., Hollenbeck, J. R., Gerhart, B., & Wright, P. M. (2004). *Fundamentals of human resource management.* New York: McGraw-Hill.

No-solicitation rule: Court says employer's actual practices discriminated against labor union. (2006, November). *Legal Eagle Eye Newsletter for the Nursing Profession,* p. 5.

Steingold, F. S. (2007). *The employer's legal handbook* (8th ed.). Berkeley, CA: Nolo.

Strode, R., & Beith, C. (2009, July). Something old is something new again: Structuring physician practice acquisitions. *Health Care Financial Management, 63*(7), 78–82.

Toland, B. (2009, July 6). Mandatory overtime for nurses now banned in PA. *Pittsburg Post-Gazette.* Retrieved from www.post-gazette.com/pg/09187/982038–28.stm

U.S. Census Bureau. (2011, November). *The older population: 2010.* doi: C2010BR-09

Wagner, C. M. (2007). Organizational commitment as a predictor variable in nursing turnover research: Literature review. *Journal of Advanced Nursing, 60,* 235–247.

Welton, J. M., Decker, M., Adam, J., & Zone-Smith, L. (2006). How far do nurses walk? *MEDSURG Nursing, 15,* 213–216.

Whistleblower lawsuit dismissed. (2008, June). *Legal Eagle Eye Newsletter for the Nursing Profession,* p. 6.

Whistleblower: Terminated staffer gets settlement. (2008, June). *Legal Eagle Eye Newsletter for the Nursing Profession,* p. 6.

Wrongful discharge: Employee refused to commit an illegal act, can sue for retaliation. (2009, January). *Legal Eagle Eye Newsletter for the Nursing Profession,* p. 2.

CHAPTER 9

About The Joint Commission. (2011, December 11). Retrieved from www.jointcommission.org/about_us/about_the_joint_commission_main.aspx

Berry, L. M. (2003). *Employee selection.* San Francisco: Wadsworth.

Bohlander, G., & Snell, S. (2010). *Managing human resources.* Mason, OH: South-Western.

Bureau of Labor Statistics. (2011, December). Economic news release. Retrieved from www.bls.gov/news.release/empsit.t08.htm

Croasdale, M. (2002). Practices must cope as more physicians work part-time hours. *American Medical News, 45,* 1–2.

Crow, S. M., Hartman, S. J., & McLendon, C. L. (2009). The realistic job preview as a partial remedy for nursing attrition and shortages: The role of nursing schools. *Journal of Continuing Education in Nursing, 40,* 317–323.

Danvers, K., & Nikolov, P. (2010). Does outsourcing affect hospital productivity? *Journal of Health Care Finance*, *37*(1), 13–29.

DerGuarahian, J. (2007). Emphasis on innovation. *Modern Healthcare*, *37*, 28–30.

DiLorenzo, L. P., & London, S. I. (2006). *Federal labor and employment laws* (7th ed.). Rochester, NY: WME Books.

Fallon, L. F., & McConnell, C. R. (2007). *Human resource management in health care: Principles and practice*. Burlington, MA: Jones & Bartlett.

Flynn, W. J., Mathis, R. L., & Jackson, J. H. (2007). *Healthcare human resource management* (2nd ed.). Mason, OH: Thomson South-Western.

Fried, B. J., & Fottler, M. D. (2011). *Fundamentals of human resources in health care*. Chicago: Health Administration Press.

Gatewood, R. D., Feild, H. S., & Barrick, M. (2008). *Human resource selection* (8th ed.). Mason, OH: South-Western.

Griggs v. Duke Power Co., 401 U.S. 424 (1971)

Hamric, A. B. (2005). *Advanced practice nursing: An integrative approach* (3rd ed.). St. Louis, MO: Elsevier Saunders.

Hauff, H. M. (2007). Where has all the staff gone? Strategies to recruit and retain quality staff. *Progress in Transplantation*, *17*(2), 89–93.

Health care staffing certification. (2010). Retrieved from www.jointcommission.org/assets/1/18/2010_Written_Documentation_Requirements.pdf

Heneman, H. G., & Judge, T. A. (2003). *Staffing organizations* (4th ed.). New York: McGraw-Hill.

Jones, C., & Gates, M. (2007). The costs and benefits of nurse turnover: A business case for nurse retention. *Online Journal of Issues in Nursing*, *12*(3). Retrieved from http://nursingworld.org/MainMenuCategories/ANAMarketplace/ANAPeriodicals/OJIN/TableofContents/Volume122007/No3Sept07/NurseRetention.html

Lewis, K., & Gardner, S. (2000). Looking for Dr. Jekyll but hiring Mr. Hyde: Preventing negligent hiring, supervision, retention, and training. *Hospital Topics: Research and Perspectives in Health Care, 78*(1), 14–22.

Mathis, R. L., & Jackson, J. H. (2009). *Human resource management: Essential perspectives.* Mason, OH: South-Western.

Moran, J. J. (2011). *Employment law* (5th ed.). Upper Saddle River, NJ: Prentice Hall.

Online help-wanted ads dipped in February, Conference Board reports. (2011, April). *HR Focus*, p. 10.

Phillips, J. M. (1998). Effects of realistic job previews on multiple organizational outcomes. *Academy of Management Journal, 41*, 673–690.

Recordkeeping guidance clarifies definition of "job applicant" for Internet and related technologies. (2004, March). Retrieved from www.eeoc.gov/eeoc/newsroom/release/3–3–04.cfm

Recruiting and marketing are top benefits of social media. (2010, January). *HR Focus*, pp. S1–S4.

Simon, A. B., & Alonzo, A. A. (2004). The demography, career pattern, and motivation of locum tenens physicians in the United States. *Journal of Healthcare Management, 49*, 363–375.

Steingold, F. S. (2007). *The employer's legal handbook* (8th ed.). Berkeley, CA: Nolo.

CHAPTER 10

Aguinis, H. (2009). *Performance management* (2nd ed.). Upper Saddle River, NJ: Prentice Hall.

Binns, C. (2009). CAVEman 3-D virtual patient is a holodeck for the human body. Retrieved from www.popsci.com/scitech/article/2009–06/our-bodies-our-holodecks

Blanchard, P. N., & Thacker, J. W. (2004). *Effective training: Systems, strategies, and practices* (2nd ed.). Upper Saddle River, NJ: Prentice Hall.

Bohlander, G., & Snell, S. (2010). *Managing human resources* (15th ed.). Mason, OH: South-Western.

Cohn, K. H., Bethancourt, B., & Simington, M. (2009). The lifelong iterative process of physician retention. *Journal of Healthcare Management, 54*, 220–226.

Dean, J. W., & Evans, J. R. (1994). *Total quality: Management, organization, and strategy*. Minneapolis, MN: West.

Deming, W. E. (1982). *Out of the crisis*. Cambridge, MA: MIT Center of Advanced Engineering Study.

Developing an e-learning package to provide chemotherapy updates. (2011, February). *Cancer nursing practice, 10*, 18–22.

Drucker, P. F. (1954). *The practice of management*. New York: HarperCollins.

Fallon, L. F., & McConnell, C. R. (2007). *Human resource management in health care: Principles and practice*. Burlington, MA: Jones & Bartlett.

Flynn, W. J., Mathis, R. L., & Jackson, J. H. (2007). *Healthcare human resource management* (2nd ed.). Mason, OH: Thomson South-Western.

Fox, A. (2009, January). Curing what ails performance reviews. *HR Magazine, 54*, 52–56.

Fried, B. J., & Fottler, M. D. (2011). *Fundamentals of human resources in healthcare*. Chicago: Health Administration Press.

Kerr, S. (1975). On the folly of rewarding A, while hoping for B. *Academy of Management Journal, 18*, 769–782.

Largest U.S. health insurer rewarded employees that cancelled coverage of sick patients. (2009, June). Retrieved from www.consumerwatchdog.org/newsrelease/largest-us-health-insurer-rewarded-employees-cancelled-coverage-sick-patients-consumer-w

Mathis, R. L., & Jackson, J. H. (2012). *Human resource management: Essential perspectives* (6th ed.). Mason, OH: South-Western.

Mills, J. F., & Mullins, A. C. (2008). The California mentor project: Every nurse deserves a mentor. *Nursing Economic$, 26*, 310–315.

Noe, R. A. (2010). *Employee training and development* (5th ed.). New York: McGraw-Hill.

Soltani, E., Van der Meer, R., Williams, T. M., & Pei-chun, L. (2006). The compatibility of performance appraisal systems with TQM principles—evidence from current practice. *International Journal of Operations & Production Management, 26*, 92–112.

Spurgeon, T. (2008). Multi-source feedback: The importance of enhanced self-reflection in the context of leadership competences. *International Journal of Clinical Leadership, 16*, 143–148.

Yellen, E., Davis, G. C., & Ricard, R. (2002). The measurement of patient satisfaction. *Journal of Nursing Care Quality, 16*, 23–29.

CHAPTER 11

About AMA: Statement of ethics. (2008). Retrieved from www.marketingpower.com/AboutAMA/Pages/Statement%20of%20Ethics.aspx

Anderson, J., & Albritton, K. (2011). Impatient patients. *Marketing Health Services, 31*(1), 6–7.

Austin, J. D., & Wilson, K. (2011). Prognosis: Convenience. *Marketing Health Services, 31*(3), 21–23.

American College of Healthcare Executives code of ethics. (2011). Retrieved from www.ache.org/ABT_ACHE/ACHECodeofEthics-2011.pdf

Beach Thielst, C. (2011). Using social media to engage patients. *Healthcare Executive, 26*(3), 66–70.

Bendinger, B., Maxwell, A., Barnes, B., Alessandri, S., Tucker, E., McGann, A., et al. (2009). *Advertising and the business of brands.* Chicago: The Copy Workshop.

Berkowitz, E. N. (2004). *Essentials of healthcare marketing.* Burlington, MA: Jones & Bartlett.

Binder, J. L., & Reeves, J. (2010). Bridging the generation gap. *Marketing Health Services, 30*(2), 22–25.

Blakeman, R. (2009). *The bare bones introduction to integrated marketing communication.* Lanham, MD: Rowman & Littlefield.

Brower, L. (2011). Care without compromise. *Marketing Health Services, 31*(2), 16–19.

Burke, T. R., & Goldstein, G. (2010). A legal primer for social media. *Marketing Health Services, 30*(3), 30–31.

Chordas, L. (2010). The "We Fit" e-Nation. *Best's Review, 110*(12), 96.

Chordas, L. (2011). Looking up. *Best's Review, 112*(1), 16.

Dancer, M., Fisher, C., & Wilcox, I. (2011). Creating customer value: New horizons on the managed markets journey. *Pharmaceutical Executive, 31*(3), 86–90.

Davila, F. (2010). The unseen subsidization of health insurance contracting and pricing methodologies. *Physician Executive, 36*(5), 60–63.

Evangelista, W. S., & Poulin, M. (2009). The new sales force. *Pharmaceutical Executive, 29*(11), 25–28.

Feinberg, D. A. (2011). Why advertise . . . and why not? *Marketing Health Services, 31*(2), 3–5.

Fell, D. (2009). The new era of connected healthcare. *Marketing Health Services, 29*(4), 17–19.

Fisher, C., Wallace, M., & Wilcox, I. (2010). Tearing up the rule book. *Pharmaceutical Executive, 30*(2), 52–58.

Flory, M. (2011). Painting the town red. *Marketing Health Services, 31*(3), 24–29.

Fredricks, D. (2011). The decline of traditional healthcare marketing. *Marketing Health Services, 31*(3), 3–5.

Galloro, V. (2011). Uncertain times: But trends look good for hospital companies. *Modern Healthcare, 41*(10), 17.

Glenn, R. (2010). Growth in a parched economy. *Marketing Health Services, 30*(2), 10–13.

Gombeski, W. R., Britt, J., Wray, T., Taylor, J., Adkins, W., & Riggs, K. (2011). Spread the word. *Marketing Health Services, 31*(1), 22–25.

Gombeski, W. R., Rudy, D., Springate, S., & DePriest, P. (2010). Competency counts. *Marketing Health Services, 30*(2), 26–29.

Gombeski, W. R., Wray, T., & Blair, G. (2011). Prepare for the ambush. *Marketing Health Services, 31*(2), 24–28.

Gronlund, J. (2010). Doing more with less. *Marketing Health Services, 30*(1), 18–21.

Igaray, M., & MacCracken, L. (2011). Talking to my generation. *Marketing Health Services, 31*(1), 10–13.

Keefe, L. (2008). Marketing defined. *Marketing News, 42*(1), 28–29.

Kochman, D., & Calabria, K. (2011). Time for answers. *Marketing Health Services, 31*(4), 22–27.

Krauss, M. (2010). Writing the book on marketing healthcare IT. *Marketing News, 44*(5), 10.

Levy, P. (2011). A healthy relationship. *Marketing News, 45*(5), 6.

Lofgren, D. G., & Cantu, D. (2010). Thrive. *Marketing Health Services, 30*(3), 8–11.

Lowenstein, M. (1997). *The customer loyalty pyramid*. Westport, CT: Quorum Books.

Maceo, B. (2011). Think big. *Marketing Health Services, 31*(1), 26–31.

Mackesy, R., & Zupa, C. (2011). Ramping up robotics. *Marketing Health Services, 31*(4), 3–5.

McDaniel, C., & Gates, R. (2004). *Marketing research essentials*. Hoboken, NJ: Wiley.

Mickelberg, L. (2010). Mobile rising to become a digital channel leader. *Medical Marketing & Media, 45*(12), 31.

Moldenhauer, S. (2010). In defense of the battered sales rep. *Pharmaceutical Executive, 30*(7), 84–85.

Moldenhauer, S. (2011). Accelerated evolution. *Pharmaceutical Executive, 31*(2), 50–52.

Nelson, W. A., & Campfield, J. (2008). The ethics of hospital marketing. *Healthcare Executive, 23*(6), 44–45.

Orozco, J., Aisen, M., Limbaga, A., Waskul, D., & Waskul, G. (2011). A world-famous rehabilitation center strengthens its brand by redefining its future. *Marketing Health Services, 31*(1), 18–21.

Paton, N. E. (2010). A new marketing playbook. *Marketing Health Services, 30*(2), 8–9.

Renfrow, J. (2009). Healthcare marketing 2.0. *Response, 17*(5), 32–39.

Reyburn, D. (2010). Ambient advertising. *Marketing Health Services, 30*(1), 8–11.

Ricci, L. (2011). Spotlight on success. *Marketing Health Services, 31*(1), 14–18.

Riedman, P. (2008). A healthy approach. *Marketing News, 42*(12), 12.

Roberts, A. (2010). Tomorrow has arrived. *Marketing Health Services, 30*(2), 30–31.

Rooney, K. (2009). Consumer-driven healthcare marketing: Using the Web to get up close and personal. *Journal of Healthcare Management, 54*, 241–251.

Segbers, R. (2010). Go where the customers are. *Marketing Health Services, 30*(10), 22–25.

Simons, T. (2009). The future of healthcare marketing: Who's in charge? *Marketing Health Services, 29*(1), 32.

Snyder, L. (2012). American College of Physicians *Ethics Manual:* Sixth edition. *Annals of Internal Medicine, 156*(Suppl.), 73–104.

Solomon, S. (2010). Yours for a song. *Marketing Health Services, 30*(3), 28–29.

Solomon, S. (2011). Going mobile? *Marketing Health Services*, *31*(4), 28–29.

Spanbauer, J. (2010). Regional marketing, national growth. *Pharmaceutical Executive*, *30*(11), 94.

Squazzo, J. (2011). Creating a culture of engagement. *Healthcare Executive*, *26*(6), 18–26.

Stahl, S. (2010). Gentle collisions in marketing. *Pharmaceutical Executive*, *30*(12), 92–93.

Steblea, I., Steblea, J., & Poklea, J. (2009). Healthcare's best-kept secret. *Marketing Health Services*, *29*(4), 12–16.

Thomas, R. K. (2005). *Marketing health services*. Chicago: Health Administration Press.

Topin, A. (2011). Blame the driver, not the car. *Pharmaceutical Executive*, *31*(5), 88–90.

Weiss, R. (2010). What is your greatest marketing challenge? *Marketing Health Services*, *30*(3), 3–6.

Weiss, R. (2011). The quest for physician engagement. *Marketing Health Services*, *31*(2), 29–31.

Wilson, L. (2010). Equal pay: All-payer system favored, survey shows. *Modern Healthcare*, *40*(43), 24–25.

Yakubik, P. (2011). Healthcare reform makes marketing more critical. *Medical Marketing & Media*, *46*(6), 29.

CHAPTER 12

Baker, S. (2011). U.S. national health spending, 2009. Retrieved from http://sambaker.com/econ/classes/nhe09/

Borger, C., Smith, S., Truffer, C., Keehan, S., Sisko, A., Poisal, J., et al. (2006). Health spending projections through 2015: Changes on the horizon, *Health Affairs*, *25*, w63–w71.

CBO projects total healthcare spending to hit 26 percent of GDP by 2035. (2010). *Health Care Financial Management*, *64*(8), 9.

Centers for Disease Control and Prevention (CDC). (1999a). Ten great
    public health achievements—United States. *Morbidity and Mortality
    Weekly Report, 48*, 241–243.

Centers for Disease Control and Prevention (CDC). (1999b). Ten great
    public health achievements—United States. *Journal of the American
    Medical Association, 281*, 1481.

Centers for Medicare & Medicaid Services (CMS). (2005). *2005 annual
    report of the boards of trustees of the federal hospital insurance and federal
    supplementary medical insurance trust funds.* Retrieved from http://.cms.
    hhs.gov/publications/trusteesreport/tr2005.pdf

Centers for Medicare & Medicaid Services (CMS). (2009). The nation's
    health dollar ($2.5 trillion), calendar year 2009: Where it went.
    Retrieved from www.cms.gov/NationalHealthExpendData/downloads/
    PieChartSourcesExpenditures2009.pdf

Chantrill, C. (2011a). Federal expenditure—$3,819 bn—United States—
    2011. Retrieved from www.usgovernmentspending.com/downchart_
    gs.php?chart=10-fed&state=US&local=

Chantrill, C. (2011b). Health care US FY 1996 to FY 2016. Retrieved
    from www.usgovernmentspending.com/spending_chart_1996_2016US
    r_13s1li111mcn_10t

Chernichovsky, D., & Leibowitz, A. (2010). Integrating public health and
    personal care in a reformed US health care system. *American Journal of
    Public Health, 100*(2), 205–211.

Cutler, N. (2010). Health insurance report from pre-1965 to post-2010.
    Journal of Financial Service Professionals, 64(4), 24–28.

Darling, H. (2010). US health care costs: The crushing burden.
    Information Knowledge Systems Management, 8, 87–104.

Davis, S., & Robinson, P. (2010). Health care providers under pressure:
    Making the most of challenging times. *Journal of Health Care Finance,
    37*(2), 49–55.

Davis, K., Schoen, C., Guterman, S., Shih, T., Schoenbaum, C., &
    Weinbaum, I. (2007). Slowing the growth of U.S. health care

expenditures: What are the options? *Commonwealth Fund, 989*, 1–34. Retrieved from www.commonwealthfund.org/usr_doc/Davis_ slowinggrowthUShltcareexpenditureswhatareoptions_989.pdf

Feldstein, P. (2007). *Health policy issues: An economic perspective.* Chicago: Health Administration Press.

Finkelstein, A. (2007). The aggregate effects of health insurance: Evidence from the introduction of Medicare. *Quarterly Journal of Economics, 122*, 1–37.

Fronstin, P. (2001). The history of employment-based health insurance: The role of managed care. *Benefits Quarterly, 17*(2), 716.

Fuchs, V. (2009). Reforming US health care. *Journal of the American Medical Association, 301*, 963–964.

Fuchs, V. (2010). Government payment for health care—causes and consequences. *New England Journal of Medicine, 363*, 2181–2183.

Fuchs, V., & Emanuel, E. (2005). Health care reform: Why? What? When? *Health Affairs, 24*, 1399–1414.

Growth of spending slows dramatically, yet GDP share keeps rising. (2011). *Health Care Financial Management, 65*(2), 13.

Hyman, M. A. (2009). Finding the money for health care reform. *Alternative Therapies in Health & Medicine, 15*(5), 20–23.

Kaiser Family Foundation (KFF). (2011). *Healthcare spending in the United States and selected OECD countries April 2011.* Retrieved from www.kff.org/insurance/snapshot/oecd042111.cfm

Macinko, J., Starfield, B., & Shi, L. (2007). Quantifying the health benefits of primary care physician supply in the United States. *International Journal of Health Services, 37*, 111–126.

Marmor, T., Oberlander, J., & White, J. (2009). The Obama administration's options for health care cost control: Hope versus reality. *Annals of Internal Medicine, 150*, 485–489.

Mirabito, A., & Berry, L. (2010). Lessons that the patient-centered medical homes can learn from the mistakes of HMOs. *Annals of Internal Medicine, 152*(3), 182–185.

Moran, D. (2005). Whence and whither health insurance? A revisionist history. *Health Affairs (Project Hope)*, *24*, 1415–1425.

Notle, E., & McKee, C. (2008). Measuring the health of nations: Updating an earlier analysis. *Health Affairs*, *27*, 58–71.

O'Neill, J., & O'Neill, D. (2007). Health status, health care and inequality: Canada vs. the U.S. *Frontiers in Health Policy Research*, *10*(1), 1–44.

Organisation for Economic Co-operation and Development (OECD). (2010). OECD health data. doi: 10.1787/data-00350-en

Pettingill, R. (2009). More access isn't enough. Reform must include health promotion, oversight board, simplification. *Modern Healthcare*, *39*(11), 18.

Rittenhouse, D., & Shortell, S. (2009). The patient-centered medical home: Will it stand the test of health reform? *Journal of the American Medical Association*, *301*, 2038–2040.

Rushton, F. (2009). US health-care crisis. *Pediatric International*, *51*, 603–605.

Sessions, S., & Lee, P. (2008). Using tax reform to drive health care reform: Putting the horse before the cart. *Journal of the American Medical Association*, *300*, 1929–1931.

Turnock, B. (2009). *Public health: What it is and how it works*. Burlington, MA: Jones & Bartlett.

Weir, M., Orloff, A., & Skopal, T. (Eds.). (1988). *The politics of social policy in the United States*. Princeton, NJ: Princeton University Press.

Witmer, A., Seifer, S. D., Finocchio, L., Leslie, J., & O'Neil, E. H. (1995). Community health workers: Integral members of the health care work force. *American Journal of Public Health*, *85*, 1055–1058.

CHAPTER 13

Ahronheim, J. C., Moreno, J. D., & Zuckerman, C. (2000). *Ethics in clinical practice* (2nd ed.). Burlington, MA: Jones & Bartlett.

American College of Healthcare Executives code of ethics. (2011). Retrieved from www.ache.org/ABT_ACHE/ACHECodeofEthics-2011.pdf

Beauchamp, T. L., & Childress, J. E. (2009). *Principles of biomedical ethics* (6th ed.). New York: Oxford University Press.

Boyle, P., DuBose, E. R., Ellingson, S. J., Guinn, D. E., & McCurdy D. B. (2001). *Organizational ethics in health care: Principles, cases, and practical solutions.* San Francisco: Jossey-Bass.

Darr, K. (2005). *Ethics in health services management* (4th ed.). Baltimore: Health Professions Press.

Davies, N. (2011). Reducing inequalities in healthcare provision for older adults. *Nursing Standard, 25*(41), 49–55.

Dosick, R. W. (2000). *The business bible: Ten commandments for creating an ethical workplace.* (2011). Vermont: Jewish Light.

Dye, C. F. (2000). *Leadership in healthcare: Values at the top.* Chicago: Health Administration Press.

Edge, R. S., & Groves, J. R. (1999). *Ethics of health care: A guide for clinical practice* (2nd ed.). Clifton Park, NY: Delmar Cengage Learning.

Frankl, V. (1971). *Man's search for meaning: An introduction to logotherapy.* New York: Pocket Books.

Gilbert, J. A. (2007). *Strengthening ethical wisdom: Tools for transforming your health care organization.* Chicago: Health Administrations Press.

Griffith, J. R. (1993). *The moral challenges of healthcare management.* Ann Arbor: Health Professions Press.

Hall, R. T. (2000). *An introduction to healthcare organizational ethics.* New York: Oxford University Press.

Hoffman, S., & Podgurski, A. (2008). Finding a cure: The case for regulation and oversight of electronic health record systems. *Harvard Journal of Law & Technology, 22,* 107.

Hsiao, C. J., Hing, E., Socey, T. C., Cai, B. (2011). *Electronic health record systems and intent to apply for meaningful use incentives among office-based physician practices: United States, 2001–2011* (NCHS Data Brief No 79). Hyattsville, MD: National Center for Health Statistics. Retrieved from www.cdc.gov/nchs/data/databriefs/db79.pdf

Institute of Medicine (IOM). (2008). *Knowing what works in health care: A road map for the nation.* Washington DC: National Academies Press.

Institute of Medicine (IOM). (2010). *A foundation for evidence-driven practice.* (Workshop summary). Washington DC: National Academies Press.

Johnson, C. E. (2009). *Meeting the ethical challenges of leadership: Casting light or shadow* (3rd ed.). Thousand Oaks, CA: Sage.

Joint Commission on Accreditation of Healthcare Organizations. (1995). *Accreditation manual for hospitals.* Oakbrook Terrace, IL: Author.

Judson, K., Harrison, C., & Hicks, S. (2006). *Law and ethics for medical careers* (4th ed.). New York: McGraw-Hill.

Lachman, V. D. (2009). *Ethical challenges in health care: Developing your moral compass.* New York: Springer.

Macklin, R. (1993). *Enemies of patients: How doctors are losing their power, and patients are losing their rights.* New York: Oxford University Press.

Monagle, J. F., & West, M. P. (2009). Hospital ethics committees: Roles, memberships, structure and difficulties. In Morrison, E. E. (Ed.), *Health care ethics: Critical issues for the 21st century* (2nd ed., pp. 293–307). Burlington, MA: Jones & Bartlett.

Morrison, E. E. (2011). *Ethics in health administration.* Burlington, MA: Jones & Bartlett.

Nwomeh, B. C., & Caniano, D.A. (2011). Emerging ethical issues in pediatric surgery. *Pediatric Surgery International, 27*, 555–562.

Pearson, S. D., Sabin, J. E., & Emanuel, E. J. (2003). *No margin, no mission: Health-care organizations and the quest for ethical excellence.* New York: Oxford University Press.

Pellegrino, E. D., & Thomasma, D. C. (1988). *For the patient's own good—the restoration of beneficence in healthcare.* New York: Oxford University Press.

Purtilo, R. B., & Criss, M. L. (2005). *Ethical dimensions in the health professions* (4th ed.). Philadelphia: Elsevier Saunders.

Sandel, S. J. (2009). *Justice: What's the right thing to do?* New York: Farrar, Straus and Giroux.

Stepanikova, I., & Cook, K. S. (2008). The effects of poverty and lack of insurance on perceptions of racial and ethnic bias in health care. *Health Services Research, 43,* 915–930.

Tauber, A. I. (2005). *Patient autonomy and the ethics of responsibility.* Cambridge, MA: MIT Press.

Timko, R. (2001). *Clinical ethics: Due care and the principle of nonmaleficence.* New York: University Press of America.

Tong, R. (2007). *New perspectives in healthcare ethics: An interdisciplinary and crosscultural approach.* Upper Saddle River, NJ: Prentice Hall.

Walter, J. K., & Klein, E. P. (Eds.). (2003). *The story of bioethics: From seminal works to contemporary explorations.* Washington DC: Georgetown University Press.

Weber, L. J. (2001). *Business ethics in healthcare: Beyond compliance.* Bloomington, IN: Indiana University Press.

Worthley, J. A. (1999). *Organizational ethics in the compliance context.* Chicago: Health Administration Press.

CHAPTER 14

Blanchard, K., & Barrett, C. (2011). *Lead with LUV: A different way to create real success.* Upper Saddle River, NJ: Pearson Education.

Branson, R. (2011). *Business stripped bare: Adventures of a global entrepreneur.* New York: Penguin Group.

Champy, J., & Greenspun, H. (2010). *Reengineering health care: A manifesto for radically rethinking health care delivery.* Upper Saddle River, NJ: Pearson Education.

Chesbrough, H. (2011). *Open services innovation: Rethinking your business to grow and compete in a new era.* San Francisco: Jossey-Bass.

Connors, R., & Smith, T. (2011). *Change the culture, change the game.* New York: Penguin Group.

Diermeier, D. (2011). *Strategies for building your company's most valuable asset: Reputation rules.* New York: McGraw-Hill.

Dlugacz, Y. D. (2010). *Value-based health care: Linking finance and quality.* San Francisco: Jossey-Bass.

Gittell, J. (2009). *High performance healthcare: Using the power of relationships to achieve quality, efficiency and resilience.* New York: McGraw-Hill.

Goldsmith, S. B. (2011). *Principles of health care management: Foundations for a changing health care system* (2nd ed.). Burlington, MA: Jones & Bartlett.

Halvorson, G. C. (2009). *Health care will not reform itself.* New York: CRC Press.

Harford, T. (2011). *Why success always starts with failure.* New York: Farrar, Straus and Giroux.

Institute of Medicine (IOM). (1999). *To err is human.* Washington DC: National Academies Press.

Lee, T. H., & Mongan, J. J. (2009). *Chaos and organization in health care.* Cambridge, MA: MIT Press.

Lombardi, D. N. (2001). *Handbook for the new health care manager* (2nd ed.). San Francisco: Jossey-Bass.

Lombardi, D., & Schermerhorn, J. (2007) *Health care management: Tools and techniques for managing in a health care environment.* Hoboken, NJ: Wiley.

Meister, J. C., & Willyerd, K. (2010). *The 2020 workplace: How innovative companies attract, develop, and keep tomorrow's employees today.* New York: HarperBusiness.

Michelli, J. A. (2011). *Prescription for excellence: Leadership lessons for creating a world-class customer experience from UCLA Health System.* New York: McGraw-Hill.

Porter, M. E. (2010). What is value in health care? *New England Journal of Medicine, 363,* 2477–2481.

Richtel, M. (2011). As doctors use more devices, potential for distraction grows. *New York Times.* Retrieved from www.nytimes. com/2011/12/15/health/as-doctors-use-more-devices-potential-for-distraction-grows.html?_r=2&nl=todaysheadlines&emc=tha23

Schein, E. H. (2004). *Organizational culture and leadership* (3rd ed.). San Francisco: Jossey-Bass.

Spear, S. J. (2009). *The high-velocity edge: How market leaders leverage operational excellence to beat the competition.* New York: McGraw-Hill.

Stevenson, J., & Kaafarani, B. (2011). *Breaking away: How great leaders create innovation that drives sustainable growth—and why others fail.* New York: McGraw-Hill.

Wiseman, L., & McKeown, G. (2010). *Multipliers: How the best leaders make everyone smarter.* New York: HarperCollins.

INDEX